Oral Health and Medicine

Oral Health and Medicine

Editor: Edward Thomas

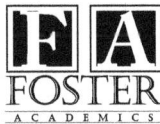

FA
FOSTER
ACADEMICS

www.fosteracademics.com

www.fosteracademics.com

FA
FOSTER
ACADEMICS

Cataloging-in-Publication Data

Oral health and medicine / edited by Edward Thomas.
    p. cm.
Includes bibliographical references and index.
ISBN 978-1-63242-616-1
1. Mouth--Care and hygiene. 2. Oral medicine. 3. Dental care.
4. Dental public health. 5. Dentistry. I. Thomas, Edward.
RK60.7 .O73 2019
617.601--dc23

© Foster Academics, 2019

Foster Academics,
118-35 Queens Blvd., Suite 400,
Forest Hills, NY 11375, USA

ISBN 978-1-63242-616-1 (Hardback)

Contents

Preface VII

Chapter 1   **Oral Health Related Quality of Life** 1
Javier de la Fuente Hernández, Fátima del Carmen Aguilar Díaz
and María del Carmen Villanueva Vilchis

Chapter 2   **Dental Implants** 26
Dongliang Zhang and Lei Zheng

Chapter 3   **Drug-Induced Oral Reactions** 48
Ana Pejcic

Chapter 4   **Narrow Diameter and Mini Dental Implant Overdentures** 62
Elena Preoteasa, Marina Imre, Henriette Lerner, Ana Maria Tancu
and Cristina Teodora Preoteasa

Chapter 5   **Are the Approximal Caries Lesions in Primary Teeth a Challenge
to Deal With? — A Critical Appraisal of Recent Evidences in this
Field** 86
Mariana Minatel Braga, Isabela Floriano, Fernanda Rosche Ferreira,
Juliana Mattos Silveira, Alessandra Reyes, Tamara Kerber Tedesco,
Daniela Prócida Raggio, José Carlos Pettorossi Imparato
and Fausto Medeiros Mendes

Chapter 6   **Factors Associated with the Presence of Teeth in the Adult
and Elderly Xukuru Indigenous Population** 120
Cecilia Santiago Araujo de Lima and Rafael da Silveira Moreira

Chapter 7   **Pain Evaluation Between Stainless Steel and Nickel Titanium
Arches in Orthodontic Treatment** 138
M. Larrea, N. Zamora, R. Cibrian, J. L. Gandia and V. Paredes

Chapter 8   **Advances in Radiographic Techniques used in Dentistry** 163
Zühre Zafersoy Akarslan and Ilkay Peker

Chapter 9   **Dental Caries and Quality of Life among Preschool Children** 200
Joana Ramos-Jorge, Maria Letícia Ramos-Jorge, Saul Martins de Paiva,
Leandro Silva Marques and Isabela Almeida Pordeus

Permissions

List of Contributors

Index

Preface

Oral infections and inflammations can affect the overall health of the oral cavity. Dentists strongly recommend the maintenance of oral hygiene for the prevention of oral diseases. General guidelines of ensuring good oral health include brushing twice daily and using flossettes, floss and interdental brushes. Regular checkups for professional evaluation and cleaning are highly recommended. The most common types of dental disease are gum diseases and tooth decay. Limiting the intake of snacks and eating a balanced diet can help prevent periodontal disease and tooth decay. Vitamin C-rich foods, vegetables, yogurt, cheese, etc. have proven benefits in oral care. The mouth may be affected by several cutaneous and gastrointestinal conditions. Pathological conditions in the biofilm surrounding the teeth lead to plaque-induced diseases. Oral medicine aims to treat lichen planus, pemphigus vulgaris and Behçet's disease. The diagnosis and follow-up care of pre-malignant lesions of the oral cavity, chronic and acute pain conditions relative to myofascial pain, paroxysmal neuralgias and atypical facial pain, among others. It also involves the management of temporomandibular joint disorder, trigeminal neuralgia, Sjögren's syndrome, etc. This book is a clinical guide to oral health and medicine and unravels the recent studies in these disciplines. The topics included herein are of utmost significance and bound to provide incredible insights to readers. Researchers and students in this field will be assisted by this book.

After months of intensive research and writing, this book is the end result of all who devoted their time and efforts in the initiation and progress of this book. It will surely be a source of reference in enhancing the required knowledge of the new developments in the area. During the course of developing this book, certain measures such as accuracy, authenticity and research focused analytical studies were given preference in order to produce a comprehensive book in the area of study.

This book would not have been possible without the efforts of the authors and the publisher. I extend my sincere thanks to them. Secondly, I express my gratitude to my family and well-wishers. And most importantly, I thank my students for constantly expressing their willingness and curiosity in enhancing their knowledge in the field, which encourages me to take up further research projects for the advancement of the area.

Editor

Oral Health Related Quality of Life

Javier de la Fuente Hernández,
Fátima del Carmen Aguilar Díaz and
María del Carmen Villanueva Vilchis

1. Introduction

Data about the impacts on people´s life caused by oral condition has been gathered recently in the last decades. Functional consequences of oral disease have been documented and also the emotional and social ones. It is accepted and recognized by dental community that oral health status can cause considerable pain and suffering, if oral symptoms remain untreated would be a major source of diminished quality of life; disturbing people´s food choices or their speech, or may lead to sleep deprivation, depression, and multiple adverse psychosocial outcomes. Influencing how people grow, enjoy life, chew, taste food and socialize, as well as their feelings of social well-being. There are so many oral affections that impact negatively on quality of life like caries, periodontal disease, tooth loss, cancer, dental injuries, dental fluorosis, and dental anomalies, craniofacial disorders among others. In fact not only dental disease but also treatment experience can negatively affect the oral health related quality of life. The relationship among these anomalies or conditions with quality of life are recently findings in literature in different populations. To evaluate these impacts different instruments have been developed for pediatric and adult population.

2. Oral health concept

2.1. Health

If there are complexities in defining disease, there are even more in defining health. Definitions have evolved over time. In the biomedical perspective, early definitions of health focused on the theme of the body's ability to function; health was seen as a state of normal function that could be disrupted from time to time by disease. An example of such a definition of health is: "a state characterized by anatomic, physiologic, and psychological integrity; ability to perform personally, in family, work, and in community roles; ability to deal with physical, biologic, psychological, and social stress". Then, in 1948, the World Health Organization (WHO) proposed a definition that aimed higher, linking health to well-being, in terms of "physical, mental, and social well-being, and not merely the absence of disease and infirmity". Although this definition is most accepted one it is also criticized as being vague, excessively broad, and unmeasurable.

This brought in a new conception of health, not as a state, but in dynamic terms, in other words, as "a resource for living". [1] The WHO in 1984 revised the concept of health and defined it as "the extent to which an individual or group is able to realize aspirations and satisfy needs, and to change or cope with the environment. Health is a resource for everyday life, not the objective of living; it is a positive concept, emphasizing social and personal resources, as well as physical capacities". [2] Thus, health referred to the ability to maintain homeostasis and recover from illness. Mental, intellectual, emotional, and social health referred to a person's ability to handle stress, to acquire skills, to maintain relationships, which are important for resources for resiliency and independent living. As seen the concept of health is wide and the way we define health also depends on individual perception, religious beliefs, cultural values, norms, and social class.

2.2. Oral health

As in 1948 WHO expanded the definition of health to mean "a complete state of physical, mental, and social well-being, and not just the absence of infirmity", oral health concept followed this change aiming not minimized oral health as having or not caries. So the concept of oral health (OH) has changed over time, going from a biologist approach, in which the oral cavity contributes to protect the body from infections by chewing and swallowing, to a social and psychological approaches, that take into account other roles of the oral cavity as the contribution that it has in self-esteem, communication and interaction and facial aesthetics. There is a concept of oral health defined by Dolan, who mention that OH means "a comfortable and functional dentition which allows individuals to continue in their desired social role." [3]. This definition already includes the role of OH in the performance of daily activities of the individual. With this we see that oral health is not just a medical condition, but an aggregate of aspects such as the impact that pain may have in daily or the degree of disability or dysfunction. Nowadays the importance of the oral cavity is recognized, as vital part of the human body. It is conceptualized as not only the teeth but others structures as gums, supporting tissues, ligaments, bone, hard and soft palate, soft mucosal tissue tongue, lips, salivary glands, chewing muscles, jaws, and the temporomandibular joints.

Similarly, the Canadian Dental Association defines oral health as "a state of the oral and related tissues and structures that contributes positively to physical, mental and social well-being and enjoyment of life's possibilities, by allowing the individual to speak, eat and socialize unhindered by pain, discomfort or embarrassment". Oral Health and oral cavity should be viewed as a part of a complete body, we must see human beings and their activities and not teeth and tooth decay, thus to recognized the play that oral health has on daily life activities. Clearly, there is an interaction between how we experience quality of life and how we perceive our oral health.

3. Health Related Quality of Life (HRQoL)

The term "quality of life" (QoL) was first used by the British economist Arthur Cecil Pigou in 1920. Later, after World War II, this term was expanded into other areas such as sociology, politics [4] and health, among others. Within the area of health the concept of quality of life was introduced and initially applied in patients with neoplastic disease [5], having a peak in the 90s and essentially incorporating the patient's perception. 4

The World Health Organization (WHO) in 1952 defined the concept of QoL, as "the proper and correct perception that a person has of itself in the cultural context and values on which it is embedded, in relation to its objectives, standards, hopes and concerns. [6]

This perception may be influenced by their physical, psychological, level of independence and social relationships. [7] Later it was considered good health and quality of life to "the absence of disease or defect and the sense of physical, mental and social well-being" or "personal sense of well-being and life satisfaction." Another proposal definition in 2003 by Ventegodt is "to have a nice life and live a life of high quality." [8] Later on it was postulated that "the quality of life has to do with the degree to which an individual can enjoy the possibilities of life". This concept was proposed by the Centre for Health Promotion, University of Toronto. [9]

The variety of definitions and the lack of consensus lead us to think that the term quality of life is only understood on a personal level or as Campbell mentioned: "The QoL is a vague and ethereal concept, something that many people talk about but anybody knows clearly what it really means. [10]

On the other hand, all the above definitions are general definitions of quality of life and not quality of life related to health (HRQoL). Furthermore, it becomes evident that these terms within the medical field have been used interchangeably. Strictly research in the field of health should address processes or limit the scope of the study quality of life related to health, which refers to the effects that the sufferings directly or these treatments can occur in people. [11, 12] HRQoL is the quality of life that relates directly to the state of health of the individual. It is clear and recognized that HRQoL refers to something much broader than health.

The HRQoL assessment in a patient represents the impact that a disease and its subsequent treatment has on the patient's perception of their well-being. One of the existing definitions consider HRQoL as "the subjective assessment of the influence of health status, health care and health promotion on an individual's ability to maintain a level of functioning that allows him to perform activities that are important, and affect overall welfare." [8]

Or, as Patrick and Erickson proposed, HRQoL is the "extent to which the value assigned to duration of life in terms of the perception of physical, psychological, social and diminishing opportunities limitations because of illness value is changed, its sequelae, treatment and / or health policy ". It has also been conceptualized as "the subjective perception, influenced by the current health status, ability to perform those activities important for the individual".4

For this assessment it has been proposed that the most important dimensions of HRQoL are: social, physical and cognitive functioning, mobility and personal care and emotional wellbeing.

HRQoL is an important subjective component so it will depend on the relationship that each individual has with his life. This concept will vary and depend largely on the perception that people has about their physical, mental, social and spiritual state, largely depending on their own values, convictions and beliefs, as well as their personal cultural context and history. [13]

Given the above, to assess HRQoL should be considered the values in which each person lives, that is, the cultural context in which he is immersed, and in the individual expectations and achievements. Similarly, the perception of HRQoL is not equal over time because people change their expectations and aspirations adjusting them to different circumstances.

Clinicians interested in knowing the effects of interventions or treatments also find useful information on HRQoL, as it evaluates the final result of medical interventions at one point, not assessing only according to biological or physiological standards but at emotional and social functional level, it means to evaluate everything that a person represents.

Similarly, this information is also relevant to patients and family members making them aware of areas where their performance is affected by their health, identifying where they may need further help or therapy or supporting them to choose between various options of treatments. Moreover, it has been identified that the assessment of HRQoL in children can be used as a predictor of costs of health care and can help to identify risk groups or to evaluate health services. [14, 15].

4. Oral Health Related Quality of Life (OHRQoL)

Although oral health problems are rarely a matter of life and death they remain a major public health problem because of its prevalence and there are significant indications that oral health problems have social, economic and psychological consequences, this means that they have impact of quality of life.

Nowadays there is a growing interest in recognizing oral health as a component of quality of life, currently the dental research efforts are not only focus on rehabilitating oral-dental diseases, but in exploring the relationship between oral health status and quality of life, in order to evaluate it, improve it and maintain it. In fact, OHRQoL is an integral part of general health and well-being and is recognized by the WHO as an important segment of the Global Oral Health Program. [16]

Oral health-related quality of life was defined as a "self-report specifically pertaining to oral health–capturing both the functional, social and psychological impacts of oral disease" [17]

There is another definition that conceptualizes OHRQoL mentioning that it "reflects people's comfort when eating, sleeping and engaging in social interaction; their self-esteem; and their satisfaction with respect to their oral health". Locker suggested that it is the result of an interaction between and among oral health conditions, social and contextual factors [18] and the rest of the body as Atchison mentioned. [19]

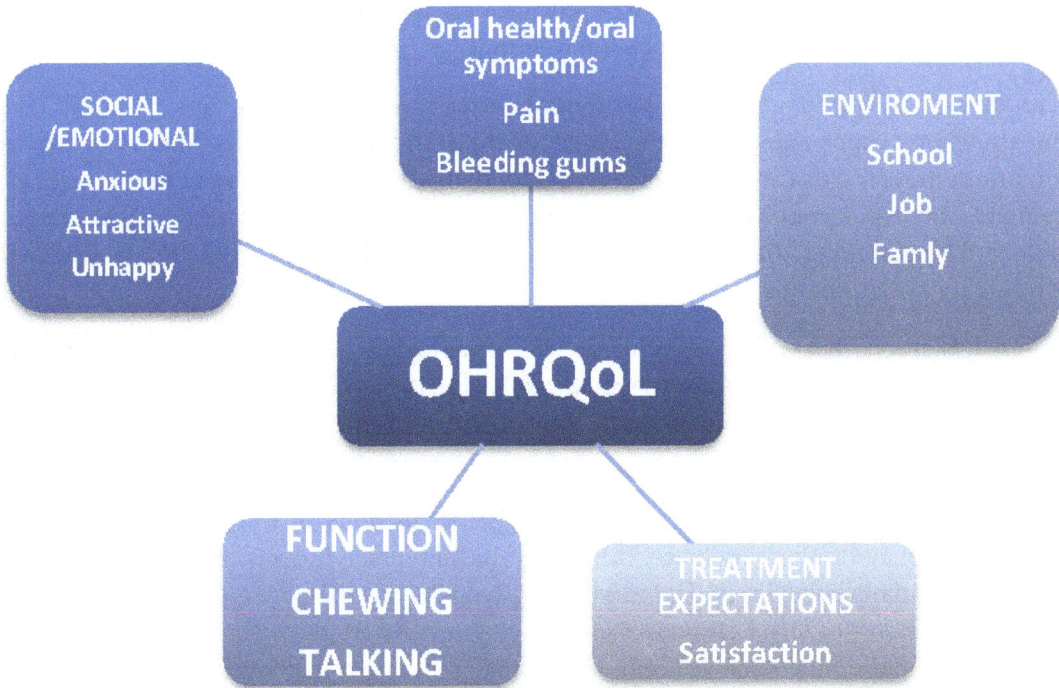

We must keep in mind that OHRQoL deals with conditions that vary in intensity and importance, some of them are life-threatening (e.g. oral cancers) some chronic (caries, periodontitis, etc.) some other dealing with aesthetics (fluorosis, dental anomalies, etc) and other are related to oral pain (pulpitis, dental treatments etc.).

As HRQoL oral health related quality of life is highly subjective and has to be assessed within the framework of patients' conditions, sociocultural environments and own experiences and states of mind: because OHRQoL is related to daily life and is unique to each individual, even patients with severe conditions can report having good quality of life. Furthermore, Quality of Life is by itself multi-faceted, showing variation over time for each individual. [20]

A long the time several oral conditions have been reported in literature as conditions having impact on OHRQoL. An example is **edentulism**, condition that can affect masticatory function, dietary choice, and nutritional level. It has been reported that wearing dentures may interfere with the ability to eat satisfactorily, talk clearly, and laugh freely.

Tooth loss is one of the worst types of damage to oral health, causing esthetic and functional problems. In addition to the biological causes of tooth loss, socioeconomic factors contribute to oral health associated with tooth loss. Socioeconomic status is related to inequalities in health, and socioeconomically disadvantaged people have higher risks of disease and suffer more from health conditions. [21] Several studies have reported an association between tooth loss and OHRQoL.

Some other common oral conditions, such as caries, periodontal disease, which are almost universal in prevalence, and which are chronic but with acute recurring episodes, also impact on QoL. In the same way other condition that might not be as common as the ones mentioned before but which prevalence cannot be considered low as dental fluorosis, craniofacial disorders and oral cancer which can be life treating.

There are several reports showing that **dental caries** has negative impacts on OHRQoL in populations of various ages across the globe, in children [22] and adults. Specially, children with caries whose scores can be about 50% greater than scores for children without caries [23]. Among toddlers and preschool-age early childhood caries (ECC) is one of the most common health problems among children with periodontal disease have lower OHRQoL compared with the general population

Another alteration that affects quality of life is **malocclusio**n. Authors as Onyeaso and Aderinokun in 2003, who conducted a study involving 614 Nigerian children aged 12-18 years, found a correlation between the malocclusion severity and the perception that children have about their dental appearance.

There is an association between the presence of malocclusion with worse OHRoQL. Particularly the one related to lack of space, facial pain has adversely effects of body image, social interaction and daily behavior of the individual. Given the fact that face and mouth appearance influence judgments of facial attractiveness, playing an important role in the development of social and occupational goals. Not only malocclusion but also its treatment has an effect on OHRQoL may also affect QoL through their effect on function and esthetics.

For instance, reports have been made demonstrating striking changes in self-concept and emotional health after **orthodontic and/or surgical treatment** of malocclusions and orofacial defects.

Another alteration that has an impacto n OHRQoL is severe **hypodontia**. It was associated with worse quality of life. Wong and cols. observed that 100% of children reported having impact in the area of oral symptoms, functional limitations in 88%, 55% to 100% emotional and social welfare. The number of missing teeth was associated moderately with the level of impact. One of the main impacts of OHQRL noted in literature was the difficulty chewing, especially among the elderly.

In Uganda, a study aiming to describe the OHRQoL in 12 years of age rural children showed that more than half of them reported oral impact "often" or "every day". Authors concluded that the presence of caries experience or treatment were associated with higher impacts on quality of life. The socially significant fluorosis was associated with greater number of impacts, but not with higher total scores. Despite low levels of oral problems these children experienced impacts on quality of life due to oral problems. Finding that most responsible for these impacts is the presence of caries and fluorosis a lower level. Also **severe fluorosis** can have a negative effect on smile aesthetics and produce functional problems, affecting self-confidence, causing discomfort, and probably disturbing social roles from a young age. [24]

Also **craniofacial disorders** cause impact on OHRQoL including limitations in verbal and nonverbal communication, social interaction, and intimacy. Individuals with facial disfigurements due to craniofacial diseases and conditions and their treatments may experience loss of self-image and self-esteem, anxiety, depression, and social stigma; these in turn may limit educational, career, and marital opportunities and affect other social relations. Diet, nutrition, sleep, psychological status, social interaction, school, and work are affected by impaired oral and craniofacial health.

Documented data, reported in Thailand, suggest that in ninety per cent of pre-adolescents have an impact related to oral health, 74% of 35–44-year olds had daily performances affected by their oral state; 46% reported their emotional stability was affected. Earlier, end points such as recurrence rates and survival were used to evaluate the efficacy of various therapeutic measures in head and neck cancer while patient's quality of life was usually ignored. Presently, the multitudinal impact of maxillofacial tumors on a patient's life has been recognized, which led various researchers to investigate the quality of life of those patients. However, studies evaluating the quality of life of patients with maxillectomy defects and the effect of prosthodontic therapy with obturator prostheses on their quality of life remain rare. A obturator prosthesis is a highly positive and non-invasive approach to improve the quality of life of patients with maxillectomy defects. [25]

Andiappan and cols. performed a meta-analysis and revealed that those receiving treatment for malocclusion and in individuals without malocclusion have significantly better OHRQoL compared to those with such condition [26]

Recent studies of the impact on OHRQoL on children's under general anesthesia treatment have shown significant improvement in oral health and psychological, social and overall wellbeing as well as a positive impact on the family.

Besides clinical conditions, there are other factors that contributed in the impact on OHRQoL as lower family income and sex. In general, women reported a greater impact on OHRQoL than men, although no differences are observed between clinical conditions present in each gender. Differences in the perception of OHRQoL between the genders may be caused by individual and subjective concepts related to beauty and personal esthetic standards, imposed by the social demands and personal needs [27].

5. Instruments to assess OHRQoL

As aforementioned, in the literature has been identified OHRQoL as a multidimensional construct containing physical, social and psychological domains. [28] The clinical indexes do not evaluate these aspects, they only measure the presence and severity of illness, and give scarce consideration to the functionality of the oral cavity as a whole, or to the impact of the symptoms on the patients' quality of life. So the clinical indexes that are commonly used to establish the presence and severity of pathological conditions should be complemented with indicators of social and emotional aspects related to the individual experience and subjective perception of changes in the patients' physical, mental, and social health. [29]

Over the years several socio-dental indicators have been developed, since Cohen and Jago first advocated the development of sociodental indicators. These indicators range from single item to composite inventories or scoring systems, covering the aforementioned OHRQoL domains. So since the 70's, several authors have been given the task to develop and test instruments that may assess the functional, emotional and social effects of oral abnormalities.

All these questionnaires around the world have been developed to measure the impact of oral disease on quality of life which comprising different domains including: pain and inability to perform normal functions of the mouth, sleep disturbances, loss of school days, degree of emotional and social wellbeing. These questionnaires could also potentially be a valuable outcome for evaluating oral health promotion programs and/or service initiatives. 30

5.1. OHRQoL instruments for adults

5.1.1. The Social Impacts of Dental Disease (SIDD) [31]

The SIDD developed in the early 1980s, was one of first socio-dental indicators. Created under a model that defines dental health status in socio-dental terms; the clinical indicators are largely determined by vulnerability whilst the social elements are more directly linked with the degree of social and psychological impact arising from dental diseases. The indicator was tested on large randomly selected samples of industrial workers in Warrington, in the North of England and skilled manual workers and their wives in the South of England.

It was developed as a component of a much broader socio-dental model of dental disease and health behavior so that both the clinical and socio-psychological aspects could be considered within an integrated framework. The model assumes that an individual's present oral health status and treatment needs are influenced by an interplay of three 'dimensions' of background and behavioural factors, namely vulnerability, motivational and preventive dimensions. The score for each individual was constructed from responses to questions relating to those five categories. A total impact score is derived by adding the number of categories. A score of 1 is given to the impact category if a positive response has been given to any of the questions in the category. Two total impact scores were used, one including (total score 0-5) and one excluding discomfort (totaL score 0-4) to see the difference if this relatively common problem was excluded.

5.1.2. Geriatric (General) Oral Health Assessment Index (GOHAI) [32]

The GOHAI is one of the most commonly used scales in assessment of OHRQoL it was developed by Kathryn Atchison and Dolan in 1990 in the USA for use with elderly populations. It is compounded by 12-items developed with three months' time reference, with five (six in the original) Likert scale options, scoring as 'often', always', 'seldom 'or 'sometimes' and 'never' reflecting the aspects that are considered to have an impact upon the quality of life of the older population. Nonetheless it was created for geriatric populations some author have used it with younger adult populations, which is reflected in the interchangeable us of the names Geriatric or General Oral Health Assessment Index. It was developed to evaluate three dimensions of OHRQoL including physical functions like eating, chewing, speech, swallowing; psychosocial functions like worry, limitations and discomfort with social contacts, dissatisfaction with appearance; and self-consciousness about oral health, pain or discomfort including the use of medication or discomfort from the mouth. The GOHAI score is determined by summing the final score of each of the12 items.

The GOHAI gives a greater weight to functional limitations or pain and discomfort. According to the research of Hassel et al., the GOHAI seems to be more appropriate when focusing on subjective oral health with minor clinical changes and immediate clinical aspects. [33]

This questionnarie has been tested on a variety of sample of subjects, of different ages, races and the reliability testes show that this instrument is acceptable in all samples tested thus far. It has also been translated and validated to a wide range of languages.

5.1.3. The Dental Impact Profile (DIP) [34]

This instrument was developed by Ronald Strauss. It consist in twenty-five items that have been placed in non-apparent order and respondents are offered three ordinal response choices (good effect, bad effect, no effect) about whether teeth or dentures have had an effect on various aspects of life. A response of "good effect" was seen as likely to be most socially acceptable and the potential for response bias in the positive direction exists. While "good effect" and "bad effect" response categories have meaning independently, they may be combined in the estimation of dental impact. Dental impact is noted for an item if teeth are seen to have an effect on that aspect of life, whether that effect is positive or negative. Responses of "no effect" are seen as indication of no dental impact. The four subscales and component items were:

1. Eating Subscale: Eating, Chewing and Biting, Enjoyment of eating, Food choice, Tasting

2. Health/Well-Being Subscale: Feeling comfortable, Enjoyment of life, General happiness, General health, Appetite, Weight, Living a long life

3. Social Relations Subscale: Facial appearance to other people, Facial appearance (to self), Smiling and laughing, Moods, Speech, Breath, Confidence around others, Attendance at activities, Success at work

4. Romance Subscale: Social Life, Romantic relationships, Having sex appeal, Kissing,

5.1.4. Dental impact on daily living (DIDL) [35]

Developed by Leao & Sheiham in 1996. The Dental Impact on Daily Living (DIDL) is a socio-dental measure which assesses five dimensions of quality of life comfort, appearance, pain, daily activities, eating. Comfort, related to complaints such as bleeding gums and food packing; Appearance, consisting of self-image; Pain; Performance, the ability to carry out daily activities and to interact with people; and Eating restriction, relating to difficulties in biting and chewing. The measure consists of a questionnaire of 36 items, which assesses the oral impacts on daily living, and a scale, which is a graphical representation of a method developed by Leao to assess the importance respondents attribute to the different dimensions involved. Items are summed into a score for each dimension. To compute the score, coded responses within each dimension were summed and divided by the number of items, resulting in a dimension score (For example, Appearance has four questions. The score for this dimension would be the sum of coded responses for all four questions divided by four). Impacts were coded as '+1' for positive impacts, 0 for impacts not totally negatives and '-1' for negative impacts. To construct a final score, questions within each category are summed and divided by the number of items, giving a score for each dimension. Before adding the different dimensions, they receive the respective weight attributed on the scale, otherwise it would be assumed that they were equally important. Then the five dimensions are finally added to give a final score.

One aspect to be highlighted in DIDL is the degree of flexibility offered in terms of aggregating and disaggregating data (either individual items, dimension scores or total score). Although criticized, a total score reproduces the total impact subjects are experiencing, and since dimensions sometimes may not impact separately, it appears important to have this view of the individual as a whole. Another point to be stressed is that in the total score generated by DIDL, weights attributed to dimensions (by each respondent) are personal. That is, the importance attributed to a dimension by a given individual is directly associated with his or her own impacts on that dimension. [36]

5.1.5. Oral health quality of life inventory

Developed by Cornell et al. in 1997, they included 56 questions divided 4 domains: oral health, nutrition, self-rated oral health, overall quality of life. It is part of a larger home-based interview, the Oral Health Quality of Life Interview (OHQOLI)*. In addition to the OH-QoL, OHQOLI includes self-report assessments of oral health and functional status (SROH), a Nutrition Quality of Life Index (NutQoL), and an interview version of the Quality of Life Inventory (QOLI). [37] The final OHQOLI interview has 40 SROH items, 15 OH-QoL items, and 9 NutQoL items. The OH-QoL items are distributed among the related SROH items. Thus, the subjective well-being items appear immediately following the related objective functional status items in the questionnaire. The overall format of the OHQOLI is designed for interviewer administration.

5.1.6. Oral Health Impact Profile (OHIP) [38]

The OHIP, developed by Slade & Spencer is the most widely used OHRQoL questionnaire. It is based on Locker's adaptation of the World Health Organisation's classification of impairments, disabilities and handicaps (Locker, 1988). The OHIP contains 49 assessing seven dimensions of impacts of oral conditions on people's OHRQoL including functional limitation, physical pain, psychological discomfort, physical disability, psychological disability, social disability and handicap.

A short version, OHIP-14, was later developed based on a subset of 2 questions for each of the 7 dimensions. [39] It is patient-centered, gives a greater weight to psychological and behavioral outcomes, is better at detecting psychosocial impacts among individuals and groups, and better meets the main criteria for the measurement of OHRQoL.[33] The OHIP 14 responses, "never", "hardly ever", "occasionally", "fairly often", and "very often", were codified from 0 to 4, respectively. Each of the 14 questions was assigned a score of 0 if the response was "never," and a score of 1 if the response was "hardly ever", "occasionally", "fairly often," or "very often," dichotomizing responses into no impact versus some impact. The scores assigned to the responses to the 14 questions are added to obtain values between 0 and 14. [40]

There also exist the OHIP-aesthetic which is a modified short form of the OHIP derived (OHIP-conceptual) that is most favorable in discriminating dental aesthetics, showing to be reliable and most sensitive to the dental aesthetics intervention-tooth whitening. [41]

5.1.7. Oral Impacts on Daily Performance (OIDP)

The OIDP aims to provide an alternative sociodental indicator which focuses on measuring the serious oral impacts on the person's ability to perform daily activities. It is one of many self-reported inventories to assess OHRQoL in terms of adverse impacts that oral conditions can have on everyday life experiences.

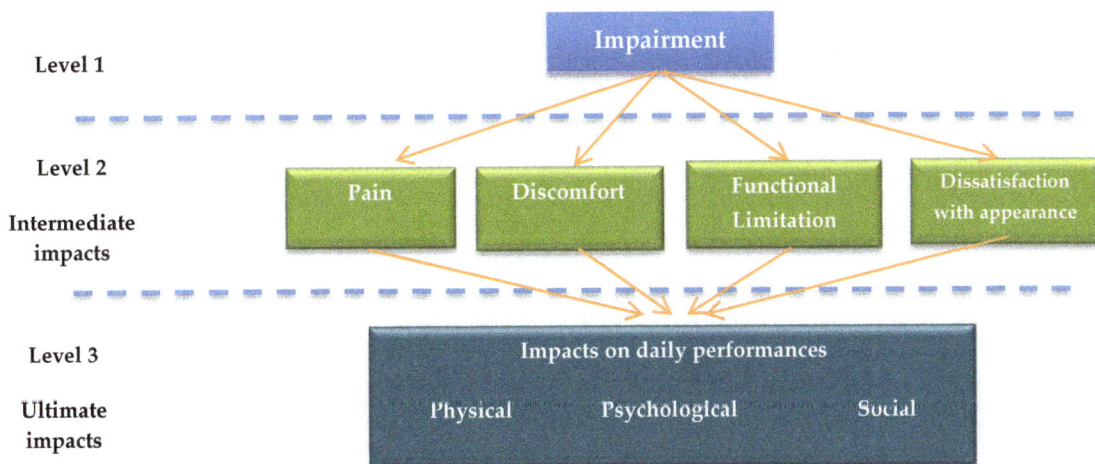

Figure 1. Theoretical framework of consequences of oral impacts

The theoretical framework of OIDP is presented in Figure 1. This is a modified model from the WHO International Classification of Impairments, Disabilities and Handicaps amended for dentistry by Locker. [42] In this modification different levels of consequence variables were established. The first level refers to the oral status, including oral impairments, which most clinical indices attempt to measure. The second level, "the intermediate impacts", includes the possible earliest negative impacts caused by oral health status: pain, discomfort or functional limitation. Dissatisfaction with appearance was added in this level since studies indicated that it was a major dimension of oral health outcomes. In addition, functional limitation may cause pain, discomfort or dissatisfaction with appearance and vice versa. The third level, or the "ultimate impacts" represents impacts on ability to perform daily activities which consists of physical, psychological and social performances. Any of the dimensions in the second level may impact on performance ability. This third level is equivalent to disability and handicap dimensions in the WHO model. The OIDP concentrates only on the measurement of "ultimate" oral impacts, thus covering the fields of disability and handicap.

The OIDP has been demonstrated to have appropriate psychometric properties when applied in population based cross-sectional surveys of elderly in Norway 43, Sweden 44, Greece and UK, Tanzania, Bosnia 45, Brazil, Thailand, among others. Studies have shown that OIDP is associated in the expected direction with self-reported oral health and clinical indicators and that personal-, socio-demographic-, and health care service related factors modify those relationships.

There are other questionnaires adapted to specific conditions/domains as the Orthognathic QOL Questionnaire, SOOQ for orthodontic surgery, OHRQOL for Dental Hygiene, The prosthetic quality of life (PQL), Quality of Life with Implant-Prostheses' (QoLIP-10)

5.1.8. The prosthetic quality of life (PQL) [46]

The PQL, created by Javier Montero and collaborators, is compounded by 11 items and can be applied in epidemiological studies or clinical trials with no special cost as regards the time required for exploration. It has a bipolar design of the responses of the items of the PQL that allows both negative and positive impacts to be recorded, such that the assessment of the physical, psychological and social well-being deriving from the use of dental prostheses, condition that makes it more complete than questionnaires limited to evaluating the presence of negative impact. Responses: Yes, a lot (1),Yes, slightly (2), It's more or less the same (3), I think it's worse (4), It's much worse (5).

5.1.9. Quality of Life with Implant-Prostheses' (QoLIP-10) [47]

Preciado and colaborators designed this instrumet of the 10-item scale that gather information on global oral satisfaction, socio-demographic, health-behavioural, clinical and prosthetic-related data. This questionnaire has shown to be reliable and valid. The factor analysis confirmed the existence of three dimensions and meaningful inter-correlations among the 10 items. The QoLIP-10 index confirmed its psychometric capacity for assessing the OHRQoL of implant overdenture and hybrid prosthesis wearers. Authors suggest that this instrument may be recommended for determining the influence of implant-retained overdentures and hybrid prostheses on the well-being of future patients.

5.2. OHRQoL instruments for children

During the past decade, several instruments have been developed to detect the impact of oral health on children´s quality of life.

Questionnaire	Abbreviation	Original Language	Year	Validated in other languages as
Social Impacts of Dental Disease	SIDD	English	1980	
Sickness Impact Profile	SIP	English	1985	
The General (Geriatric) Oral Health Assessment	GOHAI	English	1990	French [48], German [49], Mandarin Chinese [50], Arabic [51], Swedish [52], Malay [53], Arabic [54], Turkey [55], Hindi [56] Spanish [57], Portuguese [58]
Dental Impact Profile	DIP	English	1993	
Oral Health Impact Profile	OHIP	English	1994	Korean, Chinese. Swedish, Portuguese, Japanese, Hungarian, Dutch, German, Hebrew, Croatian, Slovenian, Sinhalese, Persian, Italian
Dental Impact on Daily Living	DDIDL	English	1996	
Oral Impact Daily Performance	OIDP	English	2011	Portugues, Greece, Thai, Kannada [59], Swedish, Bosnian, Norwegian
	OIDP abreviado		2012	India [60], Albanian
Prosthetic quality of life questionnaire	PQL	English	2007	
Quality of Life with Implant-Prostheses'	QoLIP-10	English	2013	

Table 1. Questionnaires to asses OHRQoL in adults

5.2.1. Child Perception Questionnaire (CPQ11–14) [61]

In 2002, Jokovic et al. developed the Child Perceptions Questionnaire (CPQ), which is one of the first instruments used to evaluate OHRQoL in children. In addition to the CPQ, there is a Parent's Perceptions Questionnaire (P-CPQ) [62] and a Family Impact Scale (FIS) [63], which is compound a battery of instruments that provide information at different levels and perspectives for OHRQoL in children.

The CPQ has two versions, one is the CPQ_{11-14} for children from 11 to 14 years of age; the other, which is the CPQ_{8-10}, is for children aged 8 to 10 years. Both aim to evaluate the impact of oral and orofacial conditions in children at a functional, emotional, and social level.

The CPQ_{11-14} was constructed using a systematic multistage process based on the theory of measurement and scale development. It is one of the most used instruments which is composed of 37 items divided into four domains or subscales: oral symptoms (n=6), functional limitations (n=9), emotional well-being (n=9) and social well-being (n=13). The questions ask about the frequency of events in the previous three months in relation to the child's oral/oro-facial condition. The response options are: 'Never'=0; 'Once/twice'=1; 'Sometimes'=2; 'Often'=3;

'Everyday/almost every day'=4. The questionnaire also contains global ratings of the child's oral health and the extent to which the oral/oro-facial condition affected his/her overall well-being. They are worded as follows: "Would you say that the health of your teeth, lips, jaws and mouth is..." and "How much does the condition of your teeth, lips, jaws or mouth affect your life overall?" A 5-point response format ranging from 'Excellent'=0 to 'Poor'=4 and from 'Not at all'=0 to 'Very much'=4, respectively, is offered for these ratings.

The CPQ_{11-14} performs well as a discriminative measure, being able to distinguish between the three groups. Jokovic and co-workers developed short-forms versions of the CPQ_{11-14} using two different approaches. This resulted in developed two short versions to facilitate the administration of the questionnaire in clinical settings (16-item short-form) and in epidemiological surveys involving general populations (8-item short-form). Important to mention is that if an 8-item version could be used as an overall scale scores but not analysis is possible at the level of the individual domains. The number of items per domain is insufficient for this purpose. [64]

5.2.2. Child Perceptions Questionnaire 8-10 (CPQ 8-10) [65]

The CPQ_{8-10} contains 29 questions. The first two relate to demographic information; the next two pertain to global items; and the remaining twenty-five are divided into four domains: oral symptoms (OS), functional limitation (FL), emotional well-being (EW), and social well-being (SW). The questionnaire registers problems occurring during a prior four-week period. The responses are recorded in a Likert scale from 0 to 4, where 0=never; 1=once or twice; 2=sometimes; 3=often; and 4=every day or almost every day. The maximum score is 100, and the minimum is 0. For the global question concerning the general perception of oral health, the possible responses are 0=very good, 1=good, 2=OK, 3=poor. Regarding the second global question: How much does oral health affect daily living? With a scale as follows: 0=not at all, 1=a little bit, 2=some, 3=a lot.

Recently Foster and cols. suggested that these two questionnaires to be acceptable to be used in younger age group, since 5 years of age. They proposed to use a single questionnaire, CPQ_{8-10} or the short CPQ_{11-14}, to evaluated OHRQoL in children from 5 to 14 years of age [66], thus facilitating the use in prospective studies following children through different life stages.

5.2.3. Parental-Caregiver Perceptions Questionnaire — P-CPQ lxii and Family Impact Scale — FIS

The P-CPQ has 31 items distributed into 4 subscales: 6 oral symptoms (OS), 8 functional limitations (FL), 7 emotional wellbeing (EWB) and 10 social wellbeing (SWB). The questions refer only to the frequency of events in the previous 3 months. The items have 5 Likert response options: 'never=0', 'once or twice=1', 'sometimes=2', 'often=3', 'every day or almost every day=4'. A 'don't know' response also was permitted and scored as 0. Global ratings of the child's oral health and impact of the oral condition on his or her overall wellbeing were obtained from the parents/caregivers. The global ratings had a 5-point response format from 'excellent=0' to 'poor=4' for oral health and 'not at all=0' to 'very much=4' for wellbeing. The P-CPQ score is calculated by summing the response codes to all 31 items and dividing this sum by the number of items for which a valid response is obtained. The P-CPQ was developed for use with younger children and provides a measure of a child's OHRQoL. Where both parental and child reports are used, the P-CPQ can be regarded as complementing the latter, thus providing a comprehensive profile of a child's health and well-being.

The FIS is included in the P-CPQ and consists of 14 items that attempted to capture the effect of a child's oral or oro-facial condition on four domains: related to parental and family activities with 5 questions, parental emotions (4questions), family conflict (4 questions) and family finances (1 question). The questions ask about the frequency of events in the previous 3 months. Response options for the four domains and the respective scores were: 'Never' (scoring 0); 'Once or twice' (1); 'Sometimes' (2); 'Often' (3); and 'Everyday' or 'Almost every day' (4). A 'Don't know' (DK) response was also allowed. The FIS scores are computed by summing all of the item scores. Scores for each of the four domains can also be computed. The final score could vary from 0 to 56, for which a higher score denoted a greater degree of the impact of child's oral conditions on the functioning of parents-caregivers and the family as a whole.

In 2013 Thomson and cols developed the short form of the P-CPQ [67] obtaining a 16-and 8-item short-form versions of the P-CPQ and FIS-8 short forms that were developed using data from two New Zealand pre/post-test interventional studies. The internal reliability, validity and responsiveness of the short-form versions were acceptable. [68]

5.2.4. Child Oral Impacts on Daily Performances [69]

The C-OIDP index is specifically designed to show the final impact of a number of oral health related conditions which can affect child's daily life. it is a short and enjoyable questionnaire, and relatively quick to administer. The modification of the OIDP included adjusting the language, changing the sequence of questions, simplifying index scales and shortening the recall period. When the index had been validated, pictures of performances were developed and tested in order to make the interview more practical. It was developed and tested among 11–12 year old Thai children. Eight activities are considered: eating, speaking, cleaning teeth, relaxing, emotion, and smiling, studying, and social contact.

The 0–5 scale was changed into 0–3 scale on the computer, by grouping together scores of 1 and 2, and scores of 4 and 5.

The index score is based on the score for each of these eight daily activities. The score for each activity is obtained by multiplying the frequency value by the severity value; the maximum score is therefore 3x3=9. Thus, the score scale for each activity is between 0 and 9. The total score is calculated by adding the scores for all activities, divided by the maximum score possible (8x9=72) and multiplying by 100. The index score ranges therefore between 0-100.

The C-OIDP has two modes of the same questionnaire: bone is interviewer-administered and the other is self-administered, and the latter is used in this validation for adolescents. Both modes have been shown to produce similar results.

5.2.5. The Child Oral Health Impact Profile [70]

The COHIP consists of 34 questions grouped into five domains measuring: oral health, functional well-being, socio-emotional well-being, school performance and self-image. This instrument was designed to measure self-reported OHRQoL in children 8-15 years of age, using both positive and negative questions. It was created by an international study and was simultaneously validated in the U.S.A., Great Britain, Spain, Portugal, China, France and Holland in 2007. Data reported suggest that this instrument has an acceptable validity and reliability (Cronbach's alpha 0.91, 0.84 CCI) to be applied in population of 8 to 15 years.

	Questionnaire	Original Language	Abbreviation	year	Validated in other languages
Child Oral Health Quality of Life Questionnaire COHQOL	Child Perception Questionnaire 11-14	English	CPQ_{11-14}	2005	Árabic, [73] Portugués [74], Chinese, [75] German [76], Italian, Cambodian [77], Danish [78]
	CPQ11-14 Short form	English		2006	Portuges, Arabic 79
	Child Perception Questionnaire 8-10	English	CPQ_{8-10}	2004	Spanish [80] Portugués, Danés, Bosnian
	Family Impact Scale	English	FIS	2007	Chinese, Portugués [81]
	Parental-Caregiver Perceptions Questionnaire	English	P-CPQ	2003	Chinese, Peruvian Spanish [82]
Child Oral Impacts of Daily Performance		English	Child-OIDP	2008	Spanish [83] Canarain Portugues, Swahilli, Malayan, French, Hebrew [84]
OIDP abreviated		English		2012	Indial [9] Albanian
Child Oral Health Impact Profile		English	COHIP[29]	2008	Spanish Persian [85] Corean [86]
Early Childhood Oral Health Impact Scale		English	ECOHIS[27]		Turkey [87], Persian [88] Chinese [89]. French [90] Lituan [91], Portugues [92]
Scale of Oral Health Outcomes		English	SOHO-5	2013	Portugues

Table 2. Questionnaires to asses OHRQoL in children

5.2.6. The Early Childhood Oral Health Impact Scale (ECOHIS) [71]

It was designed to evaluate OHRQoL of children of preschool age and younger. The ECOHIS consists of 13 questions relevant to preschool-age children. The survey questionnaire relies on parental ratings of the 13 items grouped in two main parts: the child impact section and the family impact section. The child impact section covers four domains: child symptoms (1 item), child functions (4 items), child psychology (2 items), and child self-image and social interaction (2 items). The family impact section covers two domains: parental distress (2 items) and family function (2 items). Each question asks about the frequency of an oral health-related problem and is scored on a scale from 0–5, as follows: never (score 0), hardly ever (score 1), occasionally (score 2), often (score 3), very often (score 4), don't know (score 5).

5.2.7. Scale of Oral Health Outcomes (SOHO) [72]

As dental caries is a chronic disease that can affect children from a very young age and it is important to measure its impacts on quality of life, as they may affect the psychological, social and educational development of the first self-reported OHRQoL measure among 5 year-old children. All inter-item correlations were positive and none was very high, and all item-total correlation coefficients were above the recommended level of 0.2

Cronbach's alpha was 0.74. Despite the positive initial results, the assessment of this questionnaire should be an on-going process, by extending psychometric testing to properties not evaluated so far, and assessing its applicability and performance in other populations.

6. Conclusions

Multiple definitions have been postulated to conceptualize HRQoL and OHRQoL and in spite of there are different concepts we can see in every single one that quality of life refers to something much broader than health than physical status, it promotes to see a human being and his environment.

Important to mention that the assessments in the area of health are usually performed by the "professional" and although this is deemed appropriate, they often do not reflect the complex set of feelings that patient has about having or not having good health and quality of life. Therefore, relevant information about the quality of life is of practical importance for various actors in the health sector such as the health policy makers, health services researchers, epidemiologists, health program evaluators, who should underpin and complement their decisions based on this information. The evaluation of these concepts should not substitute clinical ones; rather those should complement them so to take into account the patient's own perception of their health, expectations, desires and needs. In this sense it is accepted and recognized by dental community that oral health status can cause considerable pain and suffering, dentists should not be only focus on physical status but in subjective evaluations about how people feel and how much they are satisfied or affected with their own oral condition.

The evaluation of OHRQoL promotes a shift from traditional dental criteria assessment and care that focus on a person's social and emotional experience and physical functioning in defining appropriate treatment goals and outcomes.

Author details

Javier de la Fuente Hernández, Fátima del Carmen Aguilar Díaz* and María del Carmen Villanueva Vilchis

*Address all correspondence to: fatimaguilar@gmail.com

Escuela Nacional de Estudios Superiores Unidad León – UNAM, León, Gto, México

References

[1] World Health Organization. Ottawa charter for health promotion. 1986.

[2] World Health Organization. Health promotion: a discussion document; 1984. 1984.

[3] Dolan T. Identification of appropriate outcomes for an aging population. SpecCare-Dent 1993;13(1):35–9.

[4] Schawartzmann L. Calidad de vida relacionada a la salud: aspectos conceptuales. Ciencia y Enfermería IX (2):9.21, 2003.

[5] Leplege A, Hunt S. The problem of quality of Life in Medicine. JAMA. 1997;278(1): 47-50.

[6] The World Health Organization Quality of Life assessment (WHOQOL): position paper from the World Health Organization. SocSci Med 1995;41:1403-9.

[7] World Health Organization, Concepts and methods of community-based initiatives. Community-Based Initiatives Series, Geneva: World Health Organization; 2003.

[8] Monés J. ¿Se puede medir la calidad de vida? ¿Cuál es su importancia?. CirEsp 2004; 76(2):71-1.

[9] Slade Gary D. Measuring Oral Health and Quality of Life, Department of Dental Ecology, School of Dentistry, University of North Carolina, September, 1997.

[10] Palomino B, López PG. (Programa de la Socialdemocracia Alemania 1974:58), Nota crítica: Reflexiones sobre la Calidad de Vida y el Desarrollo, Región y Sociedad, Ene-Jun, vol XI, número 17, El colegio de Sonora, pp.171-185.

[11] Testa MA, Simonson DC. Assessment of quality of life outcomes. N Enl J Med 1996;334:835-840.

[12] Gill T, Feinstein A. A critical appraisal of the quality of life measurements. JAMA 1994;272:619-625.

[13] Locker, D. Measuring Oral Health And Quality Of Life: Concepts Of Oral Health, Disease And Quality Of Life; University of North Carolina, Canada; 1997; 11-24.

[14] Williams J, Wake M, Hesketh. Health–Related Quality of Life of Overweight and Obese Children. JAMA. 2005;293(1):70-6

[15] Seid M, Varna JW, Segall D, Kurtin PS. Health-related quality of life as a predictor of pediatric healthcare costs: a two year prospective cohort analysis. Health and Quality of Life Outcomes. 2004, 2:48.

[16] WHO (2003). The World Oral Health Report 2003: continuous improvement of oral health in the 21st century—the approach of the WHO Global Oral Health Pro-gramme. Geneva, Switzerland: World Health Organization

[17] Gift HC, Atchison KA. Oral health, health, and health-related quality of life. Medical Care 1995; 33:NS57-NS77.

[18] Locker D, Jokovic A, Tompson B (2005). Health-related quality of life of children aged 11 to 14 years with orofacial conditions. Cleft Palate Craniofac J 42:260-266

[19] Atchison KA, Shetty V, Belin TR, Der-Martirosian C, Leathers R, Black E, et al. (2006). Using patient self-report data to evaluate orofacial surgical outcomes. Community Dent Oral Epidemiol34:93-102.

[20] Jean-Louis SixoubHow to make a link between Oral Health-Related Quality of Life and dentin hypersensitivity in the dental office?Clin Oral Investig. 2013 March; 17(Suppl 1): 41–44. Published online 2012 December 23. doi: 10.1007/s00784-012-0915-x

[21] Sheiham A, Alexander D, Cohen L, Marinho V, Moysés S, Petersen PE, et al. Global Oral Health Inequalities: Task Group-Implementation and delivery of oral health strategies. Adv Dent Res. 2011May;23(2):259-67.

[22] Lee, G. H., McGrath, C., Yiu, C. K., & King, N. M. (2010). A comparison of a generic and oral health-specific measure in assessing the impact of early childhood caries on quality of life. Community Dentistry and Oral Epidemiology, 38, 333–339.

[23] Huntington, N. L., Spetter, D., Jones, J. A., Rich, S. E., Garcia, R. I., & Spiro, A, 3rd. (2011). Development and validation of a measure of pediatric oral health-related quality of life: the POQL. Journal of Public Health Dentistry, 71, 185–193.

[24] Robinson, P.G., Nalweyiso, N., Busingye, J., Whitworth, J. (2005). Subjective impacts of dental caries and fluorosis in rural Uganda children. Community Dental Health, 22(4), 231-236.

[25] Pradeep Kumar, Habib Ahmad Alvi, JitendraRao, BalendraPratap Singh, Sunit Kumar Jurel, Lakshya Kumar, Himanshi Aggarwal. Assessment of the quality of life in maxillectomy patients: A longitudinal study. J AdvProsthodont 2013;5:29-35

[26] Andiappan M, Gao W, Bernabé E, Kandala NB, Donaldson AN, Malocclusion, orthodontic treatment, and the Oral health Impact Profile (OHIP-14) Systematic review and meta-analysis.Angle Orthod. 2014 Aug 26. [Epub ahead of print]

[27] BATISTA, MariliaJesus, PERIANES, Lílian Berta Rihs, HILGERT, Juliana Balbinot, HUGO, Fernando Neves, & SOUSA, Maria da Luz Rosário de. (2014). The impacts of oral health on quality of life in working adults. Brazilian Oral Research, 28(1), 1-6. Epub August 26, 2014. Retrieved September 15, 2014, from http://www.scielo.br/scielo.php?script=sci_arttext&pid=S1806-83242014000100249&lng=en&tlng=en. 10.1590/1807-3107BOR-2014.vol28.0040

[28] Slade GD, Assessing oral health outcomes: Measuring oral health and quality of life : proceedings of a conference held June 13-14, at the University of North Carolina-Chapel Hill, North Carolina. Chapel Hill, N.C., Department of Dental Ecology, School of Dentistry, University of North Carolina; 1997:IX, 160 s.

[29] Gherunpong S, Tsakos G, Sheiham A. A sociodental approach to assessing dental needs of children: Concept and models. Int J PaediatrDent. 2006;16:81-8.

[30] Sischo L, Broder HL.Oral health-related quality of life: what, why, how, and future implications.J Dent Res. 2011 Nov;90(11):1264-70. doi: 10.1177/0022034511399918. Epub 2011 Mar 21.

[31] Aubrey Sheiham, Annie M. Cushing, Joan Maizels M.A.,THE SOCIAL IMPACTS OF DENTAL DISEASE. MEASURING ORAL HEALTH AND QUALITY OF LIFE, 1996

[32] Atchison KA, Dolan TA: Development of the Geriatric Oral Health Assessment Index. J Dent Educ 1990, 54:680-687. /

[33] Locker D, Matear D, Stephens M, Lawrence H, Payne B: Comparison of the GOHAI and OHIP-14 as measures of the oral health-related quality of life of the elderly. Community Dent Oral Epidemiol 2001, 29:373-381

[34] Strauss RP, Hunt RJ. Understanding the value of teeth to older adults: Influences on quality of life. Journal of Am. Dent. Assoc. 1993; 124: 105-110.

[35] Leao AT, Sheilam A. The development of a socio-dental measure of dental impacts on daily living. Community Dent. Health 1996; 13: 22-26.

[36] Aubrey Sheiham, Anna T. Leao. THE DENTAL IMPACT ON DAILY LIVING..Measuring Oral Health and Quality of Life, 1996;98:1351–87.

[37] Frisch MB, Cornell J, Villanueva M, Retzlaff PJ. Clinical Validation of the quality of life inventory: A measure of life satisfaction for use in treatment planning and outcome assessment. Psychological Assessment

[38] Slade G D, Spencer A S: Development and evaluation of the oral health impact profile. Community Dent Health 11: 3–11 (1994)

[39] Slade, G.D.Derivation and validation of a short-form oral health impact profile. Community Dentistry Oral Epidemiology 1997 25: 284-290

[40] Locker D, Allen PF. Developing short-form measures of oral health-related quality of life. J Public Health Dent. 2002 Winter; 62(1):13-20

[41] Wong AH, Cheung CS, McGrath C. Developing a short form of Oral Health Impact Profile (OHIP) for dental aesthetics: OHIP-aesthetic.Community Dent Oral Epidemiol. 2007 Feb;35(1):64-72.

[42] Locker D. Measuring oral health: A conceptual framework. Community Dent Health 1988; 5:3-18.

[43] Astrom AN, Haugejorden O, Skaret E, Trovik TA, Klock KS: Oral Impacts on Daily Performance in Norwegian adults: the influence of age, number of missing teeth, and socio-demographic factors.Eur J Oral Sci 2006, 114(2):115-121.

[44] Ostberg AL, Andersson P, Hakeberg M: Cross-cultural adaptation and validation of the oral Iimpacts on daily performances (OIDP) in Swedish. Swed Dent J 2008, 32(4): 187-195

[45] Eric J, Stancic I, Sojic LT, JelenkovicPopovac A, Tsakos G: Validity and reliability of the Oral Impacts on Daily Performance (OIDP) scale in the elderly population of Bosnia and Herzegovina.Gerodontology 2012, 29(2):e902-e908

[46] Montero J, Bravo M, Lo´pez-Valverde A. Development of a specific indicator of the well-being of wearers of removable dentures. Community Dent Oral Epidemiol 2011; 39: 515–524

[47] Preciado A1, Del Río J, Lynch CD, Castillo-Oyagüe R. A new, short, specific questionnaire (QoLIP-10) for evaluating the oral health-related quality of life of implant-retained overdenture and hybrid prosthesis wearers J Dent. 2013 Sep;41(9):753-63. doi: 10.1016/j.jdent.2013.06.014. Epub 2013 Jul 2.

[48] Tubert-Jeannin S, Riordan PJ, Morel-Papernot A, Porcheray S, Saby-Collet S: Validation of an oral health quality of life index (GOHAI) in France. Community Dent Oral Epidemiol 2003, 31:275-284.

[49] Hassel AJ, Rolko C, Koke U, Leisen J, RammelsbergP.Community Dent Oral Epidemiol. 2008 Feb;36(1):34-42. doi: 10.1111/j.1600-0528.2007.00351.

[50] A-Dan W, Jun-Qi L. Factors associated with the oral health-related quality of life in elderly persons in dental clinic: validation of a Mandarin Chinese version of GOHAI. Gerodontology. 2011 Sep;28(3):184–91.

[51] AtiehMA.Gerodontology. 2008 Mar;25(1):34-41. doi: 10.1111/j.1741-2358.2007.00195.x. Epub 2008 Jan 13.

[52] Hägglin C, Berggren U, Lundgren J. A Swedish version of the GOHAI index. Psycho-
      metric properties and validation. Swed Dent J. 2005;29(3):113–24.

[53] Othman WN, Muttalib KA, Bakri R, Doss JG, Jaafar N, Salleh NC, et al. Validation of
      the Geriatric Oral Health Assessment Index (GOHAI) in the Malay language. J Public
      Health Dent. 2006 Ago 18;66(3):199-204.

[54] Daradkeh S, Khader YS. Translation and validation of the Arabic version of the Geri-
      atric Oral Health Assessment Index (GOHAI). J Oral Sci. 2008 Dec;50(4):453–9.

[55] Ergül S, Akar GC. Reliability and validity of the Geriatric Oral Health Assessment In-
      dex in Turkey. J GerontolNurs. 2008 Sep;34(9):33–9.

[56] Deshmukh SP, Radke UM. Translation and validation of the Hindi version of the
      Geriatric Oral Health Assessment Index. Gerodontology. 2012 Jun;29(2):e1052–8.

[57] Sánchez-García S, Heredia-Ponce E, Juárez-Cedillo T, Gallegos-Carrillo K, Espinel-
      Bermúdez C, de la Fuente-Hernández J et al. Psychometric properties of the General
      Oral Health Assessment Index (GOHAI) and dental status of an elderly Mexican
      population. J PublicHealthDent. 2010;70(4):300–7.

[58] CAMPOS, Juliana Alvares Duarte Bonini, CARRASCOSA, AndréaCorrêa, ZUCOLO-
      TO, MirianeLucindo, & MAROCO, João. (2014). Validation of a measuring instru-
      ment for the perception of oral health in women. Brazilian Oral Research, 28(1), 1-7.
      Epub August 18, 2014. Retrieved September 12, 2014, from http://www.scielo.br/scie-
      lo.php?script=sci_arttext&pid=S1806-83242014000100244&lng=en&tlng=en.
      10.1590/1807-3107BOR-2014.vol28.0033.

[59] Agrawal N, Pushpanjali K, GargAK.The cross cultural adaptation and validity of the
      child-OIDP scale among school children in Karnataka, South India. Community Dent
      Health. 2013 Jun;30(2):124-6

[60] Usha GV, Thippeswamy HM, Nagesh L. Validity and reliability of Oral Impacts on
      Daily Performances Frequency Scale: a cross-sectional survey among adolescents. J
      ClinPediatr Dent. 2012 Spring;36(3):251-6.

[61] Jokovic A, Locker D, Stephens M, Kenny D, Tompson B, Guyatt G. Validity and relia-
      bility of a questionnaire for measuring child oral-health-related quality of life. J Dent
      Res. 2002 Jul; 81(7):459-63.

[62] Jokovic A, Locker D, Stephens M, Kenny D,Tompson B, Guyatt G. Measuring paren-
      tal perceptions of child oral health-related quality of life.J Public Health Dent.
      2003;63:67-72.

[63] Locker D, Jokovic A, Stephens M, Kenny D, Tompson B, Guyatt G. Family impact of
      child oral and oro-facial conditions. Community Dent Oral Epidemiol. 2002;30:438-48

[64] Jokovic A, Locker D, Guyatt G. Short forms of the Child Perceptions Questionnaire
      for 11–14-year-old children (CPQ11–14): Development and initial evaluation. Health

Qual Life Outcomes. 2006; 4: 4.Published online Jan 19, 2006. doi: 10.1186/1477-7525-4-4

[65] Jokovic A, Locker D, Tompson B, Guyatt G. Questionnaire for measuring oral health-related quality of life in eight-to ten-year-old children. Pediatr Dent. 2004;26:512-8.

[66] Foster Page et al. Do we need more than one Child Perceptions Questionnaire for children and adolescents? BMC Oral Health 2013, 13:26

[67] Thomson WM, Foster Page LA, Gaynor WN, Malden PE. Short-form versions of the Parental-Caregivers Perceptions Questionnaire and the Family Impact Scale. Community Dent Oral Epidemiol 2013; 41: 441–450.

[68] Thomson WM, Foster Page LA, Gaynor WN, Malden PE. Short-form versions of the Parental-Caregivers Perceptions Questionnaire and the Family Impact Scale. Community Dent Oral Epidemiol 2013; 41: 441–450.

[69] Gherunpong S, Tsakos G, Sheiham A: Developing and evaluating an oral health-related quality of life index for children; the CHILD-OIDP. Community Dent Health 2004, 21(2):161-169.

[70] Broder HL, McGrath C, Cisneros GJ, Questionnaire development: face validity and item impact testing of the Child Oral Health Impact Profile. Community Dent Oral Epidemiol 2007; 35 (Suppl.1): 8-19.

[71] Pahel BT, Rozier RG, Slade GD: Parental perceptions of children's oral health: the Early Childhood Oral Health Impact Scale (ECOHIS). Health Qual Life Outcomes 2007, 5:6.

[72] Tsakos et al.: Developing a new self-reported scale of oral health outcomes for 5-year-old children (SOHO-5). Health and Quality of Life Outcomes 2012 10:62

[73] Brown A, Al-Khayal Z: Validity and reliability of the Arabic translation of the child oral health related quality of life questionnaire (CPQ11-14) in Saudi Arabia.Int J Paediatr Dent 2006, 16:405-411

[74] Goursand D, Paiva SM, Zarzar PM, Ramos-Jorge ML, Cornacchia GM, Pordeus IA, Allison PJ: Cross-cultural adaptation of the Child Perceptions Questionnaire 11–14 (CPQ11-14) for the Brazilian Portuguese language.HealthQual Life Outcomes 2008, 14:2

[75] McGrath C, Pang HN, Lo EC, King NM, Hägg U, Samman N: Translation and evaluation of a Chinese version of the Child Oral Health-related Quality of Life measure. Int J PaediatrDent 2008, 18:267-274.

[76] The German version of the Child Perceptions Questionnaire (CPQ-G11-14): translation process, reliability, and validity in the general population.Bekes K, John MT, Zyriax R, Schaller HG, Hirsch

[77] Turton BJ, Thomson WM, Foster Page LA, Saub RB, Razak IA Validation of an Oral Health-Related Quality of Life Measure for Cambodian Children.. Asia Pac J Public Health. 2013 Oct 4. [Epub ahead of print]

[78] Wogelius P, Gjørup H, Haubek D, Lopez R, Poulsen S. Development of Danish version of child oral-health-related quality of life questionnaires (CPQ8-10 and CPQ11-14).BMC Oral Health. 2009 Apr 22;9:11. doi: 10.1186/1472-6831-9-11

[79] Bhayat A, Ali MA Validity and reliability of the Arabic short version of the child oral health-related quality of life questionnaire (CPQ 11-14) in Medina, Saudi Arabia..EastMediterr Health J. 2014 Aug 19;20(8):409-14

[80] del Carmen Aguilar-Díaz F, Irigoyen-Camacho ME. Validation of the CPQ8-10ESP in Mexican school children in urban areas. Med Oral Patol Oral Cir Bucal. 2011 May 1;16(3):e430-5.

[81] Goursand D, Paiva SM, Zarzar PM, Pordeus IA, Allison PJ..Family Impact Scale (FIS): psychometric properties of the Brazilian Portuguese language version.Eur J Paediatr Dent. 2009 Sep;10(3):141-6.

[82] Albites U, Abanto J, Bönecker M, Paiva SM, Aguilar-Gálvez D, Castillo JL. Parental-caregiver perceptions of child oral health-related quality of life (P-CPQ): Psychometric properties for the peruvianspanish language.

[83] Bernabé E, Sheiham A, Tsakos G. A comprehensive evaluation of the validity of Child-OIDP: further evidence from Peru.Community Dent Oral Epidemiol. 2008 Aug;36(4):317-25.

[84] Kushnir D, Natapov L, Ram D, Shapira J, Gabai A, Zusman SP. Validation of a Hebrew Version of the Child-OIDP Index, an Oral Health-related Quality of Life Measure for Children. Oral Health Prev Dent. 2013 Jul 18. doi: 10.3290/j.ohpd.a30173. [Epub ahead of print]

[85] Asgari I, Ahmady AE, Broder H, Eslamipour F, Wilson-Genderson M. Assessing the oral health-related quality of life in Iranian adolescents: validity of the Persian version of the Child Oral Health Impact Profile (COHIP). Oral Health Prev Dent. 2013;11(2):147-54. doi: 10.3290/j.ohpd.a29367.

[86] Ahn YS, Kim HY, Hong SM, Patton LL, Kim JH, Noh HJ. Validation of a Korean version of the Child Oral Health Impact Profile (COHIP) among 8-to 15-year-old school children. Int J Paediatr Dent. 2012 Jul;22(4):292-301. doi: 10.1111/j.1365-263X.2011.01197.x. Epub 2011 Nov 17.

[87] Peker K, Uysal Ö, BermekG.HealthQual Life Outcomes. 2011 Dec 22;9:118. doi: 10.1186/1477-7525-9-118. Cross-cultural adaptation and preliminary validation of the Turkish version of the early childhood oral health impact scale among 5-6-year-old children.

[88] Jabarifar SE, Golkari A, Ijadi MH, Jafarzadeh M, Khadem P. Validation of a Farsi version of the early childhood oral health impact scale (F-ECOHIS).

[89] Lee GH, McGrath C, Yiu CK, King NM. Translation and validation of a Chinese language version of the Early Childhood Oral Health Impact Scale (ECOHIS).

[90] Li S, Veronneau J, Allison PJ. Validation of a French language version of the Early Childhood Oral Health Impact Scale (ECOHIS). Health Qual Life Outcomes. 2008 Jan 22;6:9. doi: 10.1186/1477-7525-6-9

[91] Jankauskienė B, Narbutaitė J, Kubilius R, Gleiznys A. Adaptation and validation of the early childhood oral health impact scale in Lithuania. Stomatologija. 2012;14(4): 108-13.

[92] Martins-Júnior PA, Ramos-Jorge J, Paiva SM, Marques LS, Ramos-Jorge ML. Validations of the Brazilian version of the Early Childhood Oral Health Impact Scale (ECOHIS). Cad SaudePublica. 2012 Feb;28(2):367-74

Dental Implants

Dongliang Zhang and Lei Zheng

1. Introduction

This chapter reviews the present and probable future need and demand for dental implants. A dental implant is defined as an artificial tooth root replacement and is used to support restorations that resemble a natural tooth or group of natural teeth.

2. The goal of modern dentistry

The goal of modern dentistry is to return patients to oral health in a predictable fashion. The partial and complete edentulous patient may be unable to recover normal function, esthetics, comfort, or speech with a traditional removable prosthesis. The patient's function when wearing a denture may be reduced to one sixth of that level formerly experienced with natural dentition; however, an implant prosthesis may return the function to near-normal limits. The esthetics of the edentulous patient are affected as a result of muscle and bone atrophy. Continued bone resorption leads to irreversible facial changes. An implant prosthesis allows normal muscle function, and the implant stimulates the bone and maintains its dimension in a manner similar to healthy natural teeth. As a result, the facial features are not compromised by lack of support as often required for removable prostheses. In addition, implant-supported restorations are positioned in relation to esthetics, function, and speech, not in neutral zones of soft tissue support. The soft tissues of the edentulous patients are tender from the effects of thinning mucosa, decreased salivary flow, and unstable or unretentive prostheses. The implant-retained restoration does not require soft tissue support and improves oral comfort. Speech is often compromised with soft tissue-borne prostheses because the tongue and perioral musculature may be compromised to limit the movement of the mandibular prosthesis. The implant prosthesis is stable and retentive without the efforts of the musculature. Implant prostheses often offer a more predictable treatment course than traditional restorations. Thus the profession and the public are becoming increasingly aware of this dental discipline. Manufacturers' sales have increased from a few million dollars to more than several hundred million dollars. Almost every professional journal now publishes refereed reports on dental implants. All U.S. dental schools now teach implant dentistry to all interfacing specialties. Implant dentistry to all interfacing specialties. Implant dentistry has finally been accepted by organized dentistry. The current trend to expand the use of implant dentistry will continue until every restorative practice uses this modality for abutment support of both fixed and removable prostheses on a regular basis as the primary option for all tooth replacement.

3. Options for replacement of lost teeth

Implants can be necessary when natural teeth are lost. When tooth loss occurs, masticatory function is diminished; when the underlying bone of the jaws is not under normal function it can slowly lose its mass and density, which can lead to fractures of the mandible and reduction of the vertical dimension of the middle face. Frequently, the physical appearance of the person is noticeably affected.

When a tooth is lost, the individual and dentist face two choices. The first choice is: should I replace the missing tooth? The second is: what is the best way to replace it? Although these decisions may seem sequential, they are interrelated in important ways. The technical options available can influence the decision to replace a tooth, and modern science has produced more and better options for tooth replacement in many circumstances. The age and general health of the patient are critical. The condition of the remaining dentition, its configuration in the mouth, and its periodontal support are very important aspects of the decision to replace. Finally, the relative cost of options can play a role, but should not be dispositive for a treatment plan. In making these decisions, the dentist and patient must evaluate all of these factors to reach the best treatment for a particular patient.

A number of restorative options for the treatment of missing teeth are recognized as accepted dental therapy, depending on particular circumstances the patient presents. These include:

1.   Tissue-supported removable partial dentures (Figure 1)

2.   Tooth-supported bridges

3.   Implant-supported teeth (Figure 2)

Likewise, there are two basic options for replacing teeth in a completely edentulous arch:

1.   Tissue-supported removable complete dentures

2.   Implant-supported over-dentures

All these therapies have their indications for use.

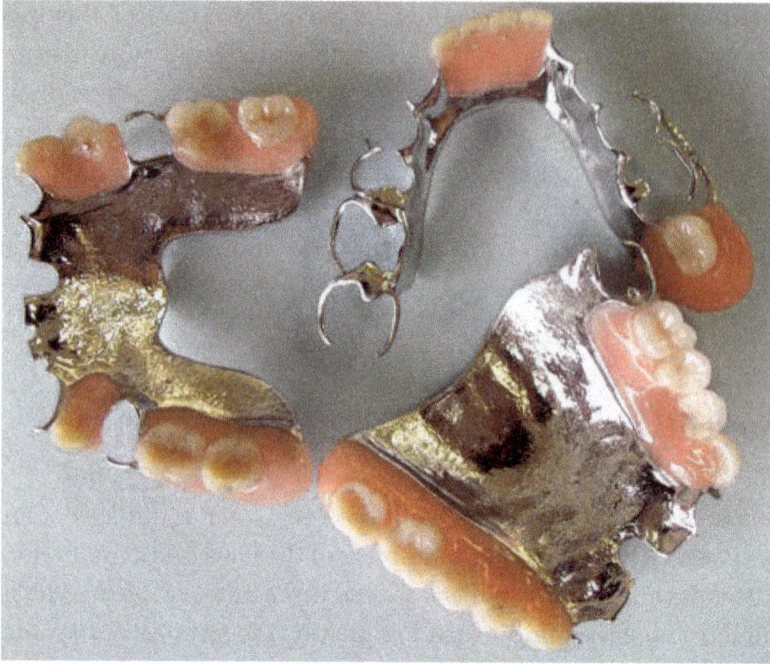

Figure 1. A typical collection of prosthetic devices, including flippers, removable partial dentures.

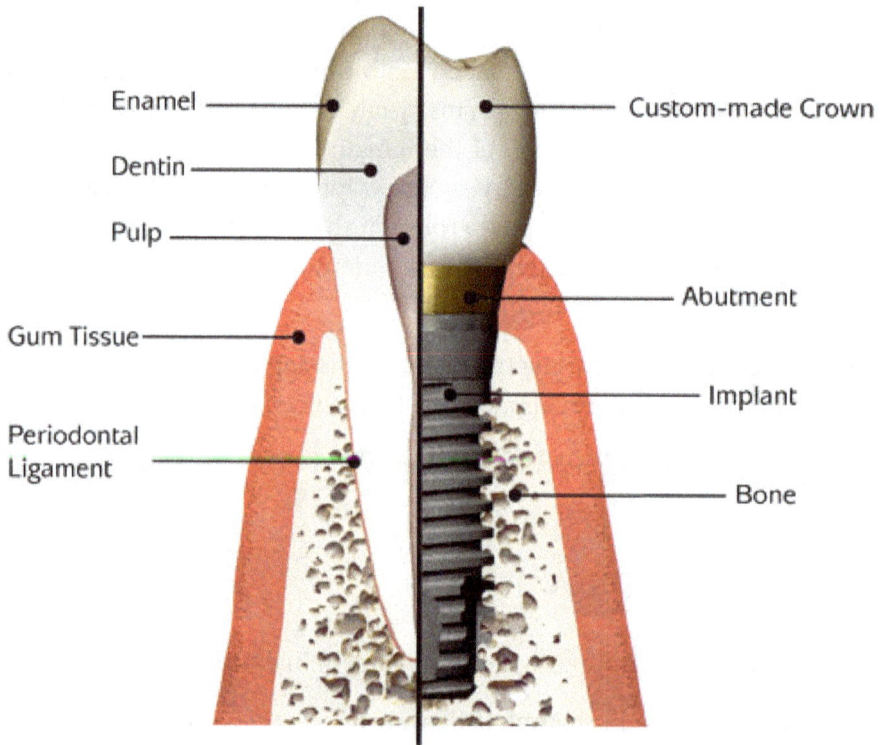

Enamel

Dentin

Pulp

Gum Tissue

Periodontal
Ligament

Custom-made Crown

Abutment

Implant

Bone

Figure 2. Comparison of natural tooth and crown with implant and crown.

4. Bone-supported prostheses

4.1. Dental implants

The implant is placed where the root of the missing tooth used to be. The replacement root is then used to attach a replacement tooth. Like the other options, dental implants are used to replace missing teeth and restore masticatory function to an individual's dentition.

The major types of dental implants are osseointegrated and fibrointegrated implants. Earlier implants, such as the subperiosteal implant and the blade implant, were usually fibrointegrated. The most widely accepted and successful implant today is the osseointegrated implant. Examples of endosseous implants (implants embedded into bone) date back over 1350 years. While excavating Mayan burial sites in Honduras in 1931, archaeologists found a fragment of mandible with an endosseous implant of Mayan origin, dating from about 600 AD.

Widespread use of osseointegrated dental implants is more recent. Modern dental implantology developed out of the landmark studies of bone healing and regeneration conducted in the 1950s and 1960s by Swedish orthopedic surgeon P.I. Brånemark. This therapy is based on the discover that titanium can be successfully fused with bone when osteoblasts grow on and into the rough surface of the implanted titanium. This forms a structural and functional connection between the living bone and the implant. A variation on the implant procedure is the implant-supported bridge, or implant-supported denture.

Today's dental implants are strong, durable, and natural in appearance. They offer a long-term solution to tooth loss. Dental implants are among the most successful procedures in dentistry. Studies have shown a 5-year success rate of 95% for lower jaw implants and 90% for upper jaw implants. The success rate for upper jaw implants is slightly lower because the upper jaw (especially the posterior section) is less dense than the lower jaw, making successful implantation and osseointegration potentially more difficult to achieve. Lower posterior implantation has the highest success rate of all dental implants.

Dental implants are less dependent than tooth-or tissue-supported prostheses on the configuration of the remaining natural teeth in the arch. They can be used to support prostheses for a completely edentulous arch, for an arch that does not have posterior tooth support, and for almost any configuration of partial edentulism with tooth support on both sides of the edentulous space.

Additionally, dental implants may be used in conjunction with other restorative procedures for maximum effectiveness. For example, a single implant can serve to support a crown replacing a single missing tooth. Implants also can be used to support a dental bridge for the replacement of multiple missing teeth, and can be used with dentures to increase stability and reduce gum tissue irritation. Another strategy for implant placement within narrow spaces is the incorporation of the mini-implant. Mini-implants may be used for small teeth and incisors.

Modern dental implants are virtually indistinguishable from natural teeth. They are typically placed in a single sitting require a period of osseointegration. This integration with the bone of the jaws takes anywhere from 3 to 6 months to anchor and heal. After that period of time a dentist places a permanent restoration for the missing crown of the tooth on the implant.

Although they demonstrate a very high success rate, dental implants may fail for a number of reasons, often related to a failure in the osseointegration process. For example, if the implant is placed in a poor position, osseointegration may not take place. Dental implants may break or become infected (like natural teeth) and crowns may become loose. Dental implants are not susceptible to caries attack, but poor oral hygiene can lead to the development of peri-implantitis around dental implants. This disease is tantamount to the development of perio-dontitis (severe gum disease) around a natural tooth.

Dental implant reconstruction may be indicated for tooth replacement any time after bone growth is complete. Certain medical conditions, such as active diabetes, cancer, or periodontal disease, may require additional treatment before the implant procedure can be performed. In some cases in which extensive bone loss has occurred in a jaw due to periodontal disease, implants may not be advised. Under proper circumstances, bone grafting may be used to augment the existing bone in a jaw prior to or in conjunction with placement.

5. Improvements in dental implant technology

New dental technology, materials, and designs have improved the dental implant procedure. Patients no longer have to wait to replace their missing teeth; the dental implant, abutment, and crown can be placed in just one visit. With immediate dental implants, the patient doesn't need to live with a space between teeth or wear a temporary crown while waiting for the dental implant to heal. With single-visit dental implants becoming more successful, more patients are inquiring about this procedure.

Using an ICAT cone beam CT scanner, a dentist can preplan dental implant surgery through 3-D imaging, creating a virtual mock-up of the mouth, which may eliminate an incision through the gums to find the bone. This, in turn, means less pain and healing time for the patient. During the planning stages, the prosthetic tooth can be fabricated by a dental labora-tory and can be ready at the time of surgery. This procedure bypasses the osseointegration period, in which the implant fuses to the bone. Although the implant still needs to heal, it can do so with the dental crown attached.

Mini-implants are a relatively recent implant technology. They are used primarily for dentures; a series of mini-implants are placed through the mucosa into the bone of the jaw. Posts are used to anchor the appliance into place. Mini-implants mean less pain and healing time, and normally cost less than traditional dental implants. These cutting-edge dental implants also eliminate the wait on the healing process for the final step. Patients can start wearing their replacement teeth right away.

Traditional dental implants meant that a new dental appliance was necessary, but some patients may be able to use existing dentures with mini-implants. Existing dentures can be fitted to attach to the posts implanted during surgery, enabling patients to return home with their repurposed dentures immediately after their surgery. Mini-implants are being used, in some indicated cases, to anchor dental crowns and dental bridges as well.

For the next 20 years the current elderly and baby-boom generations will be dominant factors in the demand for adult dental services. The former and a large portion of the latter did not experience the full benefits of modern preventive dentistry. They lost more teeth as children and young adults than the birth cohorts that follow them. Also, their dentitions suffered from greater caries attack, but they received substantial restorative care. Some of these restorations are likely to fail with time and a portion of those will require extraction, either due to the sequelae of previous restorative treatment or due to the advance of periodontal disease. Both generations have retained most of their natural teeth and are likely to want to replace those teeth they have already lost or will lose. Individuals aged 50 years and older today are likely to experience a substantial need for tooth replacement, and many of them will act on that need by choosing to have dental implants.

Over a longer time horizon, when today's young adults and children reach the age at which previous generations required substantial prosthetic replacement, their tooth loss is likely to be much less than those previous generations. That is good news. They will retain teeth, many of them sound. Hopefully, these groups will enjoy natural dentition throughout their life and will navigate old age with functioning, heal thy, natural teeth.

6. Generic prosthetic component terminology

A generic language for endosteal implants was developed by Misch and Misch in 1992. The order in which it is presented follows the chronology of insertion to restoration. In formulating the terminology, five commonly used implant system in the United States were referenced. Fifteen years later, the dramatic evolution of the U.S. implant market has resulted in changes in nearly all the implant lines and component designs. In 2000 the U.S. market alone ban to choose from more than 1300 different implant designs and 1500 abutments in various materials, shapes, sizes, diameters, lengths, surfaces, and connections. More than ever, a common language is needed. In pharmacology the variety of pharmaceutical components makes it impossible to list them all by proprietary names, but a list by category of drugs is useful. Likewise, implant components still can be classified into broad application categories, and the practitioner should be able to recognize a certain component category and know its indications and limitations.

This book incorporates a generic terminology, first introduced by Misch and Misch for endosteal implants, that blends a continuity and familiarity of many implant systems with established definitions from the terms of the Illustrated Dictionary of Dentistry and the glossaries from Terms of The Academy of Prosthodontics, American Implantologists.

7. Generic implant body terminology

Root from implant are a category of endosteal implants designed to use a vertical column of bone, similar to the root of a natural tooth. Although many names have been applied, the 1988 National Institutes of Health consensus statement on dental implants and the American Academy of Implant Dentistry recognized the term root form. The exponential growth of implant use over the last 20 years has been paralleled by an explosion of the implant manufacturing field. There are currently more than 90 implant body designs available, offering countless combinations of design features: screws, baskets, plateaus, ball, cylinders, diameters, lengths, prosthetic connections, and surface conditions.

The most common root form design combines a separate implant body and prosthodontic abutment abutment to permit only the implant body placement during bone healing. A second procedure is required to attach the implant abutment. The design and surgical philosophy is to achieve clinical rigid fixation that corresponds to a microscopic direct bone-to-implant interface without intervening fibrous tissue occurring over any significant portion of the implant body before the prosthetic phase of the procedure. Over the years, three different surgical approaches have been used for the two-piece implant systems: one stage, two stage, and immediate restoration.The two-stage surgical process places the implant body below the soft tissue, until the initial bone healing has occurred. During a second-stage surgery, the soft tissues are reflected to attach a permucosal element or abutment. During a one-stage surgical approach, the implant body and the permucosal abutment above the soft tissue are both placed until initial bone maturation has occurred. The abutment of the implant then replaces the permucosal element without the need for a secondary soft tissue surgery.

The immediate restoration approach places the implant body and the prosthetic abutment at the initial surgery. A restoration is then attached to the abutment (out of occlusal contacts in partially edentulous patients) at the appointment.

An implant body especially designed for one surgical method may also be selected. For example, a permucosal element may already be attached to the implant body by the manufacturer to facilitate a one-stage surgical approach. An implant body also may have a prosthetic abutment, which may be part of the inserted and restored at the initial surgery. This was the original concept first introduced by Strock in the 1930s.

There are three primary types of root form body endosteal implant based on design, cylinder, screw, or combination.

Cylinder (press-fit) root form implants depend on a coating or surface condition to provide microscopic retention to the bone. Most often the surface is either coated with a rough material (e.g., hydroxyapatite, titanium plasma spray) or a macro retentive design (e.g., sintered balls). Cylinder implant are usually pushed or tapped into a prepared bone site. They can be a paralleled wall cylinder or a tapered implant design. Screw root forms are threaded into a slightly smaller prepared bone site and have the macroscopic retentive elements of a thread for initial bone fixation. They may be machined, textured, or coated. There are three basic screw-thread geometries: V-thread, buttress (or reverse buttress) thread, and power (square) thread designs. Threaded implants are primarily available in a parallel cylinder or tapered cylinder design. Micro or macro thread features, variable thread pitch, depth, and angle, as well as self-tapping features, can be combined to create a myriad of implant designs. Combination root forms have macroscopic features from both the cylinder and screw root forms. The combination root form design also may benefit from microscopic retention to bone through varied surface treatments (machined, textured, and the addition of coatings).

Root forms also have been described by their means of insertion, healing, surgical requirements, surface characteristics, and interface.

8. Implant body regions

The implant body may be divided into a crest module (cervical geometry), a body, and an apex Each section of an implant has features that are of benefit in the surgical or prosthetic application of the implant

8.1. Implant body

An implant body is primarily designed for either surgical ease or prosthetic loading to the implant bone interface. Year ago, the implant body was the primary design feature. A round implant permits round surgical drills to prepare the bone. A smooth-walled cylinder implant allows the implant to be pressed or tapped into position, similar to a nail into a piece of wood. A tapered cylinder fits into the top of the osteotomy for further ease of placement.

A cylinder implant design system offers the advantage of ease of placement, even in difficult access locations. The cover screw of the implant also may be attached to the implant before implant placement. For example, in the very soft D4 bone the posterior regions of the maxilla, the surgeon must rotate a threaded implant design into place. Very soft bone may strip during threaded implant insertion. This may result in lack of initial fixation, and the implant will not be rigid. A tapered cylinder implant may be pressed by hand into soft bone and can be initially fixated more easily, The speed of implant rotation during insertion and the amount of apical force in implant insertion soft bone are less relevant for a press-fit cylinder. The cylinder system also presents some benefits for the single-tooth implant application, especially if adjacent to teeth with tall clinical crowns. Thread extenders are needed for the screw implant in these situations, as well as additional tools to insert the cover screw of the implant. In dense bone, cylinder systems also are easier and faster to place because bone tapping is not required

Most cylinder implants are essentially smooth-sided and bullet-shaped implants that require a bioactive or increased surface area coating for retention in the bone. When these materials are placed on an implant, the surface area of bone contact increases more than 30%. The greater the functional surface area of the bone implant contact, the better the support system for the prosthesis.

A solid screw implant body design is the most commonly reported in the literature. A solid screw body is defined as an implant of a circular cross section without penetrating any vents or holes. A number of manufactures provide this design (e.g., Nobel Biocare, Biomet, Zimmer, ITI, BioHorizons, LifeCroe, Bio-Lok). The thread may be V-shaped, buttress, reverse buttress, or square (power thread) in design. The V-shaped threaded screw has the longest history of clinical use. The most common outer thread diameter is 3.75mm, with 0.38-mm thread depth, and a 0.6-mm thread pitch (distance). The carious body lengths usually range from 7 to 16 mm, although lengths from 5 mm to 45 mm are available. Similar body designs are offered in a variety of diameters (narrow, standard, wide) to respond to the mechanical, esthetic, and anatomical requirements in different areas of the mouth.

A solid screw implant body permits the osteotomy and placement of the implant in dense cortical bone as well as in fine trabecular bone. The surgery may be easily modified to accommodate both extremes in bone density, The solid screw permits the implant removal at the time of surgery if placement is not ideal. It also permits implant removal at the Stage II surgery if angulation or crestal bony contours are not deemed adequate for long-term prosthesis success. The solid screw implant body may be machined or roughened to increase marginally the functional surface area or to take advantage of biochemical properties related to the surface coating (e, g., bone bonding or bone growth factors).

A threaded implant body is primarily designed to increase the bone-implant surface area and to decrease the stresses at the interface during occlusal loading. The functional surface area of a threaded implant is greater than a cylinder implant by a minimum of 30% and may exceed 500% depending on the thread geometry. This increase in functional implant surface area decreases the stress imposed on the implant-bone interface and is directly related to the thread geometry.

8.2. Crest module

The crest module of an implant body is that portion designed to retain the prosthetic component in a one-piece or two-piece implant system. It also represents the transition zone from the implant body design to the transosteal region of the implant at the crest of the ridge. The abutment connection area usually has a platform on which the abutment is seated; the platform offers physical resistance to axial occlusal loads. An antirotation feature also is included on the platform (external hex) or extends within the implant body (internal hex, octagon, Mores taper or cone screw, internal grooves or cam tube, and pin slots). The implant body has a design to transfer stress/strain to the bone during occlusal loads (e, g., threads or large spheres), whereas the crest module often is designed to reduce bacterial invasion. (e. g., smoother to impair plaque retention if crestal bone loss occurs). Its smoother dimension varies greatly from one system to another (0.5 to 0.5 mm). When the crest module is smooth, polished metal, it is often called a cervical collar.

A high-precision fit of the external or internal anti-rotational component (flat to flat dimension) is para-mount to the stability of the implant body/abutment connection. The prosthetic connection to the crest module is received by slip-fit or friction-fit with a butt or bevel joint. All prosthetic connections aim at providing a precise mating of the two components with minimal tolerance.

Another antirotational feature of an implant body may be flat sides or grooves along the body or apical region of the implant body. When bone grows against the flat or groove regions, the bone is placed in compression with rotational loads. The apical end of each implant should be flat rather than pointed. This allows for the entire length of the implant to incorporate design features that maximize desired strain profiles. Additionally, if an opposing cortical plate is perforated, a sharp, V-shaped apex may irritate or inflame the soft tissues if any movement occurs (e. g., the inferior border of the mandible).

9. Implant surgery

At the of insertion of a two-stage implant body (stage I surgery), a frost-stage cover screw is placed into the top of the implant to prevent bone, soft tissue, or debris from invading the abutment connection area during healing.

After a prescribed healing period sufficient to allow a supporting bone interface to develop, a second-stage procedure may be performed to expose the two-stage implant or to attach a transepithelial portion. This transepitthelial portions is termed a permucosal extension because it extends the implant above the soft tissue and results in the development of a permucosal seal around the implant. This implant component has also been called a healing abutment because stage II uncovery surgery often uses this device for initial soft tissue healing.

In the case of a one-stage procedure, the surgeon may have placed the permucosal extension at the time of implant insertion or may have selected an implant body design with a cervical collar of sufficient height to be supragingival. In the case of immediate load, the permucosal healing abutment may not be used at all if a temporary prosthesis is delivered on the day of surgery or may be sued until the suture removal appointment and the temporary teeth delivery. The permucosal extension is available in multiple heights to accommodate soft tissue variations. It also can be straight, flared, or anatomical to assist in the initial contour of the soft tissue healing.

9.1. Prosthetic attachments

The abutment is the portion of the implant that supports or retains a prosthesis or implant superstructure. A superstructure is defined as a metal framework that attaches to the implant abutment(s) and provides either retention for a removable prosthesis (e, g., a cast bar retaining an overdenture with attachments) or the framework for a fixed prosthesis. Three main categories of implant abutments are described, according to the method by which the prosthesis or superstructure is retained to the abutment; (1) an abutment for screw retention uses a screw to retain the prosthesis or superstructure, (2) an abutment for cement retention uses dental cement to retain the prosthesis or superstructure, and (3) an abutment for attachment uses an attachment device to retain a removable prosthesis(such as an O-ring attachment).The abutment for cement/screw/attachment may be screwed or cemented into the implant body, but this aspect is not delineated within the generic terminology

Each of three abutment types may be further classified as straight or angled abutments, describing the axial relationship between the implant body and the abutment. An abutment for screw retention uses a hygiene cover screw placed over the abutment to prevent debris and calculus from invading the internally threaded portion of the abutment retention during prosthesis fabrication between prosthetic appointments.

The lack of abutment design of a decade ago has been replaced by a variety of options. The expansion of implant dentistry, is applications for esthetic dentistry, and the creativity of manufacturers in this very competitive market is responsible today. In the abutment for cement category, the doctor may choose from one-and two-piece abutments; UCLA type(plastic castable, machined/plastic castable, gold sleeve castable); two-piece esthetic; two-piece anatomical; two-piece shoulder; preangled (several angulations); or ceramic, Zirconia, or computer-assisted custom design. The abutment for screw category also has been enlarged with one-and two-piece overdenture abutments of different contours and heights.

Many manufacturers classify the prosthesis as fixed whenever cement retains the prostheses, fixed/removable when screws retain a fixed prosthesis, and removable when the restoration is removed by the patient. This description implies that only screw-retained description, because a fixed, cemented prosthesis also may be removed by the dentist (especially when a temporary cement is used). The generic language in this chapter separates prostheses into either fixed or removable in a method similar to traditional prosthetics.

9.2. Prosthesis fabrication

An impression is necessary to transfer the position and design of the implant or abutment to a master cast for prosthesis fabrication. A transfer coping is used in traditional prosthetics to position a die in an impression. Most implant manufacturers use the terms transfer and coping to describe the component used for the final impression. Therefore a transfer coping is used to position an analog in an impression and is defined by the portion of the implant it transfers to the master cast, either the implant body transfer or the abutment transfer coping.

Two basic implant restorative techniques are used to make a master impression, and each uses a different design transfer coping, based on the transfer technique performed. An indirect transfer coping uses an impression material requiring elastic properties. The indirect transfer coping is screw into the abutment or implant body and remains in place when a traditional "closed tray" impression is set and removed from the mouth. The indirect transfer coping is usually slightly tapered to allow ease in removal of the impression and often has flat sides or smooth undercuts to facilitate reorientation in the impression after it is removed.

A direct transfer, often square, and a long central screw to secure it to the abutment or implant body and may be used a pick-up implant coping. An "open tray" impression tray is used to permit direct access to the long central screw securing the indirect transfer coping. After the impression material is set, the direct transfer coping screw is unthreaded to allow removal of the impression from the mouth, direct transfer copings take advantage of impression materials having rigid properties and eliminate the error of permanent deformation because they remain within the impression until the master model is poured and separated.

9.3. Laboratory fabrication

An analog is defined as something that is analogous or similar to something else. An implant analog is used in the fabrication of the master cast to replicate the retentive portion of the implant body or abutment (implant body analog, implant abutment analog). After the master impression is obtained, the corresponding analog (e, g., implant body, abutment for screw) is attached to the transfer coping and the assembly is poured in stone to fabricate the master cast.

A prosthetic coping is a thin covering, usually designed to fit the implant abutment for screw retention. It serves as the connection between the abutment and the prosthesis or superstructure. A prefabricated coping usually is a metal component machined precisely to fit the abutment. A castable coping usually is a plastic pattern cast in the same metal as the superstructure or prosthesis. A screw-retained prosthesis or superstructure is secured to the implant body or abutment with a prosthetic screw.

10. Prosthetic options in implant dentistry

Implant dentistry is similar to all aspects of medicine in that treatment begins with a diagnosis of the patient's condition. Many treatment options stem from the diagnostic information. Traditional dentistry provides limited treatment options for the edentulous patient. Because the dentist cannot add abutments, the restoration design is directly related to the existing oral condition. On the other hand, implant dentistry can provide. On the other hand, implant dentistry can provide a range of additional abutment locations. Bone augmentation may further modify the existing edentulous condition in both the partial and total edentulous arch and therefore also affects the final prosthetic design. As a result, a number of treatment options are available to most partially and completely, the implant treatment plan of choice at a par particular moment is patient and problem based. Not all patients should be treated with the same restoration type or design.

Almost all man-made creations, whether art, building, or prostheses, require the end result to be visualized and precisely planned for optimal results. Blueprints indicate the finest details for buildings. The end result should be clearly identified before the project begins, yet implant dentist often forget this simple but fundamental axiom. Historically in implant dentistry, bone available for implant insertion dictated the number and locations of dental implants. The prosthesis then was often determined after the position and number of implants were selected.

The goals of implant dentistry are to replace a patient's missing teeth to normal contour, comfort, function, esthetics, speech, and health, regardless of the previous atrophy, disease, or injury of the stomatognathic system. It is the final restoration, not the implant, that accomplish these goals. In other words, patients are missing teeth, not implants. To satisfy predictably a patient's needs and desires, the prosthesis should first be designed. In the stress treatment theorem, the final restoration is first planned, similar to the architect designing a building before making the foundation foundation. Only after this is accomplished can the abutments necessary to support the specific predetermined restoration be designed.

11. Completely edentulous prosthesis design

The completely edentulous patient is too often treated as though cost were the primary factor in establishing a treatment plan. However, the doctor and staff should specifically ask about the patient's desires. Some patients have a strong psychologic need to have a fixed prosthesis as similar to natural teeth as possible. On the other hand, some patients do not express serious concerns whether the restoration is fixed or removable as long as prosthetic problems are addressed. To assess the ideal final prosthetic design, the existing anatomy is evaluated after restoration is desired.

An axiom of implant treatment is not provide the most predictable, most cost-effective treatment that will satisfy the patient's anatomical needs and personal desires. In the completely edentulous patient, a removable implant. Supported prosthesis offers several advantages over a fixed-implant restoration.(Box 1).

BOX 1. Advantages of Removable Implant-supported Prostheses in the Completely Edentulous Patient

*facial esthetics can be enhanced with labial flanges and denture teeth compared with customized metal or porcelain teeth. The labial contours of the removable restoration can replace lost bone width and height and support the labial soft tissues without hygienic compromise.

*The prosthesis can be removed at night to manage nocturnal parafunction.

*Fewer implants may be required.

*Less bone augmentation may be necessary before implant insertion.

*Shorter treatment if no bone augmentation is required.

*The treatment may be expensive for the patient.

*Long-term treatment of complications is facilitated.

*Daily home care is easier.

However, some completely edentulous patients require a fixed restoration because of desire or because their oral condition makes the fabrication of teeth difficult if a superstructure and removable prosthesis are planned. For example, when the patient has abundant bone and implants have already been placed, the lack of crown height space may not permit a removable prosthesis.

Too often, treatment plans for completely edentulous patients consist of a maxillary denture and a mandibular overdenture with two implants. However, in the long term, this treatment option may prove a disservice to the patient. The maxillary arch will continue to lose bone, and the bone loss may even be accelerated in the premaxilla. Once this dimension is lost, the patient will have much more difficulty with retention and stability of the restoration. In addition, the lack of posterior implant support in the mandible will allow posterior bone loss to continue. Paresthesia, facial changes, and reduced posterior occlusion on the maxillary prosthesis are to be expected. The doctor should diagnose the amount of bone loss and its consequences on facial esthetics, function, and the psychological and overall health. Patients should be made aware of future compromises in bone loss and its associated problems with minimal treatment options, which do not address the continued loss of bone in regions where implants are not inserted.

It is even more important to visualize the final restoration at the onset with a fixed-implant restoration. After this first important step, the individual areas of ideal or key abutment support are determined to assess whether it is possible to place the implants to support the intended prosthesis. The patient's force and bone density in the region of implant support are evaluated. The additional implants to support the expected forces on the prosthesis designed may then be determined with implant size and design selected to match force and area conditions. Only then is the available bone evaluated to assess whether it is possible to place the implants to support the intended prosthesis. In inadequate natural or implant abutment situations, the existing oral conditions or the needs and desires of the patient must be altered. In other words, either the mouth must be modified by augmentation to place implants in the correct anatomical positions, or the mind of the patient must be modified to accept a different prosthesis type and its limitations. A fixed-implant restoration may be indicated for either the partially or the completely edentulous patient. The psychological advantage of fixed teeth is a major benefit, and edentulous patients often feel the implant teeth are better than their own. The improvement over their removable restoration is significant.

BOX 2. Advantages of fixed Restorations in the Partially Edentulous patient

1. psychological (feels,more like natural teeth)

2. Less food entrapment

3. Less maintenance (no attachments to change of adjust)

4. Longevity (lasts the life of the implants)

5. Similar overhead cost as completely implant-supported overdentures

---

The completely implant-supported overdenture requires the same number of implants as a fixed-implant restoration. Thus the cost of implant surgery may be similar for fixed or removable restorations. Fixed prostheses often last longer than overdentures, because attachments do not require replacement and acrylic denture teeth wear faster than porcelain to metal. The chance of food entrapment under a removable overdenture is often greater than for a fixed restoration, as soft tissue extensions and support are often required in the latter. The laboratory fees for a fixed prosthesis may be similar to a bar, coping attachments, and over denture. Because the denture or partial denture fees are much less than fixed prostheses, many clinicians charge the patient a much lower fee for removable over dentures on implants. Yet chair time and laboratory fees are often similar for fixed or removable restorations that are completely implant supported. One should consider increasing the patient fees for over dentures to a level more in line with fixed restorations.

Type	Definition
FP-1	Fixed prosthesis; replaces only the crown; looks like a natural tooth
FP-2	Fixed prosthesis; replaces the crown and a portion of the root; crown contour appears normal in the occlusal half but is elongated or hypercontoured in the gingival half
FP-3	Fixed prosthesis; replaces missing crows and gingival color and poration of the edentulous site; prosthesis most often uses denture teeth and acrylic gingival, but may be porcelain to metal
RP-4	Removable prosthesis ; overdenture supported completely by implant
RP-5	Removable prosthesis; overdenture supported by both soft tissue and implant

Table 1. Prosthodontic classification

12. Partially edentulous prosthesis design

A common axiom in traditional prosthodontics for partial edentulism is to provide a fixed partial denture whenever applicable. The fewer natural teeth missing the better the indication for a fixed partial denture. This axiom also applies to implant prostheses in the partially edentulous patient. Ideally, the fixed partial denture is completely implant supported rather than joining implants in the treatment plan. Although this may be a cost disadvantage, it is outweighed by significant intraoral health benefits. The added implants in the edentulous site result in fewer pontics, more retentive units in the restoration, and less stress to the supporting bone. As a result complications are minimized and implant and prosthesis longevity are increased (BOX 2)

13. Prosthetic options

In 1989, Misch proposed five prosthetic options for implant dentistry (Table 1). The first three options are fixed prostheses (FPs). These three options may replace partial (one tooth or several) or total dentitions and may be cemented or screw retained. They are used to communicate the appearance of the final prosthesis to all the implant team members. These options depend and the aspects of the prosthesis in the esthetic zone. Common to all foxed options is the inability of the patient to remove the prosthesis. Two types of final implant restorations are removable prostheses (RPS); they depend on the amount of implant support, not the appearance of the prosthesis.

13.1. Fixed prostheses

13.1.1. FP-1

An FP-1 is a fixed restoration and appears to the patient to replace only the anatomical crowns of the missing natural teeth. To fabricate this restoration type, there must be minimal loss of hard and soft tissues. The volume and position of the residual bone must permit ideal placement of the implant in a location similar to the root of a natural tooth. The final restoration appears very similar in size and contour to most traditional fixed prostheses used to restore or replace natural crowns of teeth.

The FP-1 prosthesis is most often desired in the maxillary anterior region, especially in the esthetic zone during smiling or speaking. The final FP-1 restoration appears to the patient to be similar to a crown on a natural tooth. However, the implant abutment can rarely be treated as a natural tooth prepared for a full crown. The cervical diameter of a maxillary central incisor is approximately 6.5 mm with an oval to triangular cross section. However, the implant abutment is usually 4 mm in diameter and round in cross section. In addition, the placement of the implant rarely corresponds exactly to the crown-root position of the original tooth. The thin labial bone lying over the facial aspect of a maxillary anterior root remodels after tooth loss and the crest width shifts to the palate, decreasing 40% within the first 2 years. The occlusal table is also usually modified in unesthetic regions to conform to the implant size and position and to direct vertical forces to the implant body, For example, posterior mandibular implant –supported prostheses have narrower occlusal tables at the expense of the buccal contour, because the implant is smaller in diameter and placed in the central fossa region of the tooth.

Because the width or height of the crestal bone is frequently lacking after the loss of multiple adjacent natural teeth, bone augmentation is often required before implant placement to achieve natural-looking crowns in the cervical region. These are no interdental papillae in edentulous ridges; therefore soft tissue augmentation also is often required to improve the interproximal gingival contour. Ignoring this step causes open "black" triangular spaces (where papillae usually be present) when the patient smiles. FP-1 prostheses are especially difficult to achieve when more than two adjacent teeth are missing. The bone loss and lack of interdental soft tissue complete the final esthetic result, especially in the cervical region of the crowns.

The restorative material of choice for an FP-1 prosthesis is porcelain to noble to noble-metal alloy. A noble-metal substructure can easily be separated and soldered in case of a nonpassive fit at the metal try-in, and noble metals in contact with implants corrode less than nonprecious alloys. Any history of exudate around a subgingival base-metal margin will dramatically increase the corrosion effect between the implant and the base metal. A single tooth FP-1 crown may use aluminum oxide cores and porcelain crowns, or ceramic abutments and porcelain crowns. However, the risk of fracture ma increase with the latter scenario, as implant forces are greater on implants than natural teeth.

13.1.2. FP-2

An FP-2 fixed prosthesis appears to restore the anatomical crown and a portion of the root of the natural tooth. The volume and topography of the available bone is more apical compared with the ideal bone position of a natural root (1 to 2 mm below the cement-enamel junction) and dictate a more apical implant placement compared with the FP-1 prosthesis. As a result, the incisal edge is in the correct position, but the gingival third of the crown is overextended, usually apical and lingual to the position of the original tooth. These restorations are similar to teeth exhibiting periodontal bone loss and gingival recession.

The patient and the clinician should be aware from the onset of treatment that the final prosthetic teeth will appear longer than healthy natural teeth (without bone loss). The esthetic zone of a patient is established during smiling in the maxillary arch and during speech of sibilant sounds for the mandibular arch. If the high lip during smiling or the low lip line longer are usually of no esthetic consequence, provided that the patient has been informed before treatment.

As the patient becomes older, the maxillary esthetic zone is altered. Only 10% of younger patients do not show any soft tissue during smiling, whereas 30% of 60 year old and 50% of 80year olds do not display gingival regions during smiling. The low lip position during speech is not affected as much as the mandibular soft tissue during speech.

A multiple-unit Fp-2 restoration does not require as specific an implant position because the cervical contour is not displayed during function. The implant position may be chosen in relation to bone width, angulation, or hygienic considerations rather than purely esthetic demands (as compared with the FP-1 prosthesis). On occasion, the implant may even be placed in an embrasure between two teeth. This often occurs for mandibular anterior teeth for full-arch fixed restorations. If this occurs, the most esthetic area usually requires the incisal two thirds of the two crowns to be ideal in width, as though the implant were not present. Only the cervical region is compromised. Although the implant is not positioned in the correct facial-lingual position, it should be placed in the correct facial-lingual position to ensure that contour, hygiene, and direction of forces are not compromised.

The material of choice for an FP-2 prosthesis is precious metal to porcelain. The amount and contour of the metal work is different than for a FP-1 restoration and is more relevant in an FP-2 prosthesis, because the amount of additional volume of tooth replacement increases the risk of unsupported porcelain in the final prosthesis, then the metal work in undercontoured.

13.1.3. FP-3

The FP-3 fixed restoration appears to replace the natural teeth crowns and has pink-colored restorative materials to replace a portion of the soft tissue. As with the FP-2 prosthesis, the original available bone height has decreased by natural resorption or osteoplasty at the time of implant placement. To place the incisal edge of the teeth in proper position for esthetics, function, lip support, and speech, the excessive vertical dimension to be restored requires teeth that are unnatural in length. However, unlike the FP-2 prosthesis, the patient may have a normal to high maxillary lip line during smiling or a low mandibular lip line during speech. The ideal high smile line displays the interdental papilla of the maxillary anterior teeth but not the soft tissue above the midcervical regions. Approximately 7% of males and 14% of females have a high smile or "gummy" smile and display more than 2 mm of gingival above the free gingival margin of the teeth.

The patient may also have greater esthetic demands even when the teeth are out of the esthetic simile and speech zones. Patients complain that the display of longer teeth appears unnatural even though they must lift or move their lips in unnatural positions to see the covered regions of the teeth. As a result of the restored gingival color of the Fp-3, the teeth have a more natural appearance in size and shape and the pink restorative material mimics the interdental papillae and cervical emergence region. The addition of gingival-tone acrylic or porcelain for a more natural fixed prosthesis appearance is often indicated with multiple implant abutments because bone loss is common with these conditions.

There are basically two approaches of denture teeth and acrylic and metal substructure or a porcelain metal restoration. The primary factor that determines the restoration material is the amount of crown height space. An excessive crown height space means a traditional porcelain-metal restoration will have a large amount of metal in the substructure, so the porcelain thickness will not be greater than 2-mm thick. Otherwise there is an increase in porcelain fracture Precious metals are indicated for implant restorations to decrease the risk of corrosion `and improve the accuracy of the casting, as nonprecious metals shrink more during the casing process. However, the large amount of metal in the substructure acts as a heat sink and complicates the application of porcelain during the fabrication of the prosthesis, In addition, as the metal cools after casting, the thinner regions of metal cool first and create porosities in the structure. This may lead to fracture of the framework after loading. Furthermore when the casting is reinserted into the oven bake the porcelain, the heat is maintained within the casting at different rates, thus the porcelain cool-down rate is variable, which increases the risk of porcelain fracture. In addition, the amount of precious metal in the casting adds to the weight and cost of the restoration. An FP-3 porcelain-to-metal restoration is more difficult to fabricate for the laboratory technician than an FP-2 prosthesis. The pink porcelain is harder to make appear as soft tissue and usually requires more baking cycles. This increases the risk of porosity or porcelain fracture.

An alternative to the traditional porcelain-metal fixed prosthesis is a hybrid restoration (see Table 2). This restoration design uses a smaller metal framework, with denture teeth and acrylic to join these elements together. This restoration is less expensive to fabricate and is highly esthetic because of the premade denture teeth and acrylic pink soft tissue replacements. In addition, the intermediary acrylic between the denture teeth and framework may reduce the impact force of dynamic occlusal loads. The hybrid prosthesis is easier to repair in porcelain fracture, as the denture tooth may be traditional porcelain-metal restoration. However, the fatigue of acrylic is greater than the traditional prosthesis; therefore repair of the restoration is more commonly needed.

The crown height space determination for a hybrid versus the traditional porcelain-metal restoration is 15 mm from the bone to the occlusal plane. When less than this dimension is available, a porcelain-to-metal is suggested. When a greater crown height space is present a hybrid restoration is often fabricated.

Consideration	Porcelain-metal	Hybrid
Occlusal Vertical Dimension	≦15 mm	≧15 mm
Technique	Same	Same
Retention	Cement or screw	Cement or Screw
Precision of fit	Same	Same
Esthetics	Same	Same
Soft tissue	Difficult	Easier
Teeh	Difficult	Easer (resin)
Time/Appointments	Same	Less
Weight	More	Less
Cost	More	Less
Impact forces	More	Less
Volume (bulk)	Same	Same
Lone term	Same	Same
Occlusion	Same	Same
Speech	Same	Same
Hygiene	Same	Same
Complications	Same	Same
Aging of materials	Less	More

Table 2. Comparison of Porcelain-to-Metal versus Hybrid Prostheses (FP-3)

Implants placed too facial, lingual, or in embrasures are easier to restore when vertical bone has been lost and an FP-2 or FP-3 prosthesis is fabricated, because even extremely high smile lip lines do not expose the implant abutments. The greater crown heights allow the correction of incisal edge positions. However, the FP-2 or FP-3 restoration has greater crown height compared with the FP-1 fixed types of prostheses; therefore a greater moment of force is placed on the implant cervical regions, especially during lateral forces(e.g., mandibular excursions or with cantilevered restorations). As a result, should be considered with these restorations.

An FP-2 or FP-3 prosthesis rarely has the patient's interdental papillae or ideal soft tissue contours around the emergence of the crown, because these restorations are used when there is more crown height space and the lip does not expose the soft tissue regions of the patient. In the maxillary arch, wide open embrasures between the implants may cause food impaction or speech problems. These complications may be solved by using a removable soft tissue replacement device or making overcontoured cervical restorations. The maxillary FP-2 or FP-3 prosthesis is often extended or juxtaposed to the maxillary soft tissue so that speech is not impaired. Hygiene is more difficult to control, although access next to each implant abutment is provided.

The mandibular restoration may be left above the tissue, similar to a sanitary pontic. This facilitates oral hygiene in the mandible, especially when the implant permucosal site is level with the floor of the mouth and the depth of the vestibule. However, if the space below the restoration is too great, the lower lip may lack support in the labiomental region.

13.2. Removable prostheses

There are two kinds of removable prostheses, based upon support of the restoration (see Table 1). Patients are able to remove the restoration, but not the implant. Supported superstructure attached to the abutments. The difference in the two categories of removable restorations is not in appearance (as it is in the fixed categories). Instead, the two removable categories are determined by the amount of implant support. The most common removable implant prostheses are over dentures for completely edentulous patients, Traditional removable partial dentures with clasps on implant abutment crowns have not been reported in the literature with any frequency. No long-term or short –term studies are currently available. On the other hand, complete removable overdentures have often been reported with predictability. As a result, the removable prosthetic options are primarily overdentures for the completely edentulous.

13.2.1. RP-4

RP-4 is a removable prosthesis completely supported be the implant, teeth, or both. the restoration is rigid when inserted: overdenture attachments usually connect the removable prosthesis to a low-profile tissue bar or superstructure that splints the implant abutments. Usually five or six implants in the mandible and six to eight implants in the maxilla are required to fabricate completely with favorable dental criteria.

The implant placement criteria for an RP-4 prosthesis is different than for a fixed prosthesis. Denture teeth more acrylic are required for the removable restoration. In addition, a super-structure and overdenture attachments must be added to the implant abutments. This requires a more lingual and apical implant placement in comparison with the implant position for a fixed prosthesis. The implants in an RP-4 prosthesis (and an FP-2 or FP-3 restoration) should be placed in the mesiodistal position for the best biomechanical and hygienic situation. On occasion, the position of an attachment on the superstructure or prosthesis may also affect the amount of spacing between the implants. For example, a Hader clip requires the implant spacing to be greater than 6 mm from edge to edge, and as a consequence reduces the number of implants that may be placed between the mental foramina. The RP-4 prosthesis may have the same appearance as an FP-1, FP-2, or FP-3 restoration. A porcelain-to-metal prosthesis with attachments in selected abutment crowns can be fabricated for patients with the cosmetic desire of a fixed prosthesis,. The overdenture attachments permit improved oral hygiene or allow the patient to sleep without the excess of nocturnal bruxism on the prosthesis.

13.2.2. RP-5

RP-5 is a removable prosthesis combining implant and soft tissue support. The amount of implant support is variable. The completely edentulous mandibular overdenture may have: (1) two anterior mandibular independent of each other; (2) splinted implants in the canine region to enhance retention; (3) three splinted implants in the premolar and central incisor areas to provide lateral stability; or (4) implants splined with a cantilevered bar to reduce soft tissue abrasions and to limit the amount of soft tissue coverage needed for prosthesis support. The primary advantage of an RP-5 restoration is the reduced cost. The prosthesis is very similar to traditional overdentures supported by natural teeth.

A preimplant treatment denture may be fabricated to ensure the patient's satisfaction. This technique is especially indicated for patients with demanding needs and desires regarding the final esthetic result. The implant dentist can also use the treatment denture as a guide for implant placement. The patient can wear the prosthesis during the healing stage. After the implants are uncovered, the superstructure is fabricated within the guidelines of the existing treatment restoration. Once this is achieved, the preimplant treatment prosthesis may be converted to the RP-4 or RP-5 restoration.

The clinician and the patient should realize that the bone will continue to resorb in the soft tissue-bone regions of the prosthesis of the prosthesis. Relines and occlusal adjustments every few years are common maintenance requirements of an RP-5 restoration. Bone resorption with RP-5restorations may occur two to three times faster than the resorption found with full dentures. This can be a factor when considering this type of treatment in young patients, despite the lesser cost and low failure rate.

Author details

Dongliang Zhang[1*] and Lei Zheng[2,3]

*Address all correspondence to: zhangdongliang@hotmail.com

1 Beijing Stomatology Hospital affiliated to Capital University of Medical science, Beijing City, P.R. China

2 Clinical director, Xinya dental, Changchun City, P.R. China

3 The department oral maxillofacial surgery, Jilin University, Chaoyang District, Changchun City, P.R. China

References

[1] Mish CE: Dental education: meeting the demands of implant dentistry, J Am Dent Assoc 121:334-338, 1990.

[2] Davarpanah M, Martinez H, Kebir M, Tecucianu JF, Lazzara RC, et al: Clinical manual of implant dentistry, London, 2003, Quintessence.

[3] Branemark PI, Hansson BO, Adell R, et al: Osseointegrated implants in the treatment of the deentulous jaw. Experience from a 10-year period, Scand J Plast Reconstr Surg 16(Suppl):1-132, 1977

[4] Misch EC, Misch CM: Generic terminology for endosseous implant prosthodontics, J Prosthet Dent 68:809-812, 1992.

[5] Strock AE: Experimental work on dental implantation in the alveolus, Am J Orthod Oral Surg 25:5, 1939.

[6] The glossary of prosthodontics terms, J Prosthet Dent 94: 10-92, 2005.

[7] Misch CE: Consideration of biomechanical stress in treatment with dental implants, Dent Today 25:80,82,84,85; quiz 85, 2006.

[8] Jacobs R, Schotte A, van Steenberghe D et al: Posterior jaw bone resorption in osseointegrated implant overdentures, Clin Oral Implants Res 2:63-70, 1992.

[9] Goodacre CJ, Bernal G, Rungcharassaeng K et al: Clinical complications with implants and implant prosthodontics, J Prosthet Dent 90:121-132, 2003.

[10] Misch CE: Posterior single tooth replacement. In Misch CE, editor: Dental implant prosthetics, St Louis, 2005, Mosby.

3

Drug-Induced Oral Reactions

Ana Pejcic

1. Introduction

Oral Medicine is a specialty that deals with the diagnosis and medical management of the complex medical disorders involving the oral mucosa. The success of any treatment depends on a proper and correct diagnosis. A successful diagnostician has to have qualities like knowledge, interest, intuition, curiosity, and patience. 99.9% of systemic diseases have one or more oral manifestations which are diagnosed by oral physician even before the general physician. Early recognition and diagnosis are important for early treatment, improving survival and for limiting the complications of therapy.

In present day the number of elderly people is on the rise. This is a rapidly growing population who has chronic medical conditions, take multiple medications and require routine, safe and appropriate oral and general healthcare, which may be challenging for the dental physician. The oral medicine specialists require careful assessment of each elderly person to help in the formulation of a strategy for their care, maintenance of comfort, self-respect and, effective and sympathetic dental care for them [1].

Several systemic factors are known to contribute to oral diseases or conditions, and among those are the intakes of drugs. The pathogenesis of oral adverse reactions related to intake of medications is not well-understood, and the prevalence is not known. They are, however, believed to be a relatively common phenomenon, although medication-induced oral reactions are often regarded by the health profession as trivial complaints [2].

Drug-induced side effects are a frequent occurrence. Many commonly available drugs can produce untoward consequences, even when used according to standard or recommended methods of administration. Such adverse drug reactions can involve every organ and system of the body and may be seen in all age group, and present in many different forms [3]. Regarding different parts of the oral system, these reactions can be categorized to oral mucosa and tongue, periodontal tissues, dental structures, salivary glands, cleft lip and palate, muscular and neurological disorders, taste disturbances, drug-induced oral infection, and facial edema. The oral drug reactions are often nonspecific, but they may mimic specific disease states such as Pemphigus vulgaris, Erythema multiforme, or Lichen planus [4,5]. The knowledge about drug-induced oral adverse effects helps health professionals to better diagnose oral disease, administer drugs, improve patient compliance during drug therapy, and may influence a more rational use of drugs [6].

Oral drug-reaction patterns with associated drugs and drug classes include:

2. Aphthous stomatitis

Aphthous stomatitis (also termed recurrent aphthous stomatitis, recurring oral aphthae or recurrent aphthous ulceration) is a common condition characterized by the repeated formation of benign and non-contagious mouth ulcers (aphthae), in otherwise healthy individuals. Aphthous–like ulcerations may occur from a variety of medications, including capropril and nonsteroidal anti-inflammatory drugs (NSAIDs), Asathiopurine, Losartan, and Gold compounds. It is unclear as to the mechanism leading to this reaction pattern [7,8].

The lesions may be single or multiple. Three clinical variations have been recognized: minor, major and herpetiforme ulcers. Minor form and herpetiforme ulcers heal without scarring in 7-12 days and major form persist for 3-6 weeks [9].

For treatment used topical steroids or, in severe cases, intralesional steroid injection or systemic steroids in low dose.

3. Burning mouth syndrome

Burning mouth syndrome (BMS) is a painful, frustrating condition often described as a scalding sensation in the tongue, lips, palate, or throughout the mouth. Signs and symptoms are: burning, scalding or tingling feeling on the tongue, lips, throat or palate, no specific lesion evident, with or without any sing of inflammation and discomfort usually worse at the end of the day. This syndrome may occur due to psychogenic factors, hormonal withdrawal, folate, iron, pyridoxine deficiency, or hypersensitivity reactions to the materials utilized in dental prostheses [10,11]. The most common medications that produce this side effect are: ACE inhibitors, antibiotics, hormone replacement therapy antidepressants and cephalosporin [12,13,14]. Possible treatments may include: replacing medication, treating existing disorder or treatment is aimed at the symptoms to try to reduce the pain associated with burning mouth syndrome.

- **Glossitis-**Glossitis is inflammation of the tongue. Signs and symptoms are: swollen intensely painful tongue, red and smooth tongue. Pain may be referred to the ears and salivation, fever and enlarged lymph nodes may develop if infection is present. Various drugs which can cause glossitis are: antibiotics, corticosteroids, methotrezole, and tricyclic antidepressants [15,16].

The goal of treatment is to reduce inflammation. Good oral hygiene is necessary, including thorough tooth brushing at least twice a day.

- **Oral ulcerations (nonspecific ulceration and mucositis)**

Oral ulcerations may occur in a different setting, including local irritation, chemotherapy, opportunistic infections and fixed drug reactions. Epithelial necrosis and ulceration may result from direct application of over-the-counter medications such as aspirin, hydrogen peroxide, potassium tablets, and phenol-containing compounds to the mucosa. [17]. Aspirin is often used by patients seeking relief from dental pain. The affected mucosa appears whitish and corrugated, with erosion and ulceration of the more severely damaged areas. The associated discomfort can be severe enough to require treatment. Oral drug reaction may be as small round /oval lesions/ with yellow or grey floor and may lead to difficulties in speck. Drugs including anti-neoplastics (methotrexate, 5-fluorouracil), barbiturates, dapsone, tetracyclines, nonsteroidal anti-inflammatory drugs (NSAIDs) (eg, indomethacin, salicylates, gold salts, naproxen), meprobamate, methyldopa, penicillamine, propranolol, spironolactone, thiazides, tolbutamide, alendronate, captopril, phenytoin, and (by direct contact) compounds containing aspirin can cause oral ulcerations. [18,19].

They are clinically diverse, but usually appear as a single, painful ulcer with a smooth red or whitish-yellow surface and a thin erythematous haloo. For treatment used removal of factors and topical steroids for a short time.

4. Vesico-bullous lesions

Oral drug reactions that bear striking clinical, histopathologic, and even immunopathologic resemblance to idiopathic Lichen planus, Erythema multiforme (EM), Pemphigoid, Pemphigus vulgaris, and Lupus erythematosus (LE) are well recognized, and the list of reactions in each category is constantly expanding. Clinically, any oral site can be affected; however, the posterior buccal mucosa (cheeks), the lateral borders of the tongue, and the alveolar mucosa are most commonly involved. Lesions may be isolated, although bilaterally symmetric involvement is not uncommon [20,21].

- Lichen planus – Lichen planus is a relatively common papulosquamous disorder involving the skin and mucous membranes. Often these lesions are asymptomatic. Lichen planus–like or lichenoid drug reactions are a heterogeneous group of lesions of the oral mucosa that show clinical and histopathological similarities to lichen planus. Lichenoid reactions have subsequently been reported in association with many agents (amalgam, composite resins, and dental restorative materials). A number of drugs have been implicated in lichen planus-like eruptions. The most common agents are nonsteroidal anti-inflammatory drugs and angiotensin converting enzyme inhibitors.

Although drug-induced lichenoid reactions tend to be erosive and unilateral compared with the typical bilateral presentation in idiopathic lichen planus, these associations are not consistently observed. Middle aged individuals are more commonly affected. The predilection sites are the buccal mucosa, tongue, and gingiva. The pathogenic mechanism by which drugs cause LP-like drug eruptions is not clear, T cell-mediated autoimmune phenomena are involved in the pathogenesis of Lichen planus [22,23,24,25].

Clinical characteristic oral lesions of the disease are white papules that usually coalesce, forming a net-work of lines (Wickham's striae). Six forms of the disease are recognized in the oral mucosa. The common forms are reticular and erosive, the less common are atrophic and hypertrophic, and the rare ere bullous and pigmented.

The disease can usually be diagnosed on clinical grounds alone. Histopathological examination is very helpful.

In treatment, topical steroids may be helpful, and intralesional injection. Systemic steroids in low doses can be used in severe and extensive cases.

- Erythema multiforme (EM) – like – Erythema multiforme is a syndrome consisting of symmetrical mucocutaneus lesions that have a predilection for the oral mucosa, hand, and feet. Initial bullae may rupture, giving rise to widespread superficial ulceration [26]. A spectrum of disease can be seen ranging from a benign cutaneus eruption to a severe mucocutaneous eruption. Steven-Johnson syndrome represents a severe manifestation of EM. Syndrome characterized by various clinical types of lesions. The lips are swollen, crusted, and bleeding. Drugs with potential to cause Erythema multiforme are: antibiotics (antimalarial, penicillin, sulfonamide, and tetracycline), allopurinol, barbiturates, protease inhibitors, and NSAIDs. Drug-induced EM represents approximately 25% of all reported cases. Drug-induced EM is frequently linked to agents such as sulfonamides, sulfonylureas, and barbiturates, among others [27,28,29].

- Pemphigoid – like – Drug-induced Pemphigoid can occur in the setting of a number of drugs. Antirheumatics (penicillamine, ibuprofen, phenacetin), cardiovascular drugs (furosemide, captopril, clonidine), antibiotics (penicillin's, sulfonamides), antimicrobials, thiol-containing drugs, and sulfonamide derivatives. Pemphigoid-like reactions can be limited to the oral mucosa, or they can affect other mucosal or cutaneous sites. Clinically, lesions appear as relatively sturdy vesicles or bullae that break down into shallow ulcerations. Generalized or multifocal involvement of the gingival tissues may be observed, with marked erythema and erosion of the superficial gingiva, a pattern that has been called Desquamative gingivitis. Thiol-containing drugs and sulfonamide derivatives are among the most commonly involved medications, as are the therapeutic classes of NSAIDs, cardiovascular agents, antimicrobials, and antirheumatics. Drug-induced pemphigoid patients may be younger and have more frequent oral involvement [30]. For treatment used steroids and, rarely, immunosuppressive drugs.

- Pemphigus – like – drug reactions have been reported to have similar clinical, histologic, and immunofluorescent patterns as Pemphigus vulgaris. Alpha-mercaptopropionylglycine, ampicillin, captopril, cephalexin, ethambutol, glibenclamide, gold, heroin, ibuprofen, penicillamine, phenobarbital, phenylbutazone, piroxicam, practolol, propranolol, pyritinol chlorohydrate, rifampin, and theobromine. Pemphigus-like reactions can have features of either pemphigus vulgaris or pemphigus foliaceous, although pemphigus foliaceous is uncommon in the oral cavity. Thiol-containing drugs are the most common cause of pemphigus-like reactions. In drug-induced pemphigus vulgaris, the relatively fragile vesicles are rarely observed at clinical examination, and most cases are characterized by irregular ulcerations with ragged borders that may coalesce to involve large areas of the mucosa. Patients may have circulating autoantibodies to the desmosomal components [31]. Treatment is used systemic steroides, immunosuppressive drugs and dapsone.

- Lupus erythematosus (LE) – like-Drug-induced LE is a well-recognized adverse reaction that is most commonly associated with procainamide and hydralazine, although more than 70 medications are implicated (Carbamazepine, chlorpromazine, ethosuximide, gold, griseofulvin, hydantoins, hydralazine, isoniazid, lithium, methyldopa, penicillamine, primidone, procainamide, quinidine, reserpine, streptomycin, thiouracils, and trimethadione.). Clinically, the oral lesions of drug-induced LE may simulate those of erosive lichen planus, with irregular areas of erythema or ulceration bordered by radiating keratotic striae. These lesions may affect the palate, buccal mucosa, and gingival or alveolar tissues. The rarity of lichen planus on the hard palate may be helpful in differentiating it from drug-induced LE [32]. In treatment used steroids and antimalarial drugs.

5. Color changes of oral mucosa and teeth (Pigmentation)

Pigmentation may by normal pigmentation which are a physiological finding, particularly in dark-skinned individuals because increased melanin production and deposition in the oral mucosa. No treatment is required. Abnormal oral pigmentation can result from a number of causes, including local and systemic medications (amiodarone, antimalarials, bisulfan, clofazimine, cyclophosphamide, estrogen). Discoloration can occur after direct contact with or following systemic absorption of a drug. Discoloration of the oral mucosa after drug use may be due to direct melanocytic stimulation, the deposition of pigmented drug metabolites, and erythrocyte degradation products. Local agents such as heavy metals (bismuth, lead) or dental amalgam (amalgam tattoo) may cause discoloration by traumatic implantation. Systemic medications may leave the patient with a bluish gray to yellowish-brown discoloration of the buccal mucosa, tongue, or hard palate. Typically, such pigmentation is most notable on the posterior regions of the hard palate, appears bluish-black to brown, and may be bilateral. Smoker's melanosis, or smoking-associated melanosis, is an abnormal melanin pigmentation of the oral mucosa [33].

Clinically, it appears as multiple brown pigmented areas, usually located on the anterior labial gingiva of the mandible. Teeth discoloration may be intrinsic or extrinsic. Intrinsic stains are caused by drugs (tetracycline) taken during development of tooth [34]. Extrinsic stains are taken up by tooth after development of tooth (tea, coffee, chlorhexidine) [35,36,37].

6. Black hairy tongue (Lingua villosa, Lingua nigra)

Hairy changes are on the upper side of the tongue (never on under side).Hairy tongue is a relatively common disorder that is due to marked accumulation of keratin on the filiforme papillae of the tongue. Lingua is black but may also be brown, white, green or pink. Normally asymptomatic and may develop secondary fungal infection (Candidosis). Hairy tongue may appear as a result of the growth of pigment-producing bacteria that colonize the elongate filiforme papillae. The black tongue may also be due to staining from food and tobacco. Black hairy tongue can be seen with the administration of oral antibiotics, corticosteroides, aldomet, sulfonamides and excessive smoking in adult's [38]. Treatment is elimination of predisposing factors, brushing of the tongue and local use of keratolytic agents.

7. Drug induced gingival enlargement

Gingival enlargement is seen in periodontitis, system disorders, and drug-induced states. The enlargement is usually generalized throughout the mouth but is more severe in maxillary and mandibular anterior regions. Drug-induced gingival overgrowth is a relatively common disorder of the gingiva due to several drugs. The drugs most commonly implicated are: Calcium channel blockers (amlodipine, diltiazem, felodipine, isradipine, nicardipine, nifedipine, nimodipine, nisoldipine, nitrendipine, oxidipine, and verapamil), other dihydropyridines (bleomycin), cyclosporine, phenytoin, and sodium valproate. Diffuse, non-neoplastic enlargement or overgrowth of the gingival tissues was initially recognized in patients who were using phenytoin. More recently, calcium channel blockers (members of the dihydropyridine class of medications), cyclosporine, and the antiepileptic drug sodium valproate have been associated with this reaction. Within the calcium channel blocker family, nifedipine, diltiazem, verapamil, and amlodipine are among the most commonly reported causative agents [39,40,41]. The gingival overgrowth is usually related to the dose of the drugs, the duration of therapy, the serum concentration, and the presence of dental plaque [42,43]. Clinically, both marginal gingiva and interdental papilla appear enlarged and firm, with a surface that may be smooth, stippled, or lobulated.

Treatment is discontinuation of the offending drug, improvement of oral hygiene and gingivectomy.

8. Xerostomia

Xerostomia, or dry mouth, is the most common adverse drug-related effect in the oral cavity. There are many causes of xerostomia. Pharmacologic therapy is a common cause. Xerostomia has been associated with more than 500 medications (antidepressants and antipsychotics, antihypertensives, antihistamines, anticholinergics, and decongestants). The synergistic effects of medications have been recognized and are increasingly common in elderly patients taking multiple medications (polypharmacy). In addition, habits such as smoking, alcohol consumption, and even long-term use of caffeinated drinks may contribute to oral dryness or the perception of dryness. Clinical signs and symptoms are: difficulty eating and swallowing, difficulty speaking and little saliva present in the mouth or may be thick stringy saliva [44,45].

9. Swelling

Several drugs can induce type I hypersensitivity reactions, or disease mediated by immuno-globulin E mast cells, that can range from isolated swelling of the oral tissues to full-blown anaphylaxis. Around the mouth, the lips are the most frequently involved site, followed by the tongue. The swelling is acute and is often transient. Lesions typically last for only several hours, but may last for days. Among the most common offending agents are ACE inhibitors, penicillin and penicillin derivatives, cephalosporins, barbiturates, and aspirin and other NSAIDs. Affected mucosa typically appears edematous and erythematous within minutes or hours after exposure to the offending drug. Similar contact reactions to latex had become increasingly problematic in oral health care settings until the recent shift towards non-latex replacement materials such as vinyl or nitrile rubber [46,47].

10. Oral thrush — Oral candidosis

The yeast, *Candida albicans* is the most common cause of infection of the oral cavity. Drug-induced oral candidosis is usually asymptomatic, but it may have an associated erythematous, ulcerated base. It is usually by *Candida albicans*, and less frequently by other fungal species. Predisposing factors may be local (xerostomia, dentures, antibiotic, poor oral hygiene) and systemic (steroids, HIV infections, immunosuppressive drugs). Clinical sing and symptoms are: Presents of creamy-white lesions on tongue, pain, slight bleeding if the lesions are rubbed or scraped, "cottony" feeling in the mouth, loss of taste (ageusia) and difficulty swallowing (if infection spreads to throat). This often follows the use of broad-spectrum antibiotics or the use of corticosteroid inhalers, and immunosuppressive agents such as cyclosporine, and cytotoxic therapies [48]. In treatment used topical antifungal agents and systemic.

11. Taste disturbance (Ageusia, Dysgeusia)

Numerous causes exist that can lead to a decreased ability to perceive taste or causing an unpleasant taste. The alteration in taste may be simply a blunting or decreased sensitivity in taste perception (hypogeusia), a total loss of the ability to taste (ageusia), or a distortion in perception of the correct taste of a substance, for example, sour for sweet (dysgeusia) [49].

The most common cause is due to an upper respiratory infection that affects olfaction, in turn, decreasing one's sense of taste. Drugs can also distort taste. Clinical signs and symptoms are:

total loss of ability to taste, complaints of metallic taste, impaired salty taste, reduced appetite and weight loss. Drugs causing taste disturbance are: antibiotics, ACE inhibitors, aspirin, diclofenac, diltiazem, metronidazole, propranolol, and sulphonamides [50].

12. Stomatitis — Contact allergy

Stomatitis or oral inflammation of the mouth is a nonspecific term that describes many oral drug reactions. This is a relatively common oral mucosal reaction to continuous contact of substances. Restorative materials, mouthwashes, dentifrices, food and other substances may be responsible. The clinical symptoms may include: nonspecific generalized inflamed gums, palate, lips, tongue and buccal mucosa, bleeding, oral lesions as ulcerations and erosions, and breathing difficulties if severe allergic reaction involving tongue. Lesions occur within 24 hours of ingesting the medication. The causative medication is withdrawn. Drugs are: antibiotics, food additives, mouthwashes, toothpastes, cosmetics, dental materials and topical steroids [51]. Stomatitis refers to an inflammatory process involving the mucous membrane of the mouth that may manifest itself through a variety of signs and symptoms including erythema, vesiculation, bulla formation, desquamation, sloughing, ulceration, pseudomembranous formation, and associated discomfort.

Stomatitis may arise due to factors that may be of either local, isolated conditions or of systemic origin. For example, a solitary oral ulcer with a history of a recurrent pattern may be classified as recurrent aphthous stomatitis, a purely local phenomenon. Another clinically-similar-appearing lesion, on the other hand, may represent an oral mucosal manifestation of a more generalized disease process such as Crohn's disease. Stomatitis may involve any site in the oral cavity, including the vermillion of the lips, labial/buccal mucosa, and dorsal/ventral tongue, floor of mouth and hard/soft palate, and gingivae [52].

The diagnosis is based on the history and clinical features.

Treatment is discontinuation of any the causative medication. In severe and extended lesions, low doses of steroids for one week help the lesions to heal.

13. Angular cheilitis

Angular cheilitis (AC), or perleche, is a common disorder of the angles of the mouth. This is soreness and cracks at the corners of the mouth. Several drugs may cause AC as a side effect, by various mechanisms, such as creating drug-induced xerostomia. Medication also contributes to the onset of cheilitis. There are certain medicines that have a side effect of dry lips which is potential for cheilitis. Less commonly, angular cheilitis is associated with primary hypervitaminosis A which can occur when as a result from an excess intake of vitamin A in the form of vitamin supplements. Drugs are: Aldomet, Zocor (statins), tetracycline and vitamin A [53,54].

The condition is characterized by erythema, maceration, fissuring, erosion, and crusting at commissures. Remissions and exacerbations are common. Diagnosis is based on the clinical findings.

Treatment is discontinuation of any the causative medication, and topical steroids.

14. Osteonecrosis

Osteonecrosis is a disease resulting from the temporary or permanent loss of blood supply to the bones. This is a serious oral complication of treatment with Bisphosphonates. Bone under teeth is exposed, usually triggered by a dental extraction. Most commonly associated with i.n. zoledronic acid. Clinical symptoms are: swelling and loosening of teeth, altered local sensation, facial pain, toothache, lose teeth, exposed bone, recurrent infection and marked oral odour [55,56].

15. Salivary glands

Salivary gland function can be affected by a variety of drugs that can by a variety of drugs that can produce xerostomia or ptyalismus. It is suggested this is due to both the reduced salivary flow rate and to a decrease in salivary calcium and phosphate concentration. Systemic drug therapy can also produce pain and swelling of the salivary glands. [57].

Salivary gland enlargement may be painless or associated with tenderness. The causes of salivary gland swelling are numerous, but they can be viewed as local causes or drug related (thiouracil, sulfonamides, NSAIDs, phenothiazines) [58].

16. Sialorrhoea

Sialorrhoea, or excessive salivation is commonly associated with many systemic conditions. Clinical signs and symptoms are: increased salivary floe, drooling or dribbling and increased swallowing. Drugs causing sialorrhorea are: pilocarpine, rivastigmin, nifedipine, lithium and dimercaptol [59,60]. The treatments currently available for sialorrhoea are unsatisfactory. Systemic anticholinergic drugs are often ineffective and produce unacceptable side effects.

17. Halitosis

Halitosis is the offensive breath resulting from poor oral hygiene, dental or oral infections, ingestion of certain foods, use of tobacco, and some systemic diseases. Halitosis, or bad breath, may have many different etiologies (alcohol, drugs, and foods, smoking). It may be association with an abnormal taste in the mouth. This association is commonly seen with smoking, various foods, alcohol, periodontal disease or other oral infection. Concern about halitosis is estimated to be the third most frequent reason for people to seek dental care, following tooth decay and gum disease) [61]. A number of systemic diseases can cause halitosis, especially cirrhosis and renal failure. In diabetic ketoacidosis, patient's breath may smell of acetone. Drugs are not frequently implicated, but disulfiram dimethylsulfoxide has been associated with halitosis. Effective treatment is not always easy to find. Gently cleaning the tongue surface twice daily is the most effective way to keep bad breath in control, than, eating a healthy breakfast with rough food and chewing gum [62].

18. Hemorrhage — Bleeding

Bleeding can occur internally, where blood leaks from blood vessels inside the body, or externally, either through a natural opening such as the mouth, nose, ear, urethra, vagina or anus, or through a break in the skin. Bleeding arises due to traumatic injury, underlying medical condition, or some drugs. Drugs such as aspirin, NSAIDS, anticoagulants which thin in the blood and drug induced thrombocytopenia as caused by chloramphenicol, penicillins, streptomycin and sulfonamides may lead to oral bleeding. Broad spectrum antibiotics such as cephalosporin's decrease Vitamin K level by altering gastrointestinal flora and may lead to bleeding disorder [63].

19. Taking care of your oral health during drug use

Some easy to prevent or reduce the adverse effects of various drug therapies are as follow:

• Use of soft bristle tooth brush

• Brush or rinse after every meal

• Use mild tooth paste

• Regular use of floss without injury in gums

• Eat dry nuts alters food that stimulate salivary flow.

• Have regular dental checkup

• Use of ice chips to decrease pain and dryness of mouth

When being prescribed a new medication, ask your doctor or pharmacist about all the possible side effects [64].

Whenever a patient comes with oral lesions ask about history of medications and if significant then either reduce to the minimum dose required or switch to alternative regimen depending upon the severity of symptoms. Sometimes active treatment of the concerned effect may also be required.

Author details

Ana Pejcic*

Address all correspondence to: dranapejcic@hotmail.com

Department of Periodontology and Oral medicine, Medical faculty, University of Nis, Serbia

References

[1] Cianco SG. Medication's impact on oral health. J Am Dent Assoc 2004; 135(10): 1440-1448.

[2] Porter SR, Scully C. Adverse drug reactions in the mouth. Clin Dermatol 2000; 18(5): 525-532.

[3] Scully C, Bagan JV. Adverse drug reactions in the orofacial region. Crit Rev Oral Biol Med 2004; 15(4): 221-239.

[4] Abdollahi M. Current opinion on drug-induced oral reactions: A comprehensive review. J Contemp Dent Pract 2008; (9)3: 001-015.

[5] Abdollahi M, Radfar M. A review of drug-induced oral reactions. J Contemp Dent Pract 2003; 4: 10-31.

[6] Abdollahi M, Radfar M. A Review of Drug-Induced Oral Reactions. J Contemp Dent Pract 2003; (4)1: 10-31.

[7] Vucicevic Boras V, Savage N, Mohamad Zaini Z. Oral aphthous-like ulceration due to tiotropiumbromide. Med Oral Patol Oral Cir Bucal 2007; 12(3): E209-210.

[8] Kharazmi M, Sjöqvist K, Warfvinge G. Oral ulcers, a little known adverse effect of alendronate: review of the literature. J Oral Maxillofacial Surg 2012; 70 (4): 830–836.

[9] Boulinguez S, Reix S, Bedane C, Debrock C, Bouyssou-GauthierML, Sparsa A, et al.). Role of drug exposure in aphthousulcers: a case-control study. Br J Dermatol 2000; 143: 1261-1265.

[10] Symour RA. Oral and dental disorders. In: Davies DM, Ferner RE, DeGlanville H. eds.,Davies'stextbook of adverse drugreactions, 5th ed., London, Chapman & Hall Medical, 1998: 234-250.

[11] Lorca SC, Minguez Serra PM, Silvestre FJ. Drug-induced burning mouth syndrome: a new etiological diagnosis.Med Oral Patol Oral Cir Bucal 2008; 13(3): E167-170.

[12] Fedele S, Fricchione G, Porter SR, Miggna MD. Burning mouth syndrome (stomatodynia). QJM 2007; 100(8): 527-530.

[13] Sardella A. An up-to-date view on burning mouth syndrome. Minerva Stomatol 2007; 56(6): 327-340.

[14] Culhane NS, Hodle AD. Burning mouth syndrome after taking clonazepam. Ann Pharmacother. 2001; 35(7-8): 874-876.

[15] Reamy BV, Derby R, Bunt CW. Common tongue conditions in primary care. Am Fam Physician 2010; 81(5): 627-634.

[16] Litt JZ. Drug eruption reference manual. London. The Parthenon Publishing Group, 2001: 274-421.

[17] Nordt SP. Tetracycline-induced oral mucosal ulcerations. Ann Pharmacother. 1996 May;30(5):547-8.

[18] Jones TA, Parmar SC: Oral mucosal ulceration due to ferrous sulphate tablets: report of a case. Dent Update 2006; 33(10): 632-633.

[19] Naranjo J, Poniachik J, Cisco D, et al.: Oral ulcers produced by mycophenolate mofetil in two liver transplant patients. Transplant Proc 2007, 39(3): 612-614.

[20] Criado PR, Brandt HR, Moure ER, Pereira GL, Sanches Júnior JA. Adverse mucocutaneous reactions related to chemotherapeutic agents: part II. An Bras Dermatol 2010; 85(5): 591-608.

[21] Scully C, Bagan JV. Adverse drug reactions in the orofacial region. Crit Rev Oral Biol Med 2004; 15: 221-239.

[22] Serrano-Sanchez P, Bagan JV, Soriano J, Sarrion G. Drug-induced oral lichenoid reactions. A literature review. J Clin Exp Dent 2010; 2(2): e71-75.

[23] Cobos-Fuentes MJ, Martínez-Sahuquillo-Márquez A, Gallardo-Castillo I, et al. Oral lichenoid lesions related to contact with dental materials: a literature review. Med Oral Patol Oral Cir Bucal 2009; 14: e514-520.

[24] Woo V, Bonks J, Borukhova L, Zegarelli D. Oral Lichenoid Drug Eruption: A Report of a Pediatric Case and Review of the Literature. Pediatric Dermatology 2009; 26: 458–464.

[25] Lage D, Juliano PB, Metze K, et al. Lichen planus and lichenoid drug-induced eruption: a histological and immunohistpchemical study. Int J Dermatol 2012; 51: 1199.

[26] Ayangco L, Rogers RS III. Oral manifestations of erythema multiforme. Dermatol Clin 2000; 321: 195-205.

[27] Joseph IT, Vergheese G, Gorge D, Sathyan P. Drug induced oral erythema multiforme: A rare and less recognized variant of erythema multiforme. J Oral Maxillofac Pathol 2012; 16: 145-148.

[28] Hazin R, Ibrahini OA, Hazin MI, et al: Stevens-Johnson syndrome: pathogenesis, diagnosis, and management. Ann Med. 2008; 40(2): 129-138.

[29] Iks R, Karakaya G, Erkin G, Kalyoncu AF. Multidrug-induced erythema multiforme. J Investig Allergol Clin Immunol 2007, 17(3):196-198.

[30] Vassileva S. Drug-induced pemphigoid: bullous and cicatricial. Clin Dermatol 1998; 16(3): 379-387.

[31] Civatte J. Drug-induced pemphigus diseases. Dermatol Monatsschr 1989; 175(1): 1-7.

[32] Rubin RL. Drug-induced lupus. Toxicology. 2005; 209(2):135-147.

[33] Eisen D. Disorders of pigmentation in the oral cavity. Clin Dermatol. 2000; 18(5): 579-587.

[34] Aschheim KW, Dale BG. Esthetic dentistry, a clinical approach to techniques and materials. 2nd ed., Phiadephia, Mosby, 2001:247-249.

[35] Eisen D. Disorders of pigmentation in the oral cavity. Clin Dermatol 2000; 18: 579-587.

[36] Sapone A, Basaglia R, Biagi GL. Drug-induced changes in the teeth and mouth. II Clin Ter. 1992; 140(6): 575-583.

[37] Meyerson MA, Cohen PR, Hymes SR. Lingual hyper pigmentation associated with minocycline therapy. Oral Surg Oral Med Oral Pathol Oral Radiol Endod 1995; 79: 180-184.

[38] Korber A, Dissemond J. Images in clinical medicine. Black hairy tongue. N Engl J Med 2006, 5; 354(1): 67.

[39] Shimizu Y, Kataoka M, Seto H, et. al. Nifedipine induces gingival epithelial hyperplasia in rats through inhibition of apoptosis. J Periodontol. 2002; 73(8): 861-867.

[40] Kataoka M, Kido J, Shinohara Y, Nagata T. Drug-induced gingival overgrowth–a review. Biol Pharm Bull 2005; 28(10):1817-1821.

[41] Nitin MN, Sandeep B, Arjun D, Surinder KS, Harsh M. Salivary gland tumor – our experience. Ind J Otolaryngol Head Neck Surg 2004; 56(1): 31-34.

[42] Pejcic A, Djordjevic V, Kojovic D, Zivkovic V, Minic I, Mirkovic D, Stojanovic M. Effectiveness of Periodontal Treatment in Renal Transplant Recipients. Medical Principles and Practice 2014; 23(2): 149-153.

[43] A Pejčić, Lj. Kesić, V. Živković, R. Obradović, M. Petrović, D. Mirković. Gingival overgrowth induced by nifedipine. Acta Stom Naissi 2011; 27: 1104-1109.

[44] Porter SR, Scully C, Hegarty AM. An update of the etiology and management of xerostomia. Oral Surg Oral Med Oral Radiol Endod 2004; 97(1): 28-46.

[45] Bardow A, Nyvad B, Nauntofte B. Relationships between medication intake, complaints of dry mouth, salivary flow rate and composition, and the rate of tooth demineralization in situ. Arch Oral Biol 2001; 46(5): 413-423.

[46] Kaplan AP, Greaves MW. Angioedema. J Am Acad Dermatol 2005; 53(3): 373-388.

[47] Bas M, Adams V, Suvorava T, Niehues T, Hoffmann TK, Kojda G. Nonallergic angioedema: role of bradykinin. Allergy 2007; 62(8):842-5.

[48] Muzyka BC. Oral fungal infections. Dent Clin North Am 2005; 49(1): 49-65.

[49] Porter SR, Scully C. Adverse drug reactions in the mouth. Clin Dermatol. 2000 SepOct;18(5):525-32.

[50] Drew H, Harasty L. Dysgeusia follow in a course of Zithromax: a case report. J N J Dent Assoc 2007; 78(2): 24-27.

[51] Tack DA, Rogers ES. Oral drug reactions. Dermatol therap 2002; 15: 236-250.

[52] P Lokesh, T Rooban Joshua Elisabeth, K Umadevi, K Ranganathan. Allergic Contact Stomatitis: A Case Report and Review of Literature. Indian J Clin Pract 2012; 22(9): 458-462.

[53] Park KK, Brodell TR, Helm ES. Angular cheilitis, Part 2: Nutritional, systemic, and drug –related causes and treatment. Cutis 2011; 88 (1): 27-32.

[54] Levin L, Laviv A, Schwartz-Arad D. Denture-related osteonecrosis of the maxilla associated with oral bisphosphonate treatment. J Am Dent Assoc 2007, 138(9): 1218-1220.

[55] Woo SB, Kalmar JR. Osteonecrosis of the jaws and bisphosphonates. Alpha Omegan 2007; 100 (4): 194-202.

[56] Knulst AC, Stengs CJ, Baart de la Faille H, et. al. Salivary gland swellingfollowingnaproxen therapy. Br J Dermatol. 1995; 133(4): 647-649.

[57] Scully C. Drug effects on salivary glands; dry mouth. Oral Dis 2003; 9: 165-176.

[58] Freudenreich O. Drug-induced sialorrhea. Drugs Today (Barc) 2005, 41(6):411-418.

[59] Comeley C, Galletly C, Ash D. Use of atropeine eye drops for clozapine induced hypersalivation. Aust NZ J psychiatry 2000; 34: 1003-1034.

[60] Yaegaki, K; Coil, JM. Examination, classification, and treatment of halitsis; clinical perspectives. Journal Canadian Dental Association 2000; 66 (5): 257–261.

[61] Zalewska, A; Zatoński, M; Jabłonka-Strom, A; Paradowska, A; Kawala, B; Litwin, A. "Halitosis--a common medical and social problem. A review on pathology, diagnosis and treatment. Acta gastro-enterologica Belgica 2012; 75 (3): 300–309.

[62] American Dental Association."How medications can affect your oral health."J Am Dent Assoc 2005; 136(6):831.

[63] Alan Tack D, Rogers S R.Oral drug reactions. Dermatologic Therapy 2002; 15: 236-250.

[64] P. Serrano-Sánchez, JV Bagán, Jiménez-Soriano, G Sarrión. Drug-induced oral lichenoid reactions. A literature review. J Clin Exp Dent. 2010; 2(2): e71-75.

4

Narrow Diameter and Mini Dental Implant Overdentures

Elena Preoteasa, Marina Imre, Henriette Lerner,
Ana Maria Tancu and Cristina Teodora Preoteasa

1. Introduction

Complete dentures are most frequently a challenge for practitioners. The complexity of this disease is often associated with general health problems, but also with the physiological ageing phenomenon, that increases the treatment difficulty. Completely edentulous patients, usually elderly, often complain about the functionality of conventional dentures, especially the mandibular ones, claiming their instability, poor retention and discomfort during wear.

Following the development of public health programs, a beneficial effect was found in terms of percentage decrease in the number of completely edentulous patients, but this was partially offset by the increased life expectancy. Consequently, complete edentulism remains a frequent medical condition that needs to be addressed through treatment alternatives that meet the needs of modern man. This aspect is integrated in the current medical perception that highlights the importance of an active aging process, with preservation of elderly participation in social and economic activities [1]. Additionally to population aging as a demographic trend, changes in the dental field have also occurred, related to the use of dental implants and implant prosthesis, but also to patients' perception and expectations regarding the prosthetic rehabilitation, demanding more stable, functional and aesthetic prosthesis.

Complete maxillary and mandibular dentures have been for over 100 years the standard treatment of complete edentulism. If complete maxillary denture wearers tolerate better the complete dentures, given the better conditions for support, retention and stability, the tolerance of mandibular prosthesis is generally lower. The relatively frequent instability of the mandibular denture, poor retention and associated discomfort were the starting point for the idea of setting the overdenture on 2 implants as first treatment alternative for the mandibular complete edentulism (according to McGill and York consensus) [2, 3, 4].

2. Concept of implant overdentures

Implant overdentures are inspired, as treatment concept, from the of the overdentures, the dental implants being used instead of tooth roots. If for teeth overdentures the attachment systems are optional, for the implant-supported ones they become mandatory. Therefore, the structural components of implant overdenture are the prosthesis (partial or complete over-denture), the dental implants and the attachment system. Using dental implants mainly aims to increase retention and/or to provide support for the prosthesis.

Considering the relation between the structural components of the implant overdentures, their interaction with the oral structures and functions, the biomechanical aspects, all with impact on implants survival and treatment success, numerous treatment options and concepts have been developped. These differ in various aspects, such as the design of the dental implants used (as diameter - conventional, narrow or mini dental implants, as length), as implant number, as technique of implant placement and loading, as attachment system, as prosthesis design and as their effect on the prosthesis balance, retention and patients satisfaction [5]. Regardless of their type, implant-supported overdentures bring a number of benefits compared to the conventional dentures, by increasing their stability and retention, improving the mastication and phonation, and ensuring a physical and psychological comfort.

Dental implants that are used for implant overdentures are made of high-strength alloy (Ti-Al-V), with good biocompatibility, with different designs and sizes that aim to address the prosthetic needs according to the oral particularities and clinical limitations of its execution. The first implants that were introduced in the dental practice were the ones with standard diameter, around 3.75mm. Later on, their diameter was increased and decreased (narrow), ranging between 3 and 6mm. Afterwards, the mini implants with one-piece design for implant overdentures appeared (IMTEC, later 3MESPE), with diameters of 1.8mm, 2.1mm and 2.4mm.

Using dental implants with a diameter under the conventional one has increased, aspect related to the extension of their clinical indications. These were firstly used for temporary retention of the interim prosthesis and for orthodontic anchorage. Nowadays there is an increased use of them for prosthesis stabilization.

Dental implants with a diameter below the conventional one, are classified mainly on their diameter, or design (i.e. one piece/two piece). Thus, implants with a diameter below the conventional one have been classified by some authors as narrow-diameter implants (3.0 to 3.5 mm) with smaller implants (3.0 to 3.25 mm), and mini-implants (<3.0mm) [6]. The mini-implants are sometimes divided in hybrid implants (2.7 to 2.9 mm) and mini implants (1.8 to 2.7mm).

Conventional Diameter Implant Overdentures (CDIO) use two-piece implants, with usually two-stage placement protocol, with larger diameters (over 3.5mm) and variable lengths

(8-16mm), in a number of minimum two for the mandibular overdenture. Its implementation requires wide ridges (over 5-6mm), condition that rather often is not met in the aged edentulous patients, therefore bone augmentation, supplemented sometimes by sinus lift being required. The protocol of conventional implant placement is with or without a flap, usually involves two phase surgery (one for implant placement and one for removal of the cover screw and abutment placement), with delayed implant loading, after the implants osseointegration (after 3-6 months). As prosthetic parameters and attachment selection, conventional implants have a wider spectrum of indications and treatment options. Implants can be splinted with bars as attachment systems, or be used unsplinted, with ball, locator, magnets and telescopes. When selecting the attachments, one must take into account the prosthetic space, as well as patient's manual dexterity and the degree of oral hygiene.

Narrow Diameter Implant Overdenture (NDIO) represents a category of implants that combines features from conventional implants and mini implants, with diameters between 3 and 3.5mm and variable lengths (10-18mm), comprising two distinctive subgroups, namely two-piece design (e.g. Seven Narrow Line implants, MIS Implants Technologies Inc. 18-00 Fair Lawn Ave. Fair Lawn, NJ 07410, UNITED STATES, mini Sky 2, Bredent Medical GmbH & Co, Germany, Straumann implant, Straumann Group SIX: STMN, Basel Switzerland) and one-piece design (e.g. uno line, MIS implants). Two-piece narrow implants can be used as the conventional implants (with delayed loading), or as one-piece mini implants (with immediate loading protocol). In relation to anatomical, functional and prosthetic case particularities, the number of dental implants used can be reduced, similar to that of the conventional implants (e.g., two narrow implants for the mandibular overdenture).

Mini Dental Implant Overdentures (MDIO) use mostly-one piece dental implants (miniSky1, Bredent, MDI 3MESPE) with diameters between 1,8mm and 3mm and variable lengths (10mm-18mm), that require one-stage surgery for implant placement, followed by prosthesis application in the same appointment, with soft material in the housing area (progressive loading) or fixation of the matrices in the denture base (immediate loading). Within the mini implants, those with a diameter between 2.7 and 3mm are classified as hybrid implants, these having sometimes a two-piece design and can be used as narrow dental implants (e.g., two narrow implants for the mandibular overdenture).

The main features of the overdentures on dental implants with a diameter below the conventional one, considering their three main categories according to their diameter, are synthesized in table 1.

The decision to use either a CDIO, NDIO or MDIO as treatment for complete edentulism, starts from the acknowledgment of patient's preferences and expectations, within the limitations of the systemic and oral health-status. In systemic alterations with indications of limited surgery or that negatively affects the healing process, NDIO and MDIO are more indicated than CDIO, due to their reduced invasiveness. Oral particularities, such as the anatomical conditions (bone quality and quantity, the shape of the alveolar ridge, skeletal class), thickness and health of the oral mucosa (e.g., denture stomatitis, candidiasis), available prosthetic restorative space (especially as vertical dimension, given the necessary space for abutment, attachments and prosthesis thickness, in order to prevent its fracture) should all be considered when choosing between the implant prosthesis alternatives.

	Conventional implant overdenture(CDIO)	Narrow diameter implant overdenture (NDIO)	Mini dental implant overdenture (MDIO)
Implant's diameter	>3.5mm	3.5 – 3.0 mm 3.0- 3.25 mm (smaller)	2.9-2.7mm (hybrid) 1.8mm – 2.7mm
Implant's length	> 8mm	> 10mm	> 10mm
Design	Two-piece implants	One- and two-piece implants	One-piece implants and two-piece (hybrid)
Number			
Maxilla	Minimum 4	Minimum 4	Minim 6 (minimum 4 for hybrid implants)
Mandible	Minimum 2	Minimum 2	Minimum 4 (minimum 2 for hybrid implants)
Surgery	Usually two-stage implant placement protocol	One- or two-stage implant placement protocol	One-stage implant placement protocol
Loading	Usually delayed loading	Immediate or delayed loading	Immediate loading
Overdenture support	Soft tissue and implant support	Soft tissue-support	Soft tissue-support
Overdenture design	Open palate maxillary denture	As a conventional complete denture	As a conventional complete denture
Attachment system	Splinted implants (bar) and unsplinted (ball, locator, magnets, telescope)	Unsplinted (ball, locator, magnets, telescope)	Unsplinted (Ball with O- ring)
Aim	improve overdenture retention, stability and support	improve overdenture retention and stability	improve overdenture retention and stability

Table 1. Main features of the overdentures on dental implants, in regard to their diameter

Patients with a high risk of developing implant or overdenture-related complications should be identified, and treatment personalized according to their nature. There are conditions with absolute contraindications of surgical procedures (e.g., recent myocardial infarction, stroke, cardiovascular surgery, and transplant; profound immunosuppression; bisphosphonate use, diabetes), but even in these cases the degree of disease-control is far more important than the nature of the systemic disorder itself [7, 8]. Behavioral aspects may increase some complication rates (e.g., implants are not indicated in heavy drinkers or smokers, more than 10 cigarettes per day). In patients with decreased manual dexterity or coordination deficiencies alternatives that promote simpler plaque control and easier overdenture placement and removal should be chosen (e.g. ball attachments are preferred to bars). Bruxism or other parafunctions with occlusal overloads associates high occlusal loading that increases the risk of implant failure, in this cases more frequent check-ups and sometimes the increase of the implant number are required. When more than two implants are used, there is a higher risk of overdenture fracture, and the reinforcement of the overdenture base is recommended [9].

The patient's expectations towards the prosthetic outcomes must be assessed in terms of functional restorations, esthetics and prosthesis retention. It is recommended to acknowledge the patient's perception and reasons of dissatisfaction toward the previous prosthesis, in order to correctly evaluate and inform him about the benefits of each particular type of implant overdenture. Additionally, financial aspects need to be explained to the patient, as comparative analysis of the additional costs of each treatment alternative, putting them in balance with the treatment benefits.

2.1. Concept of Mini Dental Implant Overdentures (MDIO)

Based on similar principles of overdentures with roots or conventional implants, using mini implants for overdenture has been suggested, as an alternative with advantages such as the less invasive surgical interventions with lower risks and lower costs, but with similar results [10, 11].

Implant overdentures are nowadays increasingly preferred to conventional dentures. Patients are more informed about the benefits of implant prosthesis, more frequently request and accept these treatment alternatives. The significant improvement in denture retention, with rapid regaining of functionality after implant placement, is an important motivating factor. The surgical and prosthetic techniques are significantly simplified, being more widely used one-stage implant placement protocol, with immediate loading, becoming a less invasive treatment that promotes rapid healing and has good treatment outcomes. MDIO fits this prosthetic treatment trend, and is seen as an appropriate option for the elderly edentulous, implants having a survival rate between 88.5% and 96%, higher in the mandible than in the maxilla [12, 6, 13]. Their use is increasing in relation to the relatively frequently reduced ridge width in the edentulous patient, that often limit using conventional implants without extensive surgical procedures for augmentation, that are usually not easily accepted, especially by the elderly patients [14].

Biomechanical studies support the use of narrow and mini implants, but draw attention to their increased risk of fracture, which should be considered. The decrease of implant diameter does not affect the implant osseointegration. Block et al. analyzed the effect of implant diameter on the pullout force required to extract the implant and proved that, after 15 weeks for osseointegration, no correlation was found to its diameter, but only with its length [15]. Clinical studies confirm that short implants were often accompanied by failure, but narrow implants have a good prognosis [16]. Therefore the narrow and mini implants used for overdenture should have at least 10mm length, in relation to their diameter, but also to the bone's height.

Given the good results obtained in vivo and in vitro, narrow and mini implants, seem to be the successors of conventional diameter implants in overdentures. Mini dental implants were originally designed by Victor Sendax [17]. At first they had diameters between 1.8- 2.4 mm, and were used for stabilization of interim prosthesis during implant osseointegration, stabilization of occlusion rims and for orthodontic anchorage. Afterwards, histological studies confirmed that these implants osseointegrate and clinical studies acknowledge a high survival rate, of about 83,9 to 97.5% [18]. Consequently, their usage expanded for definitive prosthesis both fixed (for single narrow edentulous spaces) and removable (for partial and complete denture stabilization). Mini implants, as endoosseous implants, are indicated to complete edentulous patients with narrow ridges, where the prosthetic treatment on implants is chosen, but reduced surgical invasiveness is beneficial, for example for those with general systemic risk factors [6]. It is particularly suitable for elderly patients, with multiple comorbidities and a low income, and who often do not accept complex and expensive dental interventions.

The mini implants have a number of features that have to be known and considered, both when it comes to selecting the implants, as well as during the treatment phases. Thus the mini dental implants are most commonly one-piece implants, with reduced diameter, conventional length, tapered, self-threading, made of biocompatible titan-based materials, with rough sandblasted surface treated by acid. IMTEC (currently part of 3M ESPE) developed mini dental implants with a diameter of 1.8mm to 2.4mm, supplemented recently by those with a diameter of 2.9mm (indicated especially in the maxilla), and with lengths of 10, 13, 15 and 18 mm. These implants have been designed differently, with 2.5mm transgingival collar (for thick gingiva) or without it (for thin gingiva). The upper surface of the endosteal dental implant may be polished and remain outside the bone within the mucosa, but the rough surface must be placed within the bone. Regarding the implant thread, it may be standard for D1 and D2 Misch bone densities (usually encountered in the mandible), or Max Thread, for D2 and D3 bone density (most frequently encountered in the maxilla) [19]. The implant prosthetic element, the abutment, has a spherical design like the ball attachment system, with an overall height of 4mm or 6 mm. Its gingival part has a square-profile section, with or without transgingival collar, which must remain outside the mucosa for at least half of its length. The attachment system is O-ring type, a resilient retention device composed of a metal matrix and a rubber ring, available in the following three options:

- standard: provides strong retention and tolerate a divergence of implants up to 30°;

- micro: has a 30% lower height than the standard matrix, offers an advantage for reduced prosthetic restorative spaces, provides a higher retention and compensates less for the implant divergence;

- O-Cap: provides extra-firm retention, mini-implants should be placed almost parallel, being used with delayed implant loading.

Therefore, the main coordinates of mini implant selection, according to the case particularities, are the following:

- Implant number: at least 4 in the mandible and at least 6 in the maxilla;

- Implant size, as diameter and length, is chosen according to ridge width, bone height and bone density. Usually, smaller diameter implants, of 1.8-2.1mm are used in the mandible, in bone with D1 and D2 Misch density, and mini implants with diameter of at least 2,4mm are recommended in D3 bone density in the maxilla. Implants should have a diameter with at least 2 mm less than the width of the ridge, which can be assessed using a clinical compass, or subtracting from the clinically measured width minimum 2mm corresponding to the mucosa thickness (Figure 1). The implants' length is chosen according to the bone height (at least 2 mm less than the bone height), which can be approximated by overlaying the specially designed grid on the panoramic radiography;

- Choosing between mini implants according to thread design is related to bone density (standard in the mandible and Max Thread in the maxilla);

- Choosing between mini implants with or without transgingival collar is related to the mucosa thickness.

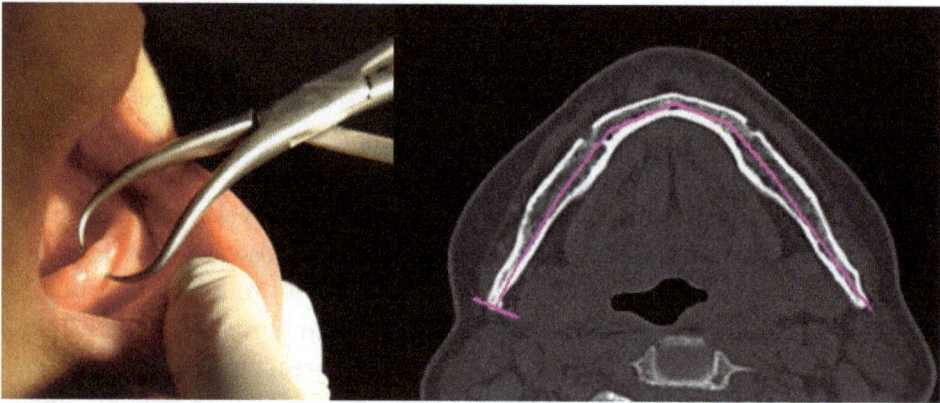

Figure 1. Clinical and radiological assessment of bone width

In case of MDIO, implants are placed without extensive augmentation procedure, through a less invasive surgical procedure, considering the anatomical limitation. In the mandible, mini implants are placed in the interforaminal region (7mm anterior to the mental foramen, to prevent damaging the inferior alveolar neurovascular bundle), and in the maxilla, anterior to the maxillary sinuses (protecting both the maxillary sinus and the nasal fosses). Within the mandible, when the mandibular canal is making a loop and the bone height allows it, implants can be placed behind the mental foramen. When placing the implants, it is recommended to keep a distance of at least 4.5 mm between them.

Most of the companies that produce implants are usually making available a line of implants with different diameters, and, for the same diameter, different corresponding implants lengths. Some of them, as mini Sky1 (Bredent Medical, Germany), that are hybrid implants, ensure a simpler implant selection and implant placement related to the implant options that differ only by implant length (10mm, 12mm and 14mm, and have the same diameter of 2.8mm, are identical as endosteal and abutment design) and have all the same simple implant placement protocol (only two drills are needed). Using hybrid implants allows, according to the bone quality and prosthetic needs, the reduction of the implant number (e.g., in the mandible only 2 mini Sky1 hybrid implants can be used instead of 4 mini implants with a diameter of 1,8-2,5 mm). Compared to the surgical implant kit of conventional denture, the one for mini implants is usually considerably simpler, containing fewer components (basically 1 or 2 drills for implant osteotomy and 2 ratchets), promoting a reduced time of the surgical phase, beneficial when considering this is a major stress for the patient.

Treatment with MDIO includes a surgical phase (implants placement) and a prosthetic phase (transformation of the denture in overdenture), both conducted in one clinical appointment.

Before implant placement some simple preoperative interventions are required, such as instruction and motivation on maintaining proper oral hygiene (antibacterial mouthwash as Chlorhexidine may be recommended), with prophylactic antibiotherapy and sedation.

For mini implant placement local anesthesia is sufficient, and a flap or flapless technique can be used, with or without a surgical guide (Figure 2).

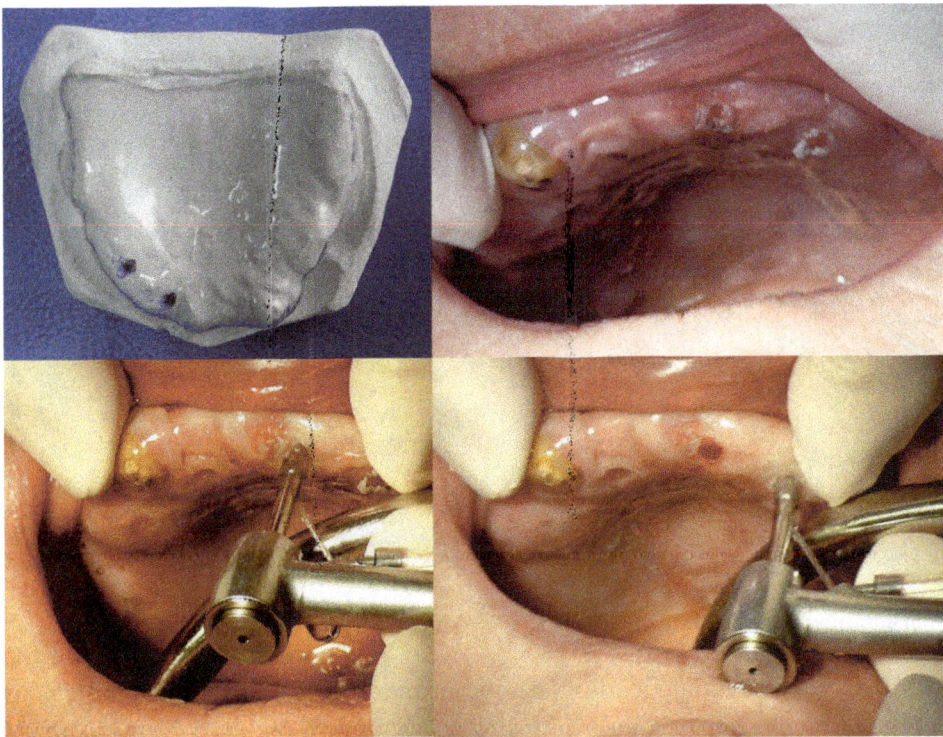

Figure 2. Implant placement using a surgical guide

For the flapless technique, the implant site is marked and the cortical bone is pierced with the same small size drill. Flap technique (Figure 3) is recommended in cases with thick mucosa or flabby ridge in order to properly asses bone offer, or in cases where 1.8 mm implants are to be placed into 3 mm narrow ridges. Initial implant osteotomy should be performed with a pilot drill with a diameter smaller than the one of the implant, in order to obtain bone condensation. Considering the positive effect of bone tapping on osseointegration, osteotomy depth varies according to bone density, about 2/3 of implant length for D1 bone density, about 1/2 of implant length for D2 bone density and about 1/3 of implant length for D3 bone density. Also, abundant irrigations with refrigerated sterile saline solution are mandatory. Implant placement should be done using slow movements, especially in high density bone, in order to avoid the heat trauma created by friction that may cause harmful effects in the bone (necrosis by heating) and also the implant fracture, which is more frequent in mini implants due to their decreased diameter. The self-tapped implant is placed and advanced into the bone by hand ratchet or headpiece and must be operated slowly, without extreme pressures. When screwing with the ratchet, the left hand finger is onto the ratchet in the mini implant's axis and the pressure is created with the right hand only on the ratchet arm, in the direction pointed by the arrow. The optimum value for the insertion torque is 35Ncm and should not exceed 45Ncm. If during the mini implant placement the torque exceeds 45Ncm it is recommended to unscrew the implant and expand the osteotomy, as depth or diameter. The implant body should be fully inserted into the bone.

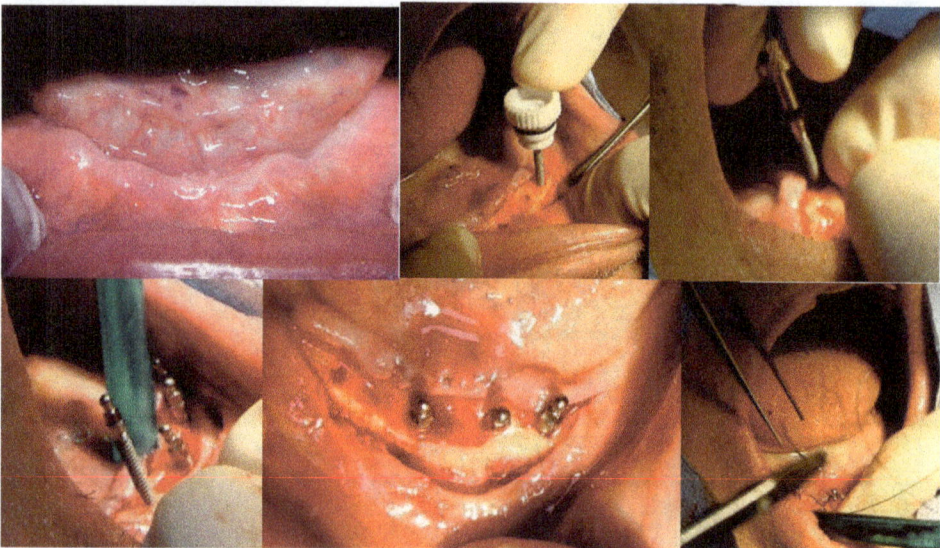

Figure 3. Mini implant placement, using a flap technique

In case of MDIO, for immediate loading, a good primary stability of the implants is required, which is related to the implant insertion torque (minimum 30 to 35 Ncm; in this respect, unfavorable situations are more frequently encountered in the maxilla, and are very rare in the mandible), bone compression and anchorage in the cortical bone. For immediate loading of the implants it is necessary to have a complete denture before the implants insertion that will be transformed into the overdenture, either as the old or newly manufactured prosthesis.

For immediate loading, the attachment caps, which contain rubber O-rings, are placed on the implants. The first clinical step is to remove the acrylic material from the inner part of the overdenture base, in the area corresponding to the implant site, quantitatively until the overdenture passive fits on the overdenture-bearing area. Fixing the housings can be done directly (by the dentist in the clinic) or indirectly (by the dental technician, in the laboratory). For housing fixing in the clinic, isolation of the gingival part of the implant abutment is done with latex materials (as piece of rubber dam or medical gloves), in order to prevent the acrylic material penetration under the O-ball head. Metal housings are placed combining rotational movements and pressure, until they fit passively. Preparing the prosthesis consists of repeatedly marking each matrix site accompanied by acrylic material removal from the corresponding denture base area. It is recommended to verify passive fit using soft silicone materials as Fit checker (GC Corporation). Afterwards, definitive metal housing fixation is done intraorally with acrylic materials, in centric occlusion. For a more accurate reproduction, before implant placement an occlusal registration can be taken and can be used during this treatment phase. Finally it is recommended to perform an accurate polishing of the denture around the metal matrices, in order to prevent plaque accumulation that favors occurence of peri-implant mucositis and peri-implantitis.

If the insertion torque is less than 35Ncm, the primary stability is not sufficient for immediate loading. Therefore, it is recommended to use progressive loading through the usage as soft lining material such as matrices during the osseointegration phase, and also to ensure weaker occlusal load in the area corresponding to the implant site. Metal housing fixation is recommended to be done after 3 to 6 months after implant placement.

A very important aspect is to verify, during the osseointegration period, the occlusion, the overdenture stability and the prosthesis of the antagonist jaw, as key elements for ensuring a good treatment prognosis.

Rubber O-rings are a part of the attachment system that wear-out over time and must be checked and periodically replaced in relation to loss of retention. Associated to the unavoidable alveolar bone resorption, denture relining or renewal are necessary over time. If overdenture renewal is desired, abutment analogues are used during impression.

MDIO has many advantages for older patients, often complete denture wearers that are dissatisfied with its retention and stability. Thus, through a reduced invasiveness surgical procedure, which requires less clinical time, with average costs, in a single session, a removable prosthesis with a good stability and with immediate functional integration can be achieved, providing the mental and physical comfort in order to carry out current social activities. At the same time, this treatment option has the advantage of an easy maintenance of oral and denture hygiene, through the unsplinted implants, an important aspect especially for elderly people, with frequent deficiencies when it comes to manual dexterity.

2.2. Concept of Narrow Diameter Implant Overdentures (NDIO)

The growing popularity of MDIO associated a general increase in the usage of implant overdentures among elderly completely edentulous patients. This is due to the clinical success of MDIO, the increase of its acceptability among edentulous patients, and the possibility for dentists to use it without extensive training in oral implantology (implant placement require one surgical intervention, relatively easy to perform. Within completely edentulous patients, narrow alveolar ridges are very common, mini and narrow implants being advantageous considering that they can be used without bone augmentations or other extensive surgical procedures, such as ridge splitting technique, being more easily accepted by elderly patients. At the same time, it is undeniable that the use of conventional diameter implants has numerous advantages, such as a reduced risk of implant fracture, reduced stress peaks at the implant-bone interface, the possibility to reduce the number of implants and the use of attachments according to the prosthetic needs, with different retention degrees [6]. Subsequently, the concept called NDIOhas developed, which uses implants with a diameter between the conventional and the mini dental implants, and is partially similar to both MDIO and CDIO. Narrow diameter implants with diameters between 3 and 3.5 mm, designed initially for fixed restorations of narrow edentulous spaces, expanded their use for implant overdentures. These can be found in different options, as size (implants with diameter between 3.0 and 3.25 are named sometimes small implants) and design (one- or two-piece implants, with different attachment systems).

NDIO, as treatment alternative has particularities common to both CDIO and MDIO, such as:

• Like the MDIO, it is mainly indicated in cases with narrow ridges (1.5-2 mm more than implant diameter) and resorbed ridges;

• Surgery is usually minimally invasive, similar to MDIO (without bone augmentation, possibility to use flapless implant insertion technique);

• The implant number can be reduced compared to MDIO, being similar to that of CDIO, due to the increased implant diameter;

• Narrow implants can be loaded immediately or delayed, depending on bone density, insertion torque, primary implant stability, being possible to use previous dentures or the ones manufactured after implant placement;

• Two-piece narrow implants allow insertion into bone with a lower density with delayed loading after 3 to 6 months, similar to CDIO;

• Two-piece narrow implants usually can be used with different attachment systems, with different retention degree, resiliency and possibility to compensate implant divergence (e.g., Locator can compensate up to 40° implant divergence);

• When compared to mini dental implants, narrow dental implants have a lower fracture risk, due to the larger diameter;

• NDIO, like MDIO, compared to CDIO, require reduced clinical time, reduced surgery (as number of appointments and complexity of the procedures), which favors a faster healing process and patient's comfort, reducing the biological and financial costs and overall being a more suitable treatment alternative for the elderly.

Narrow dental implants have diameters of 3 to 3.5 mm and are available in one- or two-piece design. Using the two-piece implants has the advantage of choosing to use either immediate or delayed loading, and for the latter either subgingival or transgingival healing. They may be placed flap or flapless, the latter the disadvantage of a less reliable assessment of the bone offer, but the advantage of promoting a faster healing. Usually, using a two-piece implant associates the possibility to choose from several attachment systems, and therefore a better treatment individualization, according to biomechanical and functional features, is available.

The increased interest towards implants designed for stabilization of the removable prosthesis is justified by the high prevalence of edentulism, which is usually treated by conventional complete dentures, alternatives that rather often have stability and retention deficiencies, problems that are more and more perceived as being unacceptable. In addition to this, more often cases with a high degree of treatment difficulty (mainly related to changes related to previous removable prosthetic treatment, as severe ridge resorption) are encountered and concerns are related to the increase of the age when edentulism occurs, that associates difficulties in generally adapting to new, and particularly to new prosthesis. Therefore, the increased use of narrow and mini implants is related to the reduced treatment invasiveness correlated to the functional benefits, which is a very important aspect for the elderly, popula-tion category in which most of the edentulous patients are encountered.

Treatment of edentulism with implant prosthesis is frequently accompanied by difficulties related to the limited bone offer – as a result of buccal or lingual bone resorption (narrow ridges) or as apical bone resorption (resorbed ridges). Narrow ridges are more often encoun-tered in skeletal class II patients with a hypodivergent pattern. Conventional removable prostheses are barely tolerated by patients with sharp ridges (sometimes associated with irregularities such as exostosis, with thin covering mucosa, sensitive to pressures) or with severe ridge resorption and imprecise peripheral boundaries, situations which are encoun-tered mainly in the mandible. Most of the completely edentulous patients that are denture wearers have severe ridge resorption, which associates difficulties both for conventional denture (through decreased support area) and CDIO (bone offer is insufficient for placement of conventional implants). Between these two treatment alternatives there are MDIO and NDIO, and when appropriate, the latter is preferred due to preserving the benefits of the first and having other important advantages (e.g., as stated before, a lower risk of implant fracture, possibility to use a reduced number of implants).

NDIO is found as a treatment option with indications similar to MDIO, in cases with narrow alveolar ridge, but it is a suitable treatment alternative also in cases of increased ridge resorp-tion, associated with denture intolerance. Similar to MDIO, for NDIO implant diameter should be chosen according to ridge width (the ridge width should be at least 2 mm larger than the implant's diameter). NDIO are more indicated than MDIO in the maxilla, as a preventive mean, considering that the survival rate of implants is lower in the maxilla than in the mandible. NDIO versus MDIO has the advantage of the possibility to use a smaller number of implants, for example for the mandibular prosthesis 2 narrow implants can be used instead of 4 mini implants (Figure 4).

Implant placement is similar for the one-piece narrow implants to that of mini implants, and for the two-piece narrow implants to conventional implants. The surgical kit includes a reduced number of drills and ranches, which should be used according to the manufacturer's instructions. In two-piece implants a one- or two-stage protocol can be used, that depends

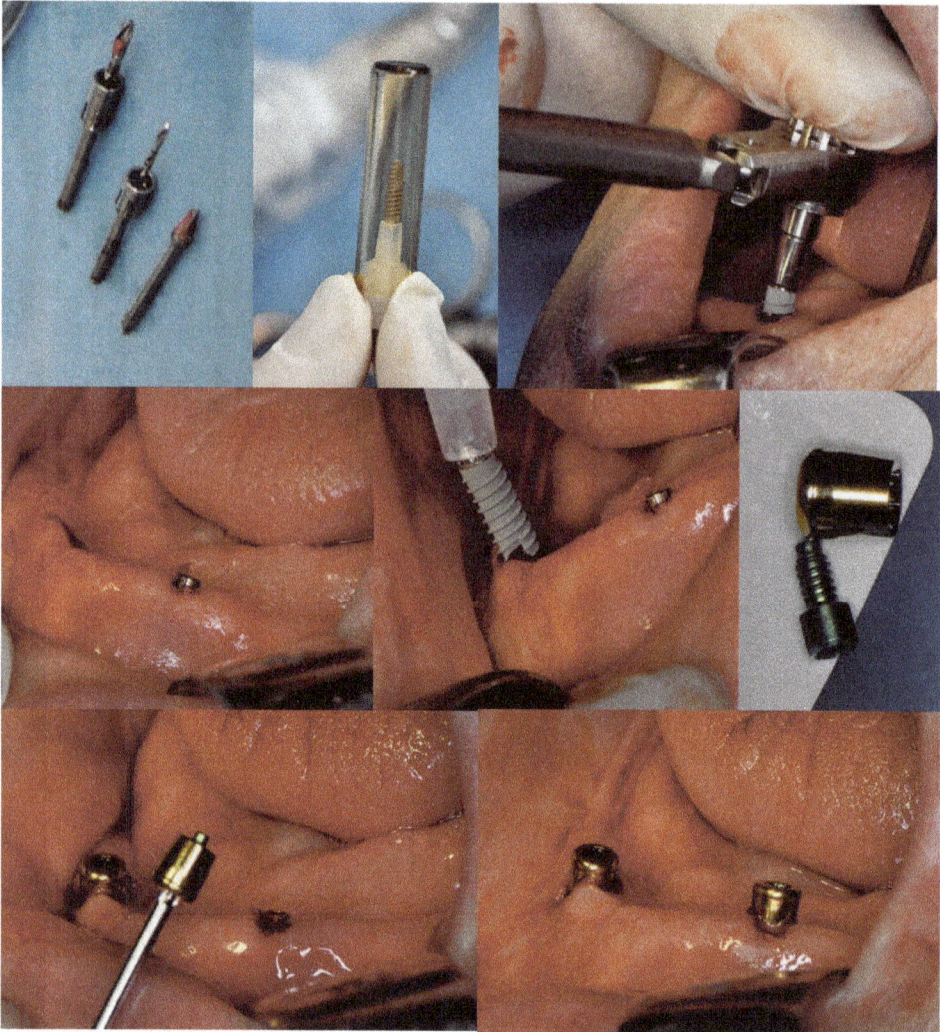

Figure 4. Narrow implant and Locator placement

mostly on the implant's primary stability. Therefore NDIO, compared to CDIO has the advantages of less surgical invasiveness and its associated benefits, overcoming some deficiencies of MDI, while preserving its advantages (good retention and stability of the overdenture, easy maintenance) [20].

Prosthesis execution differs according to the type of narrow implant used and coordination of treatment planning. Thus, when using one-piece narrow implants with one-stage surgery the process is similar to the one used for MDIO. When an attachment system with increased retention is used, like the Locator, it is recommended to use soft acrylic or silicone material as matrices during osseointegration. In this regard, silicone materials with different retention levels were developed, such as Retention.Sil (Bredent) that has 3 options according to the detachment force desired (200, 400, 600 gf). When using two-piece narrow implant with two-stage surgery, after osseointegration, the healing abutment is uncovered by a new surgical procedure, and replaced with the attachment, followed by the procedures needed in order to transform the denture into the overdenture.

3. Clinical phases of MDIO and NDIO

NDIO and MDIO are treatment options for complete edentulism, usually aiming the stabilization of the removable prosthesis. Alveolar ridge resorption, modifications of the muscle insertions and muscle tonus, neuromuscular coordination and control deficiencies increase treatment difficulties and favor occurrence of ill-fitting dentures, its retention and balance deficiencies being possible to be addressed through an implant overdenture. NDIO or MDIO have usually a mucosal support, not an implant one, the attachments only aiming to increase overdenture retention and stability. As clinical phases MDIO and NDIO are mostly similar, differences being encountered especially between one- and two-piece implants, when used with one or two-stage surgery.

Patient evaluation. Before implant placement, an accurate analysis of oral and systemic status is required. Although mini or narrow implant placement is done through surgical procedures with reduced invasiveness, the absolute contraindication should be accounted (e.g., recent myocardial infarction or stroke, profound immunosuppression, radiotherapy or bisphosphonate use) [7, 8]. Oral particularities should be accurately acknowledged through clinical and radiological examination, as anatomical and functional aspects. Considering the implant placement, ridge width should be evaluate by computed tomography or by clinical means (as using a clinical compass), the latter being sometimes confirmed by direct assessment during the surgical phase, after flap elevation. Bone height is best established using also computed tomography, but usually in the mandible only a panoramic radiography is used. Mucosa thickness is assessed by probing it with a periodontal probe.

The most commonly used radiological investigation is the panoramic radiography, which provides information on bone size and anatomical limitations (mandibular canal, mental foramen, maxillary sinus, nasal fossae). Computed tomography is indicated especially in cases with severe bone resorption, for an accurate bone offer evaluation and the establishment of implant site. Lateral cephalography can offer important data especially on skeletal relations, which associate anatomical and functional features relevant for treatment planning and prognosis.

Implants number and size. Implants are chosen according to the bone offer, the option with higher diameter and length being preferred. The higher the implant's diameter, the better it will resist to lateral forces, the longer it is, the better it will resist to vertical forces. Therefore, in order to compensate the decreased diameter of mini implants and to increase the resistance to lateral forces, a higher number of implants are placed. Usually, for mini implants 4 MDI in the mandible are placed between the mental foramens and 6 in the maxilla, anterior to the maxillary sinus. For hybrid and narrow implants their number may be reduced (2 in the mandible, 4 in the maxilla), related to the higher diameter. Bone density influences implant size selection. Therefore, 1.8 mm diameter implants can be placed in bone with D1 and D2 density, but an increased diameter, of 2.4 mm, is recommended for D3 bone density.

Implant placement. Mini- and narrow-implants are placed through a surgical procedure that is usually considered as having decreased invasiveness, and can be performed by a general dentist.

MDI and NDI insertion can be done with or without a surgical guide. The last option has the advantage of a more accurate positioning of the implants, in accordance with prosthetic aspects. Using a surgical radiological guide, manufactured based on the existing prosthesis, allows an accurate establishment of the most distal implant site, preventing the damage to anatomical proximity structures [21].

Mini and narrow diameter implants, by their design, associate bone condensation during implant placement, which favors a good primary stability. Screwing of the implant should be done slowly, with the ratchet, while performing manual control, in order to feel "the saturation point" and to avoid implant fracture.

Flap or a flapless technique may be used for mini and narrow implant placement. The flap technique, the most commonly used, has the advantage of directly visualizing the alveolar bone volume before the osteotomy, the possibility to reshape the bone and soft tissue. As a disadvantage, it is more invasive and prolongs the duration of the surgical phase, recovery and healing phase. Flapless technique is mostly done transmucosally, being a less invasive intervention, ensuring a more rapid healing, with a lower degree of patient discomfort (Figure 5). By not disturbing the periosteum layer, there is a higher chance, compared to the flap one, to maintain the alveolar bone levels [22, 23].

Last but not least, the decision to either use a flap or not is up to the practitioner, according to patient's particularities, but also to the clinician's surgical and prosthetic skills [24].The flap technique is recommended especially when interventions are needed in order to remodel the bone support (e.g., irregular alveolar bone; reduction of bone height needed due to insufficient prosthetic space) and when direct visual access is required (e.g. flabby ridge). The flapless technique is indicated when the bone width is adequate, the ridge shows no exostosis or alterations that require surgical correction, it is preferred when using immediate loading and in patients with systemic diseases that limit the extent of surgery or interfere in the healing process [24].

Implant loading protocol. Placement of mini- or narrow-dental implants can be followed by immediate-, progressive- or delayed-loading protocol, depending mainly on the implant primary stability

Immediate implant loading protocol is used when insertion torque is above 40Ncm, for D1 or D2 bone density, being a more commonly encountered in implants placed in the mandible, in the interforaminal area, especially when a flapless technique was used. In this regard previously made prosthesis are used, which are adjusted to the new situation, followed by the fixation of the matrix in the overdenture base. Occlusion analysis should be performed, considering these alterations can have a negative impact especially in the vulnerable period of osseointegration.

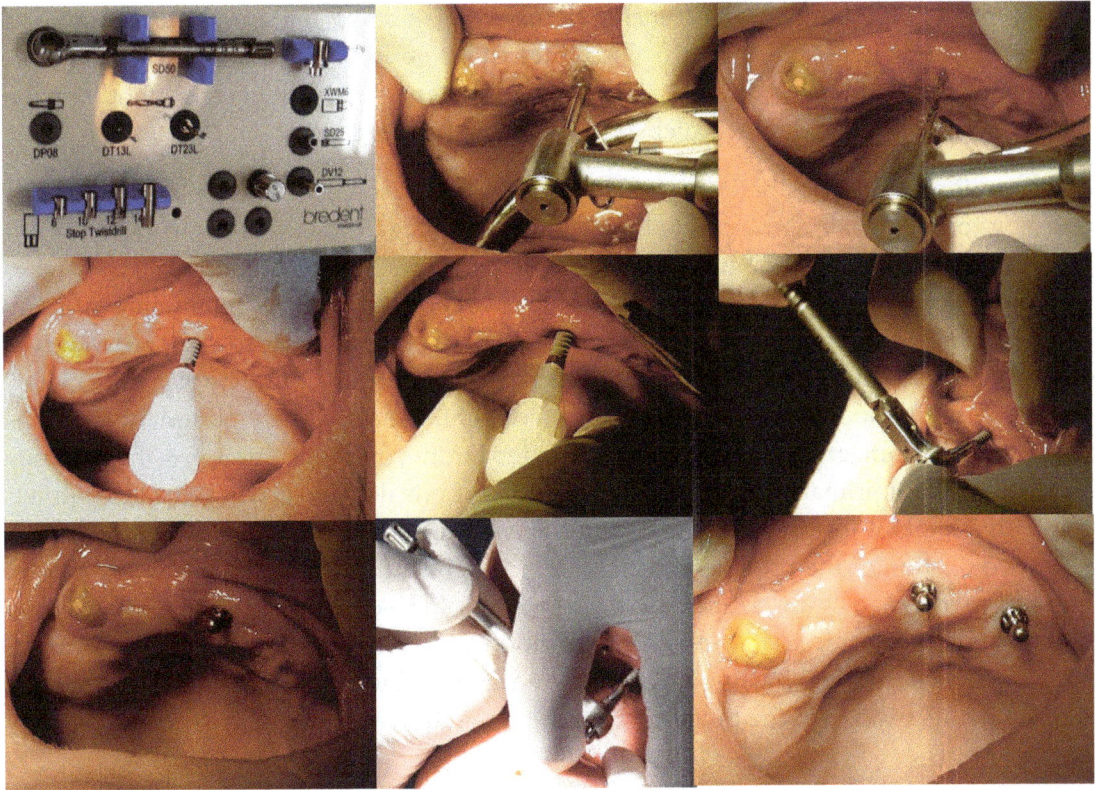

Figure 5. Hybrid implants placement, using a flapless technique

Progressive implant loading is recommended for D2 bone density and in cases with slower healing process after surgery, such as in flap techniques. Basically, for a period of 30 days postinsertion soft resilient acrylic or silicone materials are used as matrices, followed afterwards by the fixation of the matrices into the denture base.

In case of immediate and progressive loading, regular check-ups are at most importance during the osseointegration period. The overdenture must be verified in order not to exert direct pressure on the implants (only mucosal support should be noticed), as occlusal relations, as its stability and, if applicable, as the stability of the antagonist denture, as factors that may negatively influence the prognosis of the implant.

Delayed implant loading, performed at about 3 months, is indicated when the insertion torque is under 40Ncm and in patients with D3 bone density. In this case there is an additional surgical step in order to uncover the healing abutments.

Fixation of the matrices into the overdenture base. Fixing the prosthetic component of the attachment can be done in the dental office or in the dental laboratory, after verifying the denture correctness (e.g., as teeth mounting, occlusal relations, denture base extension, aesthetic and functional outcome, material status). One of the main advantages of NDIO and MDIO is related to the possibility of preserving the previous prostheses, this being related mainly to the denture correctness and patient preferences. Usually the dentures need to be renewal, most often due their deficiencies, occurred related to the improper execution or as changes in time. Even so, during the osseointegration period it is best to preserve the old denture, relined with resilient material, so that the patient can easily perceive modifications that may have a negative impact, such as the pressure on the implant.

Direct fixation of the prosthetic part of the attachment system, in the dental office, varies according to implant design, i.e. one- or two-piece implant. The clinical procedure for one-piece implants, which usually have O-ring as attachment system, is similar to that used for MDIO, previously described. For two-piece implants, applying the retention systems is different upon the implant placement protocol, i.e. one- or two-stage protocol. For one-stage protocol the procedures used are similar to those applied for one-piece implants, namely in the same clinical appointment with implant placement, the attachment abutment is applied (ball, locator, ferromagnetic metal keeper) and, depending on implant and prosthetic parameters (e.g., implant primary stability, insertion torque, bone density, occlusal loading) either a progressive implant loading (with soft material as matrices), or immediate implant loading (definitive fixation of the prosthetic attachment component, such as metal housing or ring, denture cap, magnet, in the denture base with self- or light-cured acrylic materials) is done. For two-stage protocol, after the osseointegration period, the endoosseous implants are surgically uncovered, the healing abutment are replaced by the attachment abutment, and followed by the fixation of the prosthetic attachment in the overdenture base (Figure 6).

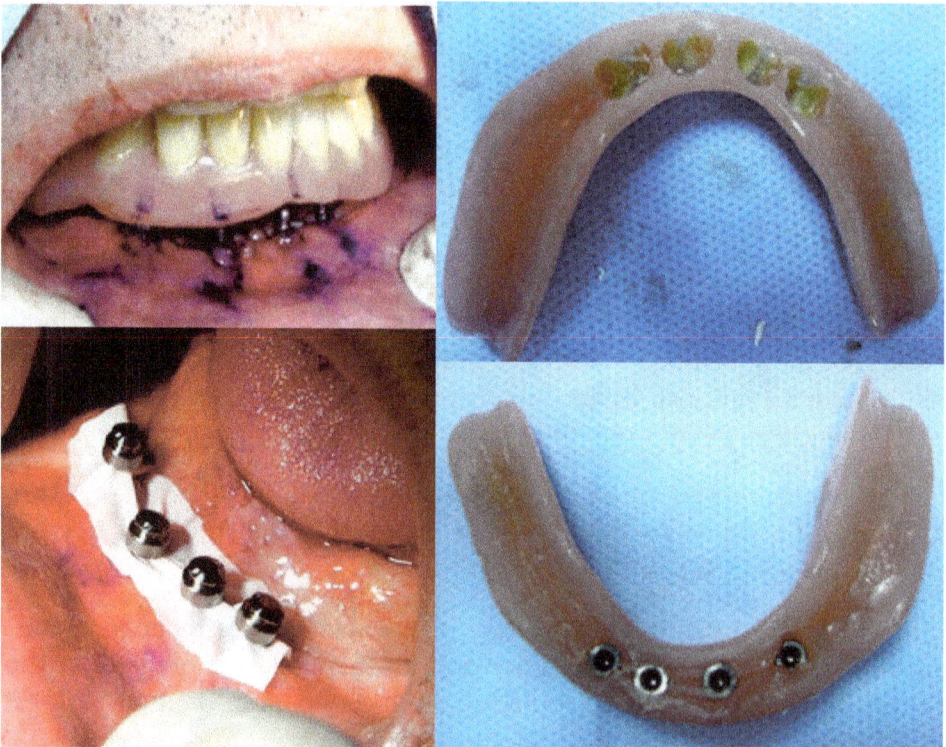

Figure 6. Direct metal housing fixing, in the dental office

Indirect fixation of the prosthetic part of the attachment system, in the dental laboratory, is mainly used when the overdenture renewal is desired. Correspondent, either impression transfer procedures after attaching the analogue, either impression taken with the prosthetic attachment component placed on the attachment abutment, can be used.

In all situations previously mentioned, overdenture adjustments and verifications are needed in order to achieve only mucosal support, passive fit on the implants and correct registrations of maxillomandibular relationship, without excessive occlusal loading. In the first 72 hours it is recommended to remove the denture only during oral and denture hygiene procedures, being highlighted to the patients the importance of a good plaque control in preventing treatment complications.

Considering that in case of MDIO and NDIO dental implants are applied in order to increase denture's retention and balance, overdenture execution should be done similar to that of conventional denture with a complete coverage of the support area, for ensuring proper retention, support and balance. Furthermore, choosing the occlusal scheme may be an important factor for treatment success, linear and lingualized occlusion being preferred for ensuring a more uniform distribution of the occlusal pressures over the bearing area, recommended especially for the mandibular overdenture. Key factors that ensure a good prognosis of conventional dentures should not be neglected in the case of MDIO and NDIO, such as the correct registration of maxillomandibular relations, at a correct vertical dimension of occlusion and centric relation.

Frequently used attachment systems for MDIO and NDIO. These types of implant prosthesis are usually retained by unsplinted implants, with attachment systems that only provide better denture retention and balance, while the prosthesis has only mucosal support. The most frequently used attachment systems are O-ring type, but also other alternatives are encountered, such as Locator, magnets, telescopes (especially double conical crowns, which are less rigid).

O-ring attachment system is used for both one- and two-piece narrow and mini dental implants. O-ring system is encountered in different designs, as the one of mini dental implant manufactured by 3M ESPE (spherical abutment with a metal matrix and rubber ring) or the one of miniSky 1 hybrid implants from Bredent Medical (spherical abutment with a metal ring and rubber ring). The metal matrix are made of Au or Ti, and can be activated, ensuring a different retention level. This attachment system has a resiliency degree, being a semi-rigid type, with positive effect on stress distribution. The system compensates for an implants divergence of about 20°-30°. Due to wearing over time, the rubber rings must be replaced periodically, when not ensuring the proper overdenture retention. This is encountered most frequently in cases with denture deficiencies that contribute to denture instability (e.g., overextended denture flanges, incorrect mounting of artificial teeth, unstable occlusal contacts).

Locator attachment systems, developed later, brought a number of advantages for NDIO. They can be used in cases with decreased vertical prosthetic space (at about 10 mm from the ridge crest to the height of the denture), generally having below 5 mm height with the denture cap in place, value that is below of that of O-ring attachment system. Also, it compensates for a higher angle of implant divergence, up to 40°. Even so, they are designed for ensuring an internal and external retention, but in order to use both, implants must be placed nearly parallel. If implants are placed under a divergent angle, only internal retention is preserved. Depending on the manufacturer, different alternatives are available according to the level of retention and gingiva thickness.

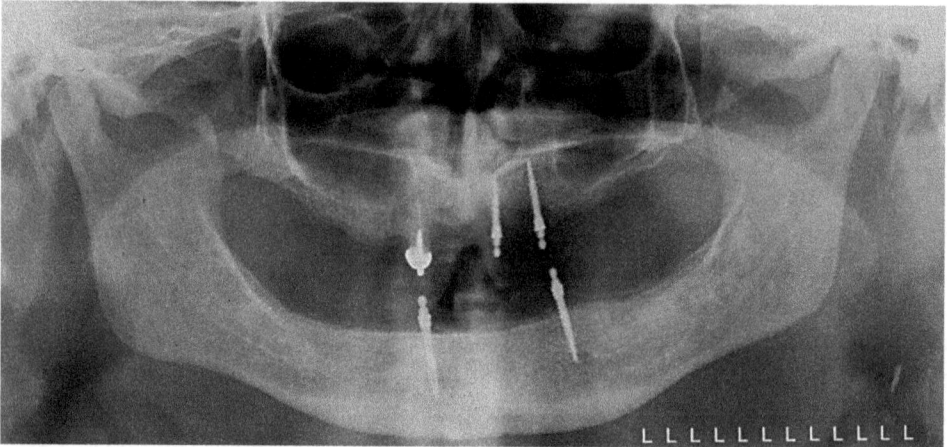

Figure 7. miniSky 1 implant overdentures – radiological examination 2 years after implant placement

4. Advantages and disadvantages of MDIO and NDIO

Implant overdentures, and especially MDIO and NDIO have registered an increased usage, which is probably related to its better treatment outcome, when compared to conventional complete denture. Among others, there can be mentioned beneficial aspects as the increased prosthesis balance and retention (especially for the mandibular denture), the improvement of oral functions (mastication, phonation) and self-confidence, with positive implications on the patient's physical and psychological comfort and on the quality of life.

MDIO and NDIO are particularly indicated in edentulous patients with an increased degree of treatment difficulty, unsatisfied by their conventional dentures (e.g., complaining about denture instability, pain and discomfort during wearing), with systemic alterations that limits the extent of the surgery or that refuse complex, prolonged, expensive medical interventions [25].

When compared to the fixed implant prosthesis, or even CDIO, MDIO and NDIO are simplified implant prosthetic treatment alternatives that have a satisfactory clinical success and are implemented through less invasive surgery, with reduced pain and trauma. These alternatives are well fitted to aged edentulous patients, who frequently have systemic comorbidities that associate a higher risk of complications, and generally have difficulties in accepting complex medical interventions in general, and implant treatment in particular. For these patients, aspects like the reduced invasiveness of surgical procedures, of the clinical time needed, of postoperatory discomfort, additionally to the relatively reduced costs required, are arguments that may convince them to accept the implant restoration. Overall costs are generally rated as being lower for MDIO and NDIO than for CDIO, due to the price differences of mini and narrow implants, the reduced clinical time with avoidance of some procedures (e.g., bone augmentation), the possibility to use the previous complete denture, when it corresponds qualitatively, through complications that are in general relatively easy and cheaper to resolve (e.g., loss of an implant can be solved by applying another one, followed by adjusting procedures to the existing denture; at CDIO using bars, implant loss is usually accompanied by extensive interventions, which almost covers the whole implant-prosthetic treatment).

By improving the denture stability, mastication efficiency increases, promoting a better nutritional status, and the denture detachment during mastication and phonation is reduced, offering the patient a psychological comfort [26]. MDIO and NDIO may be considered preventive treatments for reducing the side effects of ill-fitting conventional dentures, as an accelerated ridge resorption rate [27]. Additionally, one-piece mini implants associate a decreased peri-implant bone resorption compared to two-piece conventional implants, that was linked to the absence of the microgap between the endoosseous implant and the abutment, as well as the less physical displacement [28].

MDIO and NDIO require usage of a reduced number of implants, starting with 2 narrow or hybrid implants in the mandible and 4 in the maxilla, placed in most predictable anatomic area (interforaminal area), by simple surgical techniques, which ensures, in case of immediate loading, rapid regaining of functionality. Mini and narrow diameter implants minimize, through their design, the soft tissue and bone damaging, compared to conventional implants, favoring a shorter and better healing and osseointegration [29]. Placing the implants in the anterior maxillary area is beneficial, considering the occlusal load is decreased when compared to the posterior maxillary area, and also the possibility to use bicortical implant stabilization. The survival rate of implants placed in the anterior area of the mandible is high, above 90%, similar to that of conventional implants [30, 31, 32].

Increased use of MDIO and NDIO may be related also to the extended usage of implants the dental field. Also, in the general dental practice an increased surgical placement of implants is observed, probably related to patient's demands. However, the cost for dental practitioners for conventional implants remains high, both in terms of education and equipment needs, but are affordable for mini- and narrow-dental implants.

Although the use of either MDIO or NDIO is accompanied by many advantages, it must be considered that the treatment and maintenance is more complex than the one for conventional prosthesis, that may be regarded as a disadvantage, when considering the barriers that elderly face (e.g., financial hardship, transportation difficulties). Therefore, simpler solutions must be chosen, with complications that can be easily resolved (e.g., in elderly, unsplinted implants with O-ball attachments are preferred to bars). Also, there are behavioral aspects or systemic conditions that associate a higher complication rate (e.g., smokers are at greater risk of implant failure compared to nonsmokers).

Specifically linked to the MDIO and NDIO is the disadvantage of not being recommended to be insert mini and narrow dental implant immediately after tooth extraction.

Also, when using mandibular MDIO or NDIO, opposed by an edentulous maxilla treated by conventional denture, signs similar to those of Combination Syndrome may appear, as instability of the conventional denture and increase bone resorption rate in the anterior maxilla. These are managed usually through using implant prosthesis also in the maxilla.

5. Conclusions

Stabilization of conventional denture with mini- or narrow-dental implants is beneficial especially for the elderly, considering the improvement achieved through a relatively easy surgical intervention, with moderate treatment costs. In this regard, for mandibular denture stabilization either 4 mini implants or 2 hybrid/narrow implants can be used. Treatment success is strongly related to acknowledgement of patient anatomical and functional particularities, rigorous planning and execution of prosthetic and surgical phase, as well as ensuring an adequate maintenance.

Considering that edentulism is and most probably will continue to remain a frequent medical condition mostly found in the elderly, MDIO and NDIO overdentures, through their specific parameters, may replace in time complete dentures and may be the most used treatment alternative.

Author details

Elena Preoteasa[1*], Marina Imre[1], Henriette Lerner[2], Ana Maria Tancu[1] and Cristina Teodora Preoteasa[3]

*Address all correspondence to: dr_elena_preoteasa@yahoo.com

1 Department of Prosthodontics, Faculty of Dental Medicine, Carol Davila University of Medicine and Pharmacy, Bucharest, Romania

2 Private Practice, Baden-Baden, Germany

3 Department of Oral Diagnosis, Ergonomics, Scientific Research Methodology, Faculty of Dental Medicine, Carol Davila University of Medicine and Pharmacy, Bucharest, Romania

References

[1] WHO. Active Aging. A Policy Framework. Madrid; 2002. http://whqlibdoc.who.int/hq/2002/WHO_NMH_NPH_02.8.pdf?ua=1 (accessed 3 October 2014).

[2] Thomason JM, Kelly SA, Bendkowski A, Ellis JS. Two implant retained overden-tures--a review of the literature supporting the McGill and York consensus state-ments. Journal of Dentistry 2012;40(1) 22-34.

[3] Feine JS, Carlsson GE, Awad MA, Chehade A, Duncan WJ, Gizani S, Head T et al. The McGill Consensus Statement on Overdentures. Montreal, Quebec, Canada. May 24-25, 2002. International Journal of Prosthodont 2002;15(4) 413-4.

[4] Melescanu Imre M, Marin M, Preoteasa E, Tancu AM, Preoteasa CT.Two implant overdenture--the first alternative treatment for patients with complete edentulous mandible. Journal of Medicine and Life 2011;4(2) 207-9.

[5] Preoteasa E, Marin M, Imre M, Lerner H, Preoteasa CT. Patients' Satisfaction With Conventional Dentures and Mini Implant Anchored Overdentures. Revista Medico-Chirurgicala a Societatii de Medici si Naturisti din Iasi 2012;116(1) 310-16.

[6] Klein MO, Schiegnitz E, Al-Nawas B. Systematic review on success of narrow-diame-ter dental implants. The International Journal of Oral & Maxillofacial Implants 2014;29 Supplement 43-54.

[7] Diz P, Scully C, Sanz M. Dental Implants in the Medically Compromised Patient. Journal of Dentistry 2013;41(3) 195-206.

[8] Gomez-de Diego R, Mang-de la Rosa M, Romero-Pérez MJ, Cutando-Soriano A, Lo-pez-Valverde-Centeno A. Indications and Contraindications of Dental Implants in Medically Compromised Patients: Update. Medicina Oral Patologia Oral y Cirugia Bucal 2014;19(5):e438, -9.

[9] Preoteasa E, Murariu CM, Ionescu E, Preoteasa CT. Acrylic Resin Reinforcement With Metallic and Nonmetallic Inserts. Revista Medico-Chirurgicala a Societatii de Medici si Naturalisti din Iasi 2007; 111(2) 487-93.

[10] Lerner H. Minimal invasive implantology with small diameter implants. Implant Practice 2009, 2(1) 30-5.

[11] Preoteasa E, Meleşcanu Imre M, Preoteasa CT, Marin M, Lerner H. Aspects of oral morphology as decision factors in mini-implant supported overdenture. Romanian Journal of Morphology and Embryology 2010;51(2) 309-14.

[12] Shatkin TE, Shatkin S, Oppenheimer AJ, et al. A simplified approach to implant den-tistry with mini dental implants. Alpha Omega. 2003; 96(3) 7 15.

[13] Preoteasa E, Imre M, Preoteasa CT. A 3-Year Follow-up Study of Overdentures Re-tained by Mini–Dental Implants. The International Journal of Oral & Maxillofacial Implants 2014; 29(5) 1034-41.

[14] Sohrabi K, Mushantat A, Esfandiari S, Feine J. How successful are small-diameter im-plants? A literature review. Clinical Oral Implants Research 2012;23 (5) 515–525.

[15] Block MS1, Delgado A, Fontenot MG.The effect of diameter and length of hydroxyla-patite - coated dental implants on ultimate pullout force in dog alveolar bone. Journal of Oral and Maxillofacial Surgery 1990;48(2) 174-8.

[16] Renouard F, Nisand D. Impact of implant length and diameter on survival rates. Clinical Oral Implants Research 2006;17 (2) Supplement 35-51.

[17] Singh RD, Ramashanker, Chand P. Management of atrophic mandibular ridge with mini dental implant system. National Journal of Maxillofacial Surgery 2010;1(2) 176-8.

[18] Griffitts TC, Collins CP, Collins PC. Mini dental implants: an adjunct for retention, stability, and comfort for the edentulous patient. Oral Surgery, Oral Medicine, Oral Pathology, Oral Radiology, and Endodontology 2005;100 (5) 81-4.

[19] Misch CE. Contemporary Implant Dentistry 2nd edition. St. Louis: Mosby Inc; 1999.

[20] Rossein KD. Alternative treatment plans: implant supported mandibular dentures. Inside Dentistry 2006; 2(6) 42-43.

[21] Melescanu Imre M, Preoteasa E, Tancu A, Preoteasa CT. Imaging Technique for the Complete Edentulous Patient Treated Conventionally or With Mini Implant Overdenture. Journal of Medicine and Life 2013;6(1) 86-92.

[22] Campelo LD, Camara JR. Flapless implant surgery: A 10-year clinical retro- spective analysis. International Journal Oral Maxillofacial Implants 2002;(17) 271–276.

[23] Sunitha RV, Sapthagiri E. Flapless implant surgery: A 2-year follow-up study of 40 implants. Oral Surgery, Oral Medicine, Oral Pathology and Oral Radiology 2013;116 (4) 237–243.

[24] Scherer MD, Ingel AP, Rathi N. Flapped or Flapless Surgery for Narrow-Diameter Implant Placement for Overdentures: Advantages, Disadvantages, Indications, and Clinical Rationale. The International Journal of Periodontics & Restorative Dentistry 2014;34(3) Supplement 89-95.

[25] Christensen GJ.The 'mini'-implant has arrived. The Journal of the American Dental Association 2006;137(3) 387-90.

[26] Preoteasa E, Iosif L, Amza O, Preoteasa CT, Dumitrascu C. Thermography, an Imagistic Method in Investigation of the Oral Mucosa Status in Complete Denture Wearers. Journal of Optoelectronics and Advanced Materials 2010;12(11) 2333–4.

[27] Awad MA, Lund JP, Dufresne E, Feine JS. Comparing the efficacy of mandibular implant-retained overdentures and conventional dentures among middle-aged edentulous patients: satisfaction and functional assessment. The International Journal of Prosthodontics 2003;16, 117–22.

[28] Flanagan D, Mascolo A. The Mini Dental Implant in Fixed and Removable Prosthetics: A Review. Journal of Oral Implantology 2011;37 (1) 123-132

[29] Bulard RA. Mini implants. Part I. A solution for loose dentures. The Oklahoma Dental Association Journal. 2002;93.42-46.

[30] Dantas Ide S, Souza MB, Morais MH, Carreiro Ada F, Barbosa GA. Success and survival rates of mandibular overdentures supported by two or four implants: a systematic review, Brazilian Oral Research 2014;28(1) 74-80.

[31] Bergendal T, Engquist B. Implant-supported overdentures: a longitudinal prospective study. The International Journal of Oral & Maxillofacial Implants 1998;13 (2) 253–62.

[32] Klein MO, Schiegnitz E, Al-Nawas B. Systematic review on success of narrow-diameter dental implants. The International Journal of Oral & Maxillofacial Implants. 20

5

Are the Approximal Caries Lesions in Primary Teeth a Challenge to Deal With? — A Critical Appraisal of Recent Evidences in This Field

Mariana Minatel Braga, Isabela Floriano, Fernanda Rosche Ferreira,
Juliana Mattos Silveira, Alessandra Reyes, Tamara Kerber Tedesco,
Daniela Prócida Raggio, José Carlos Pettorossi Imparato and
Fausto Medeiros Mendes

1. Introduction

Approximal surfaces have been pointed as a challenge regarding the control of caries lesions in primary teeth, specially due to the larger area of contact between adjacent teeth and limited salivary access [1, 2]. In addition, children can present less dexterity to using dental floss and depend on parent's collaboration to remove interproximal dental plaque [3]. Therefore, poor compliance to flossing by children [4] seems to contribute to make the arrestment of approximal caries lesions more difficult. Consequently, identifying and understanding attitudes towards flossing are very important tasks to aid health professionals for flossing orientation and its incentive [4].

Several evidences have been published recently as promising alternatives in order to deal with approximal caries lesion in primary teeth and minimize the effects of poor compliance with flossing and/or repair eventual irreversible dental decay caused by caries progression.

Minimally invasive interventions have been proposed to caries lesion management, comprising early detection, preventive procedures and minimal invasion [5]. This approach also proposes to minimize the discomfort of patient [6], specially to deal with pediatric patients' dental anxiety and fear [7]. However, even considering minimal invasive treatments, there are operational differences among them that could interfere on children's discomfort and acceptability. Indeed, when exploring options for dental treatment, not only the efficacy/effectiveness but also the cost-efficacy/effectiveness and the patient's discomfort/satisfaction should also be comparatively investigated for available approaches.

Based on the exposed above, this chapter aims to present the particularities of dealing with approximal caries lesions and make a critical appraisal concerning effectiveness/efficacy, applicability, utility and clinical relevance of recent published studies and their findings. In this way, we expect to permit the clinicians to choose the best option for treating initial and advanced approximal caries lesions in primary teeth basing your decision-making process on relevant scientific evidences.

2. Approximal caries

Caries lesions (clinical signs of the disease) are developed on the biofilm-tooth interface [8-10] and the key factor of their formation is the presence acid-producing biofilm of the tooth surface [11]. Usually, minerals from oral fluids and tooth are in balance. However, when a tooth surface has biofilm accumulated for some period, changes in pH occur, caused by biofilm bacterial metabolism [8]. These pH fluctuations at biofilm-tooth interface may cause tooth mineral loss when the pH is decreasing (demineralization) or mineral gain when the pH is increasing (remineralization) [12]. When there is a prevalence of demineralization over remineralization, mineral loss is observed and this leads to a caries lesion [8, 13]. Thus, caries lesions start with mineral loss from the tooth surface and, if the biofilm is not removed, they progress until cavitation and tooth destruction.

Considering that the demineralization/remineralization processes occur on the biofilm-tooth interface, special attention should be given to the main biofilm stagnation areas, as occlusal surfaces, approximal surfaces and smooth surfaces along the gingival margin. These areas are relatively protected from mechanical wear by tongue, cheeks, abrasive food, and toothbrushing [13].

Since mechanical removal of the stagnated biofilm does not occur, the lactic acid produced by this biofilm acts on enamel and may cause demineralization. As the enamel is constituted by hydroxyapatite crystals, separated from each other by small intercrystalline spaces filled with water and organic material [14], the mineral loss due to caries results on an increase of these intercrystalline spaces, increasing the enamel porosity [15]. The mineral loss is higher in the subsurface of caries lesions and the surface layer thickness of the lesions ranged from 35 to 130 μm. The maximum mineral content in this layer corresponds to 74% to 100% of that of sound enamel [16]. This histopathological process is observed clinically as the formation of white spot lesions. The mentioned mineral loss results in the loss of translucence of the enamel and the opaque appearance of the white-spot lesion [17]. On the approximal surfaces, these lesions developed between the contact point and the gingival margin, resulting in a kidney-shaped white spot lesion (Figure 1). This area is the one most prone to biofilm accumulation on approximal surfaces (Figure 2).

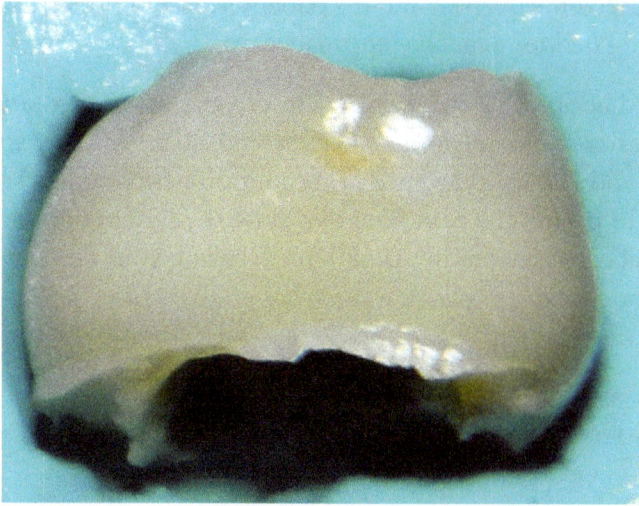

Figure 1. Approximal caries lesions. Note the shape of this lesion, located contouring the contact point, which is the area where the biofilm usually stagnates.

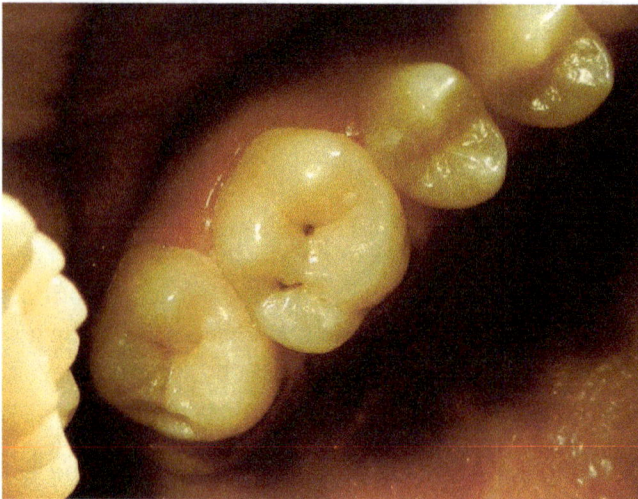

Figure 2. Biofilm accumulation on approximal surfaces. Note other dental surfaces are clean, but the biofilm remains stagnated in approximal areas.

The progression of enamel caries takes place along the enamel prisms, and in the approximal surfaces results on a conical shape [18] (Figure 3 and 4). If the plaque stagnation on caries lesions does not succeed, the lesion may reach the dentinoenamel junction and progress into the dentin [11] (Figure 3). The progression of an enamel lesion into dentine in primary teeth is faster than the observed in permanent ones [19].

There is no consensus in the literature about how does the progression of caries lesions when it reaches the dentinoenamel junction [11, 20]. Nevertheless, it is known that in lesions that reach the dentinoenamel junction, demineralized dentine is present, as part of the progression of enamel lesions [21]. On the other hand, the level of bacterial invasion is very low [22], especially because there is no cavitation. Therefore, it is expected a lower progression compared to cavitated lesions [23]. As dentine is composed of about 50% of mineral [24], caries progression into dentine tends to be faster than in enamel. As the less demineralized areas are the intertubular dentin composed of a matrix of collagen reinforced by apatite, the demineralization process tends to follow the direction of dentine tubules, resulting in the typical histology of dentine caries lesions, as you can see in Figure 3.

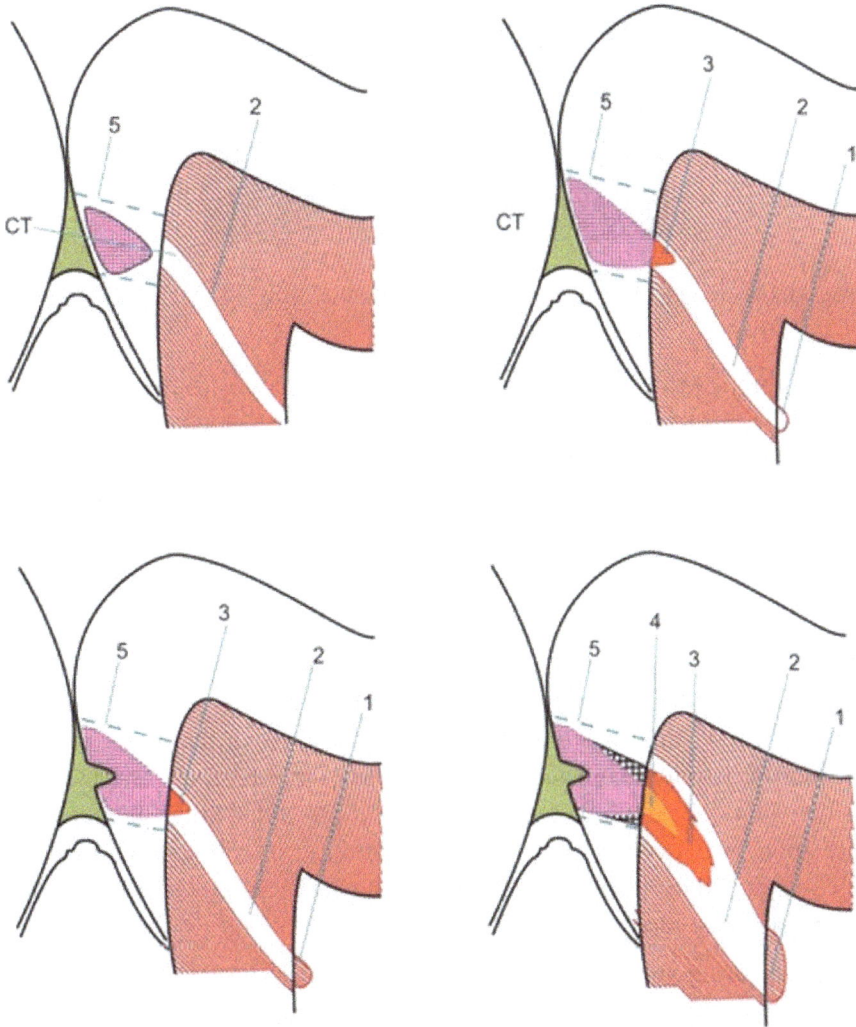

Figure 3. Schematic diagram of approximal caries progression. Different numbers symbolize different areas observed during caries lesion progression. (1- tertiary or reparative dentine, 2 - dentine tubules, 3- affected layer of carious dentine, 4-infected layer of carious dentine 5- enamel lesion) - adapted from Fejerskov et al., 2008 [14].

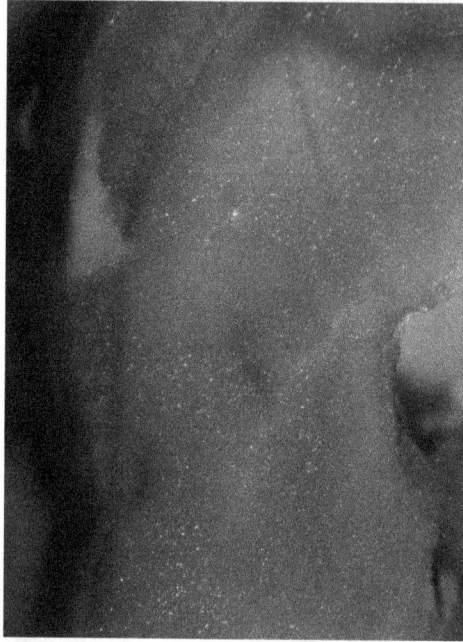

Figure 4. Histological exam of an enamel caries lesion. Note its conical shape, since progression follows the interprismatic spaces.

Substantial demineralization into dentin may be observed despite the absence of cavitation [25]. Nevertheless, if caries lesion progresses continuously into dentine, demineralized enamel may collapse and the intact surface may become cavitated. Thus, bacterial invasion into enamel and proteolytic action of bacterial enzymes mainly on the collagen may occur. If the biofilm stagnation is not controlled, an increase of the cavity size and further biofilm invasion could be expected [26]. When the cavity is present, a most infected dentine could be expected [23], which contribute to faster caries progression.

Two altered zones of dentine could be found in a dentine caries lesion: a superficial infected and a deeper affected layer [27] (Figure 3). The infected dentine consists of irreversibly acid-demineralized dentine, with its collagen degraded and highly contaminated with bacteria [28]. The affected dentine is only minimally infected and has potential to repair under suitable conditions, since their collage structure is maintained [29, 30]. Clinically, the main difference between these zones is the consistency due to the amount of collagen degradation observed in each one. The infected dentine tends to be soft and easily removed with excavators, while the affected dentine is usually harder [29] (Figure 5).

Since the progression of caries lesions is slow, the dentine may react in order to minimize the chance of occurrence of pulp exposition/inflammation. Therefore, highly mineralized peritubular dentin is secreted and reduces the tubules diameter, decreasing the dentine permeability and the chance for bacterial contamination [11]. This reaction is usually started since the caries lesion reaches the dentinoenamel junction. However, even considering the slow progression of caries lesions and pulp mechanisms for preventing pulp damage, it is not always possible to avoid the pulp exposure. When the reaction takes time to succeed, this

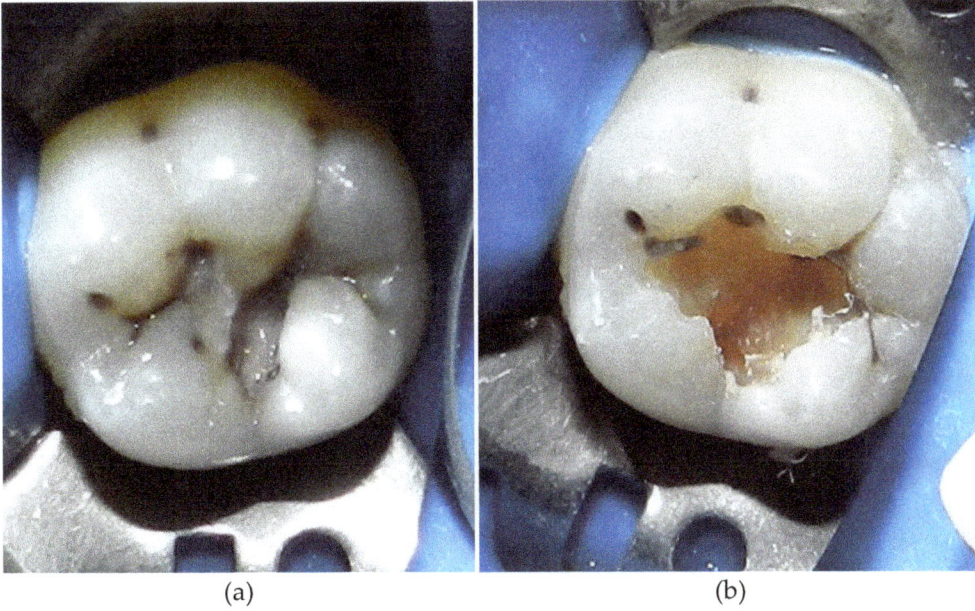

(a)   (b)

Figure 5. Clinical aspect of infected (a) and affected dentine (b) in dentine caries lesion.

highly mineralized dentine (Figure 6), also called as sclerotic dentine [31], is found in the bottom of the cavities, showing a hard consistency and usually a darker coloration.

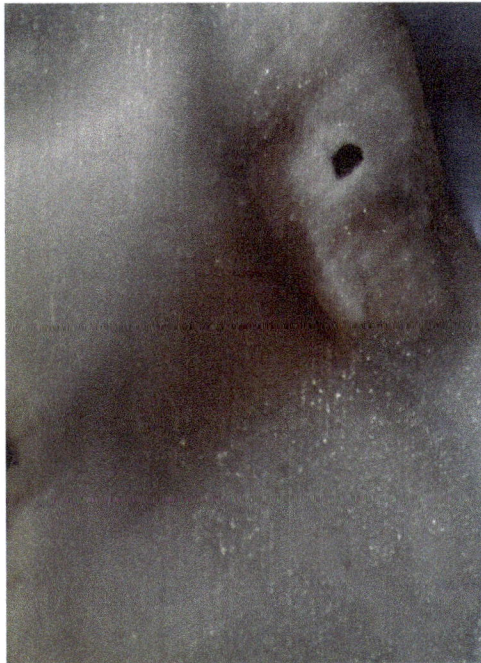

Figure 6. Histological appearance of sclerotic dentine. Note the different appearance of dentine, evidencing the hyper-mineralization of peritubular dentine.

Despite the stage of caries lesion, the presence of biofilm at the tooth surface determines caries progression [32]. Since this biofilm may be controlled, the lesion may be arrested. Therefore, both for non-cavitated and cavitated lesions, the inactivation of caries lesions would be possible, when the control of the biofilm is possible [33]. Since the biofilm control is achieved, the redeposition of mineral is facilitated. This mineral gain tend to reduce enamel porosities [34, 35]. Therefore, active lesions generally exhibits a more porous surface layer than the inactive lesions [16]. In addition, the surface wear/polishing may occur and differences in enamel surface roughness may occur [34, 35]. Due to that, active and inactive lesions tend to be different due to enamel porosity and surfaces wear/polishing (Figure 7). Besides, dentine caries may also be arrested. In these cases, there is an increase in the mineral content in the surface layer of the dentine lesions. The arrested dentine caries lesion presents more mineralized dentine, the surface is not always infected surface layer and may present sclerotic, harder

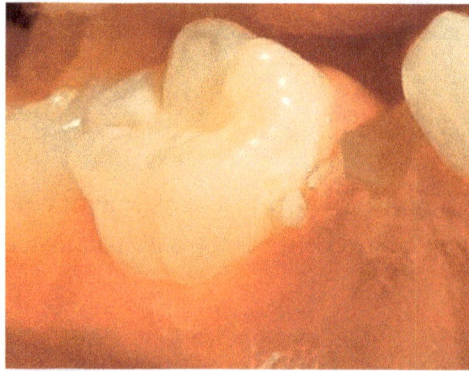

Figure 7. Active enamel caries on mesial surface of a second primary molar. Note characteristics usually associated with active lesions caused by biofilm stagnation in this area. Despite the absence of the adjacent primary molar, note the remained fragments that make the plaque removal and lesion arrestment more difficult.

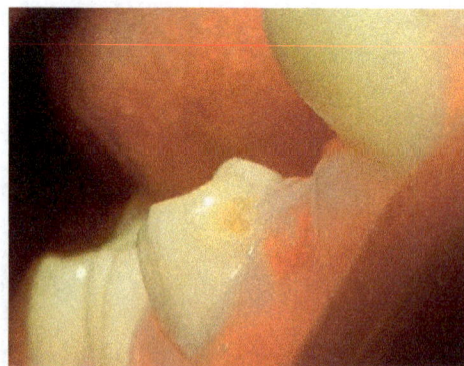

Figure 8. Active dentine caries on mesial surface of a second primary molar. Note characteristics usually associated with active lesions caused by biofilm stagnation in this area. Despite the absence of the adjacent primary molar, which will permit the mechanical control of local biofilm, this lesion did not have time enough to arrest. In this situation (absence of the adjacent tooth), this lesion tend to be arrested. That is why the picture still evidences characteristics of a dentine active lesion.

consistency and, usually, dark colour [36] (Figure 8). Changes observed in inactive dentine lesions may be detected after 6 months. However, hard consistency is usually observed after total arrestment of the lesion, which generally takes years [36].On the other hand, it is worth to state that due to difficulties in controlling the biofilm on approximal lesions, few assessed lesions present the characteristic above, as we are going to discuss in further sections of this chapter (Figures 7 and 8).

3. The challenge: Controlling approximal caries lesions

Approximal surfaces of primary molars present some particularities that expose them to a greater risk of developing caries [1, 37], and, consequently, it is a challenge when controlling caries lesion is needed.

Firstly, approximal surfaces in primary teeth present a large area of contact between them, favoring stagnation of carbohydrates and hindering biofilm removing [1, 2]. Moreover, the salivary access is limited, which contributes to further reduction of the biofilm pH compared to more accessible surfaces, promoting a more acidogenic environment and propitious to the development of caries lesions [1]. In addition, the limited salivary access reduces the exposition of these surfaces to fluorides.

Despite young children usually present wider approximal spaces [38], in most children, the anatomical conditions do not allow that approximal surfaces are cleaned only with brushing, requiring the use of dental floss to remove the biofilm. Besides, the patients' adherence to using dental floss seems to be low [39], mainly regarding children, since they could present less dexterity to flossing and depend on parent's collaboration to remove interproximal biofilm [3, 40]. In fact, a systematic review showed that interproximal caries risk decrease when children's flossing is performed by professional. However, authors suggest these findings cannot be extrapolated, since flossing has only failed when used by the children by themselves [41]. A recent study of our group showed motivational issues are more associated with non compliance with flossing by children (Figure 9).

The challenge becomes even greater when the initial lesion progresses to cavitated lesion (Figure 10). In addition, the biofilm accumulates inside the lesion and it is not possible to be removed by flossing. Consequently, the dentine inside this cavity tend to become more infected [23] and caries progression is faster. Indeed, the inactivation of cavitated lesions (only by self-removal of biofilm) is usually more observed in smooth or occlusal surfaces. We usually observe that in very small cavities or very large decays, for example. On approximal surfaces, most cavitated caries lesions hardly ever present favorable conditions to be arrested (Figure 10).

For all these reasons the approximal surfaces of primary molars are the most affected by caries lesions in some populations [1, 42]. Even in regions where this is not occurring, controlling interproximal caries lesions is still a challenge, especially due to the difficulty of the mechanical control of biofilm on such surfaces. That is why many approximal lesions are active lesions,

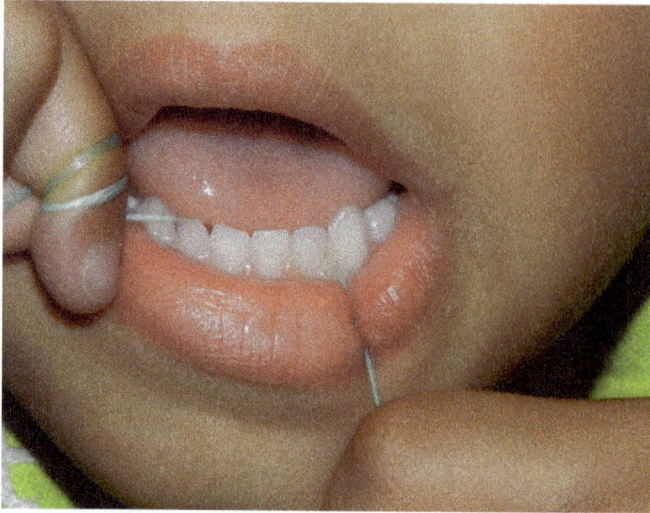

Figure 9. Child using dental floss. Sometimes, children present difficulties in dexterity for flossing. However, motivation is often the biggest problem.

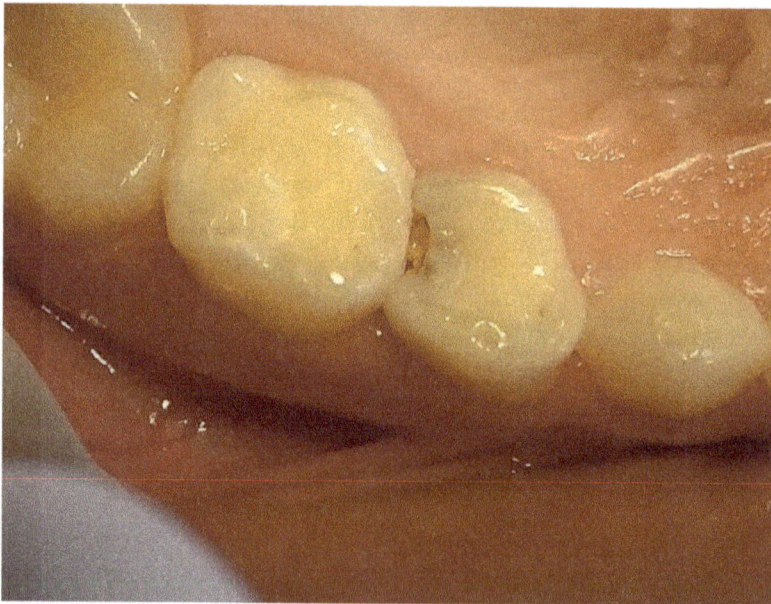

Figure 10. Cavitated lesion on distal surface of the first primary molar. Note the plaque stagnation inside the cavity, which makes difficult the control of such lesions.

although other surfaces have presented higher rates of caries progression [43]. In fact, smooth surfaces are cleaned easily [43] and lesions are easier to be controlled [44]. Besides, the occlusal surfaces, despite their morphology, are favored by the attrition [43]. In the Figure 2, it is possible to notice the remained biofilm on approximal surface, despite presenting smooth and occlusal surfaces with absence of visible plaque, complicating the control of approximal caries, even in initial stages.

Rates ranging from 70% to 90% of approximal caries progression have been shown for primary teeth after 1 or 2-year-follow-up [45, 46]. These figures have been superior to rates found for permanent teeth [47], that is comprehensible since a faster progression is expected in these teeth [48].

Based on the rationale detailed above, it is evident that controlling approximal caries lesions is really an actual challenge in pediatric clinic. Further, we will discuss about important aspects concerning detection and management of approximal caries lesions in primary teeth.

4. How may approximal caries be accurately detected? — Difficulties and important aspects

Detection of approximal caries lesions has not been a simple task. The simplest and most accepted method for caries detection among children is the visual inspection [49]. On the other hand, it is obvious that the contact between adjacent teeth makes caries detection by visual inspection more difficult. Ideally, approximal surfaces should be examined after cleaning by dental floss (Figure 11). When assessing approximal surfaces looking for caries lesions, it is important to examine, firstly, by an occlusal view. In this view, the dentist will observe the integrity and appearance of the marginal ridge. If a caries lesion is present (usually more advanced ones), cavities (Figure 10) or shadows (Figure 12) may be seen in this area. Further, the surface should be examined by buccal and lingual/palatal view. If caries lesion reaches these areas, it may be also detected by visual inspection (Figure 13). The direct examination of this surface is rare and may only occur when the adjacent tooth is not present (Figure 14).

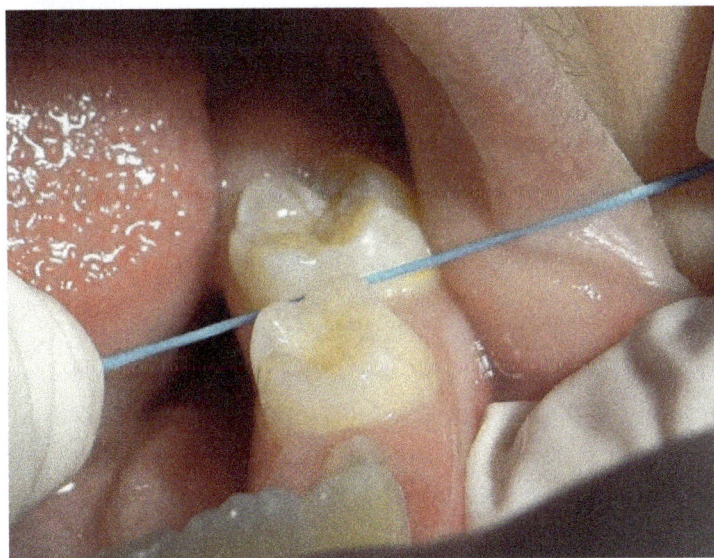

Figure 11. Cleaning the approximal surface before visual examination – note the use of dental floss.

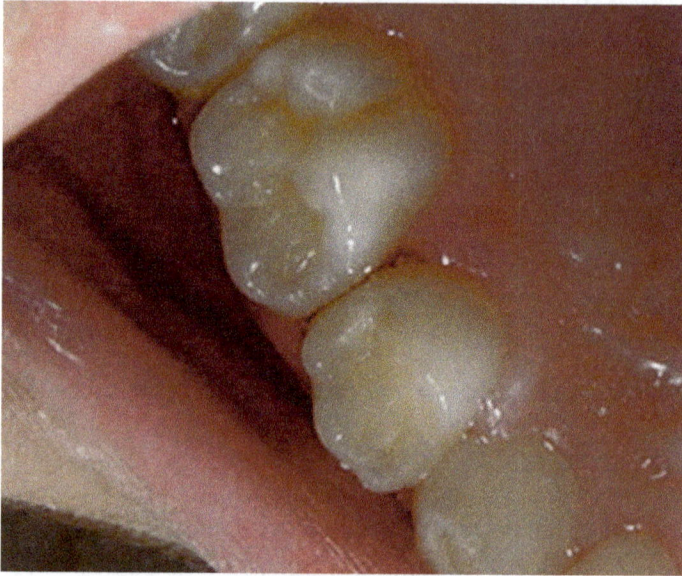

Figure 12. Approximal caries lesion evidenced by the shadow we can see above the marginal bridge.

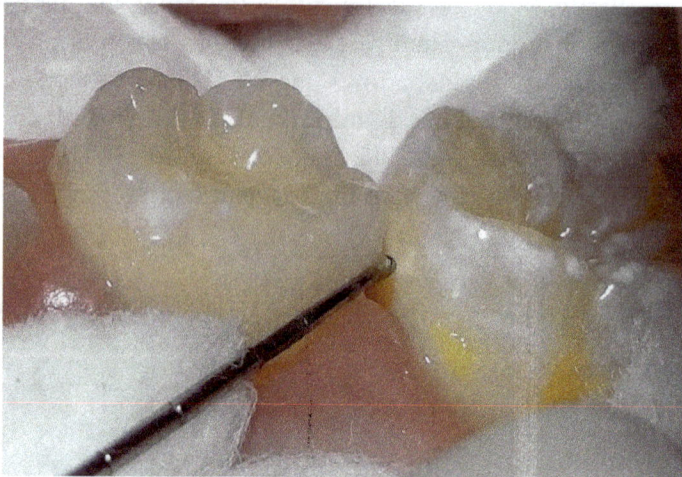

Figure 13. Buccal view – lesion may be detected since is extended from mesial into buccal surface.

The visual inspection using a scoring visual system has shown high specificity in caries detection on approximal surfaces [50]. However, lower values of sensitivity should be expected [50]. In other words, most part of non-cavitated approximal caries, as well other several cavitated lesions, cannot be detected when visual inspection is used. Radiographs have shown to increase the sensitivity of caries detection [50, 51]. On the other hand, although some clinical guidelines have recommend taking bitewing radiographs in all children to detect caries lesions in primary molars[52], its utility has been recently questioned, since no additional benefit was observed in comparison to only the visual inspection being performed [53].

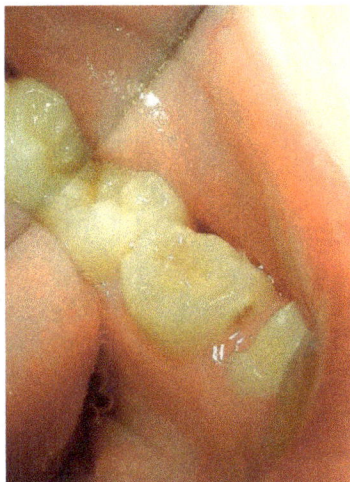

Figure 14. Direct examination of an approximal caries lesion due to the absence of the adjacent tooth.

Actually, using only visual inspection may lead to higher number of false negatives (some non-evident lesions may be missed). However, these lesions may be arrested by preventive measurements. On the other hand, the radiographs may result in higher number of false positive results, what may be worse, since it might lead to unnecessary operative treatment [53]. In addition, several non-cavitated lesions may have the radiographic appearance of a cavitated lesion (Figure 15). As a consequence of radiographic examination, they might receive unnecessary operative treatment. Weighing the pros and cons of bitewing radiographs for caries detection, it seems more useful to take bitewing radiographs in order to confirm the presence of approximal caries, in cases in which visual signs have been identified (instead of detecting non-evident caries) or to help the choice for the best option for treating an approximal caries [54]. In the last situation, radiographs may help in caries depth assessment and also, in evaluation of the periapical tissue [54].

The presence of cavities has been another concern regarding approximal caries detection, since the cavitation has been considered an important point in the prognosis of these caries lesions. As mentioned, some cavities are not detected by visual examination. Besides, radiographs do not aid in this issue, as exposed before. The temporary separation using orthodontic rubbers is an available alternative [55, 56], which permit the direct visual inspection and tactile examination of the approximal surfaces (Figures 15 to 17). This technique is well-accepted by children [49]. However, it is necessary two appointments to permit the conclusion of diagnostic using this method. Even visuo-tactile assessment of approximal surface is possible; doubts in diagnosis may remain. The interdental space created after temporary separation is around 0.8 mm [38] and may not always be large enough to guarantee there is no cavity on the surface, nor to affirm the cavity is clinically within enamel. In fact, several dentine lesions are not cavitated. Other dentine lesions may may be associated with microcavities; however, without exposing the dentine. On the other hand, we believe that some cavitations which present radiographic image into dentine may be wrongly scored as cavity clinically restricted to enamel. This is why the limited space reached after teeth separation may be not enough to the

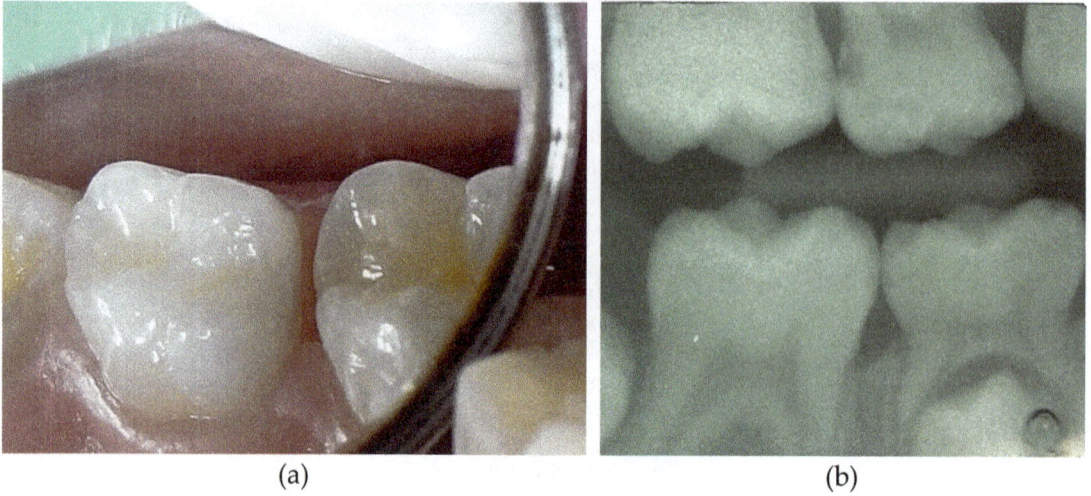

Figure 15. Direct visual inspection (a) and radiograph (b) of the same surface (distal surface of the second primary molar). Clinically, we can see a white spot on the approximal surface (absence of shadows in the marginal bridge) – (a). Radiographically, we evidence a radiolucid image suggestive of caries lesion in dentine. The image might also suggest the presence of cavity (b), that is definitely not evidenced in clinical examination (a). This case represents a false-positive result for caries in dentine that could occur in some radiographic examinations.

dentist being able to actually felt the bottom of these cavities, in order to confirm if he/she is felling enamel or dentine surface. These are limitations of this method. However, since there is no other available possibility to detect the presence of cavities, we have used the temporary separation when we suspect that a cavity is present, especially if dentine involvement is confirmed by visual signs or radiographs.

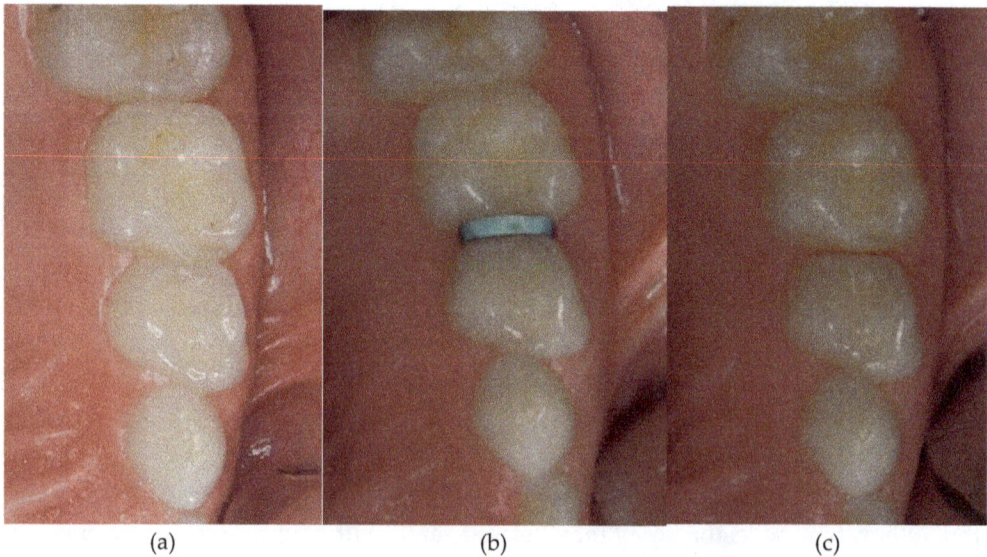

Figure 16. Temporary tooth separation using orthodontic rubbers. (a) before placing the rubber between adjacent teeth; (b) after placing the rubber; (c) after removing the rubber – note the wide space for direct examination.

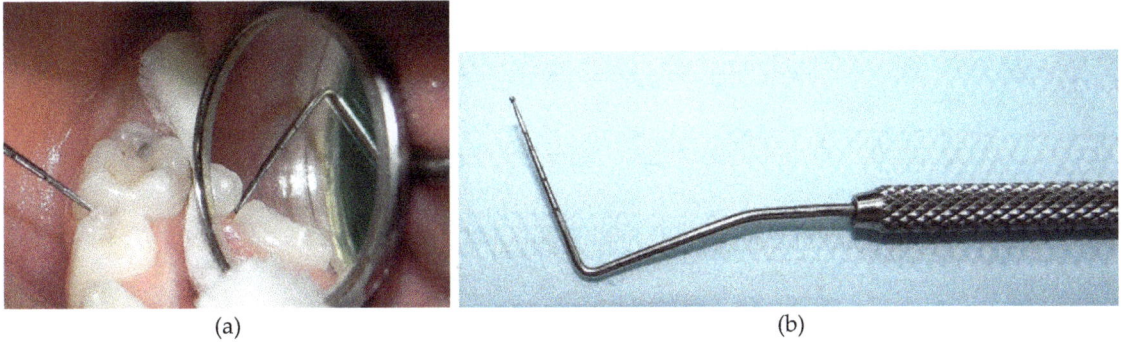

(a)   (b)

Figure 17. Temporary tooth separation using orthodontic rubbers – visual and tactile assessment of separated surfaces (a); WHO probe (ballpoint probe) used to tactile assessment of surfaces.

The activity status is not usually a differential in caries lesions assessment, especially in children. In fact, as exposed before, most part of detected approximal lesions tend to be active [43]. It is not impossible to find inactive approximal caries. However, especially among children, the interproximal plaque control is still very deficient and make the lesions arrestment more difficult. Thus, activity assessment is not a real concern in primary teeth. In some situations, when the adjacent tooth have exfoliated, we may observe a natural process of lesion inactivation of an approximal caries due to the possibility of controlling biofilm only by toothbrushing such area (see Figures 8 and 14).

5. Is it possible to control approximal caries lesions?

In theory, controlling dental caries in any surface is related to controlling of dental plaque over the lesion [32]. As the activity status of approximal caries is not usually a differential factor, we will not discuss it here. However, it is obvious that, if an approximal caries lesion is arrested, it would not demand any measure to be controlled. Considering this situation, we may guide the management of approximal caries lesions basically according to depth and severity, assessed during examination of caries lesions. The conceptual tree for managing caries lesions on approximal surfaces is presented below (Figure 18).

Non-cavitated approximal caries lesions tend to be easier to be controlled since there is no cavity to complicate biofilm removal. Besides, if these lesions are restricted to the enamel, they have a slower progression compared to dentine [45]. Therefore, several possibilities are available in order to controlling them, from the dental flossing to the use of resin infiltration.

Cavitated enamel lesions (Figure 19) are expected to progress faster than those which present intact surface. However, most part of these lesions cannot be detected clinically, neither by visual, nor by tactile assessment. If detected by tooth separation, both non-invasive and invasive treatments would be available for such cases, but there is no strong evidence of the best option in this case. Choosing the non-invasive treatment may permit to postpone invasive interventions. Otherwise, since the presence of cavity is detected, the use of restoration as a

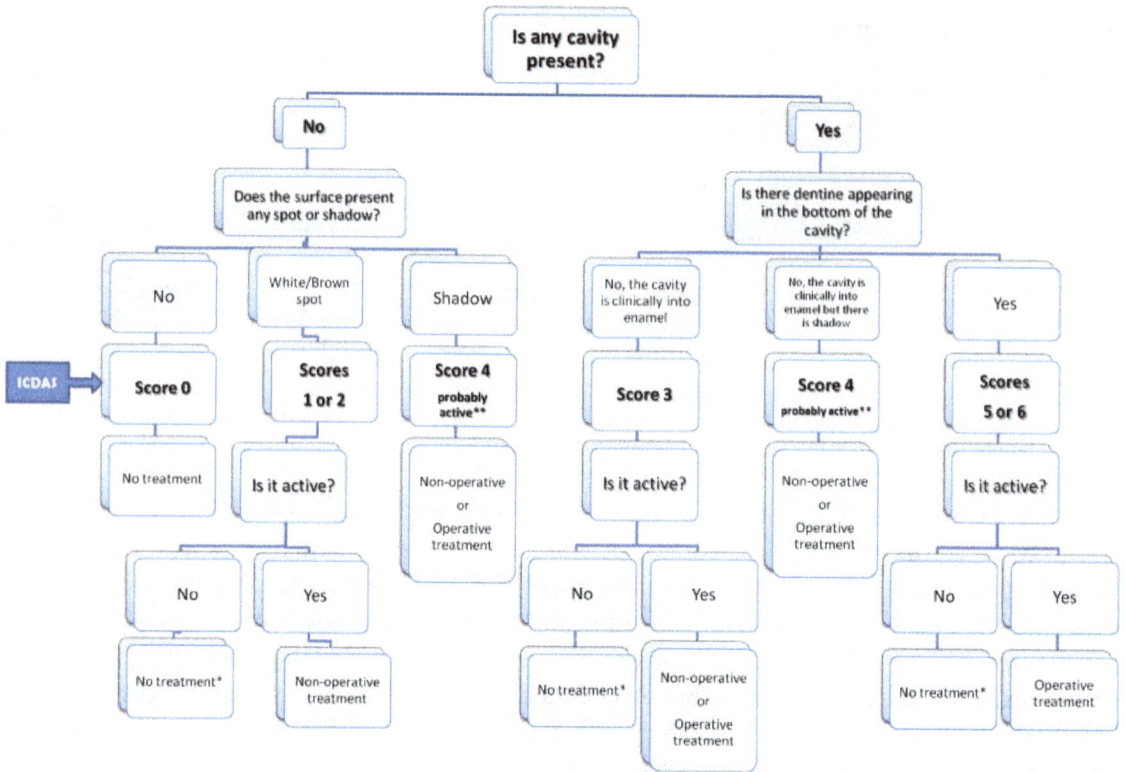

Figure 18. Conceptual tree for managing approximal caries, correlating the caries detection and activity assessment based on ICDAS and clinical decision-making. (* situations in which is usually difficult to affirm caries lesions are really inactive; ** the ICDAS activity assessment always considers lesions score 4 as probably active)

manner to control biofilm at the lesion would be necessary [57]. On the other hand, high amount of sound tissue would be acceptable in order to restore this surface adequately. Therefore, depending on patients' and professional's preferences and particularities of the clinical case, both options are possible. Considering the minimal invasive philosophy, maybe, opting for the non-restorative approach would be interesting since the children's comfort and preservation of dental structures would be maximized.

For approximal dentine caries lesions, the detection of cavities may be more relevant. If the cavitation is not easily visible or not felt by probing, the temporary separation could aid in seeking for cavities (see Figure 15). A dentine lesion progress faster than an enamel lesion. However, if the lesion is not cavitated, this progression is slower than for cavitated lesions [23], since the level of bacterial invasion is very low [22]. Based on that, we may argue the control of several outer non-cavitated dentine lesions would be possible. However, this is not so frequent. Actually, most dentine caries lesions in primary teeth are cavitated [58]. On the other hand, when the cavity is present, some approach that avoids the stagnation of the biofilm over the lesion seems to be indispensable. In this sense, any intervention which prevents biofilm accumulation on these lesions or facilitates is removal could be useful. Otherwise, it is important to clarify that mechanical removal of biofilm by flossing might not be a good choice in these cases, since the cavity may hide the plaque and interfere with caries lesion control.

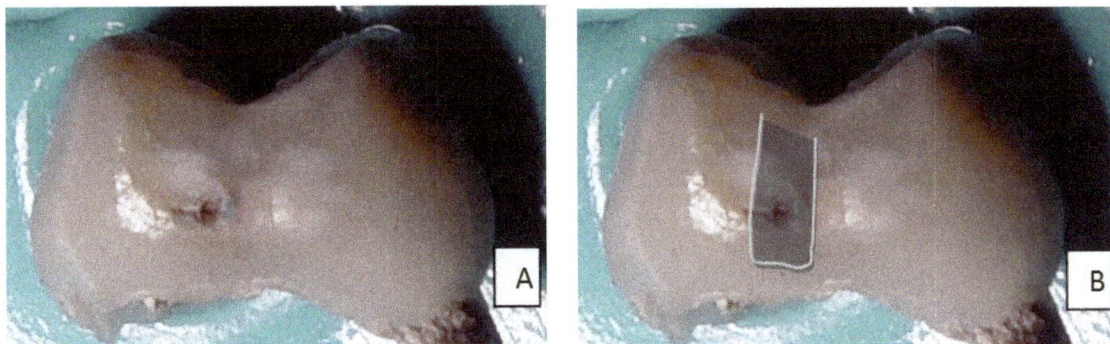

Figure 19. a) Cavitated caries lesion into enamel (direct examination). This cavity probably would not be seen when surface was assessed in the oral cavity due to the presence of the adjacent tooth. Using the temporary separation might help in detecting this cavity. Regarding treatment, we have to ponder if this lesion was detected and the option was operative treatment, a high amount of sound tissue would have to be removed. (b) Schematic representation of how accessing the mentioned cavity if the tooth was actually in the arch.

6. Options (interventions) to control initial approximal caries

Despite flossing is the most suitable method for mechanical removal of biofilm from the interproximal area [59, 60], controlling approximal caries just by flossing has not been shown to be effective [41], probably because its flossing by children and adolescents is not constant and adequate [4]. Controlling approximal caries by just flossing is a simple intervention, however, patient might be instructed and constantly motivated by professional [61]. Although dentist should never give up instructing and motivating to floss, choosing only this approach could be not enough for some approximal caries lesions. In fact, depending on children's compliance with flossing this option may not succeed, especially considering problems with motivation to flossing discussed earlier in this chapter. Thus, early interventions to initial caries lesions become even more important to arrest these lesions and prevent cavitations or lesions progression into dentine.

Initial caries lesion may be managed by remineralizing agents. A recent systematic review has shown the fluorides, in its different vehicles, present the most consistent benefit in controlling progression of initial caries lesions [62]. However, this review did not include any study which had used fluorides for approximal caries lesions in primary teeth. Actually, few studies have been performed aiming to investigate the management of initial caries in primary teeth and the evidence is inconclusive when we consider the most effective vehicle to be used, the frequence of use and the cost-effectiveness of using fluorides in primary teeth[63]. The fluoride varnish reduced in 25% the caries progression on approximal caries of primary molars [45] (Figure 20). Other fluorides vehicles, as gels and foams, have been associated with caries reduction on approximal surfaces [64]. However, they were tested in permanent teeth. The use of interdental brush or dental floss dipped in fluoride gel has been also advocated to using fluorides for approximal areas [65, 66] (Figure 21).

Another option tested for the same purpose was an association AgF followed by SnF2, resulting in a arrestment of 74% of approximal caries lesions [46]. At the moment, our group is testing

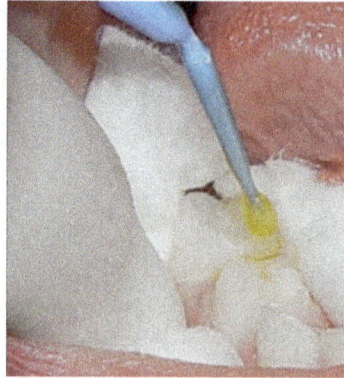

Figure 20. Application of fluoride varnish on approximal surfaces which present initial caries lesions.

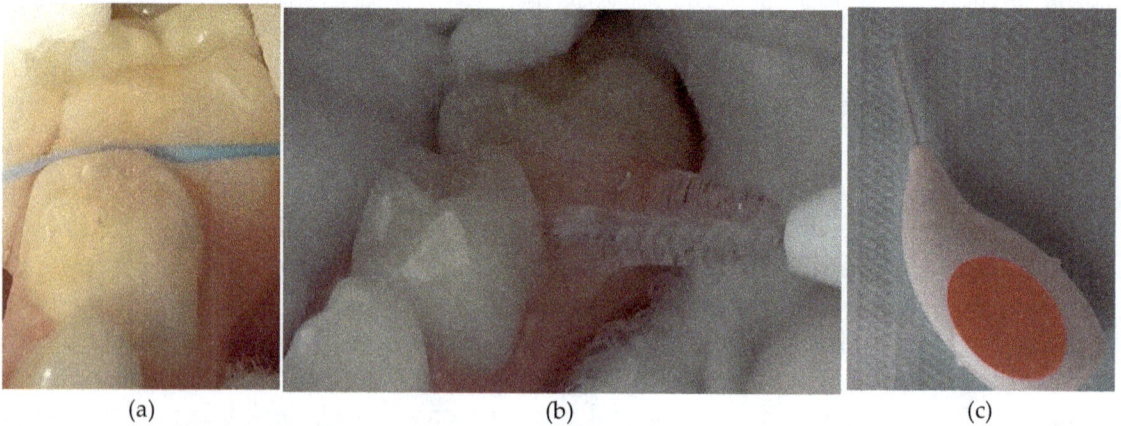

(a)   (b)   (c)

Figure 21. Use of fluoride gel on approximal initial caries lesions. (a) dental floss dipped in fluoride gel. (b) interdental toothbrush dipped in fluoride gel. (c) interdental toothbrush (note some natural space/separation is need for its introduction into approximal areas.

the use of the silver diamine fluoride (SDF) to control approximal caries in primary teeth [67] (Figure 22 and 23). A previous study of our group pointed to the possibility of using the silver diamine fluoride (SDF) in children for arrestment of enamel caries lesions on occlusal surfaces of permanent erupting molar [68]. As erupting occlusal surfaces, approximal surfaces challenge by making the mechanical control biofilm more difficult. In addition, some studies have shown that the SDF is more effective than fluoride varnish to prevent and arrest caries [69-71]. Even showing success since 1960 [69], its effectiveness had not been tested in approximal lesions of primary teeth. It is expected after SDF application, some staining may be seen on treated surfaces. The staining is probably caused by the precipitation of insoluble silver phosphates [72] (Figure 23).

Besides the remineralizing agents, another possibility in order to treat initial caries is sealing or infiltrating caries lesions [74]. Sealants have been used for several years in prevention of dental caries [75]. However, its therapeutic effect may be more expressive than the preventive one [76]. Sealing a caries lesion avoid its contact with biofilm, permitting its arrestment.

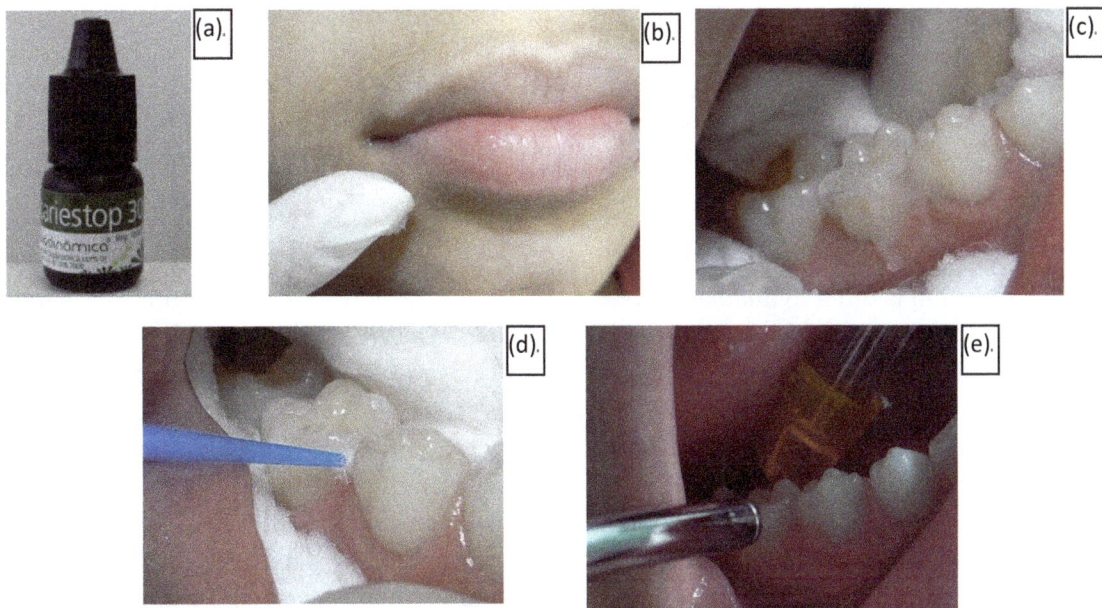

Figure 22. Application of silver diamine fluoride (SDF) in approximal caries lesions of primary teeth. (a) 30% SDF (Cariestop 30%,Biodinâmica Química e Farmacêutica LTDA, Ibiporã, Paraná, Brazil); (b) and (c) Extra-oral and intra-oral protection of soft tissues with petroleum jelly to avoid staining and mucosal irritation [73]; (d) application of SDF using a small disposable brush for 3 min – moisture was controlled by using cotton rolls and saliva ejectors. (e) washing for 30s to remove soluble final products of reaction between SDF and hydroxapatite.

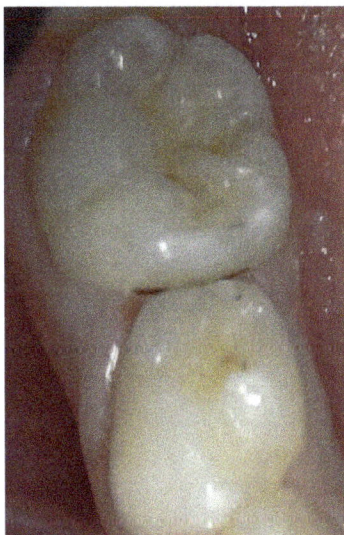

Figure 23. Staining caused by the SDF application after follow-up. The staining is probably due to deposition of silver phosphate that is a insoluble salt, responsible to the dark colour when exposed to the light [72]. Note the staining is hardly visible on treated approximal surfaces.

Sealants were initially devised for occlusal surfaces, which present a complex morphology and difficult mechanical plaque removal, especially in non-motivated or collaborative patients.

However, the principle of sealing has been extended to other surfaces in which controlling the biofilm is a challenge, as approximal surfaces [77]. The idea is the same: preventing caries lesion progression by eliminating the direct contact between the lesion and the biofilm. A previous study showed a 25% reduction in caries progression on approximal surfaces of primary teeth when sealed (comparatively to surfaces in which patients only flossed) [42]. These findings were comprehensible since when sealants are used, the poor children's compliance with flossing tends to be minimized.

Resin infiltration is other available option to "seal" caries lesions [78]. The infiltrant is a low-viscosity resin that promotes sealing into the lesion [78]. Differently from sealing, for infiltrating caries lesions, the superficial layer of caries lesion is removed by acid conditioning. Further, the lesion is infiltrated with a low-viscosity resin. Therefore, the barrier against biofilm would be created inside the lesions, instead of in the surface of caries lesions [79]. In addition, the tooth separation is not required for infiltrating caries lesions. On the other hand, if tooth separation is not performed, some doubts concerning diagnosis may remain. Besides, a kit for resin infiltration is sold containing all products used in the process and specifically designed applicators for approximal surfaces. (Figure 24). Despite these differences compared to the traditional sealants, we believe they exert similar roles in controlling caries lesions progression, since the contact between lesion and biofilm is avoided. Infiltration has been showed as an efficacious treatment for permanent teeth [79-81], but only one study was conducted in primary teeth [82]. In this study, resin infiltration was more efficacious than fluoride varnish in the arrestment of proximal lesions [82]. Although no study has compared sealing and infiltrating caries lesions on approximal surfaces of primary teeth, results in permanent teeth permit to guess that sealants and infiltrants tend to have similar efficacy when the deal is treating initial caries lesions [81].

Besides effectiveness/efficacy in controlling caries lesions, the patients' acceptance regarding the available treatments should be considered in clinical decision-making, especially treating children. Few studies have assessed patient-centered outcomes related to enamel caries lesions treatments. Sealing using relative isolation was well-accepted by most children [42]. In this study, the non-use of rubber dam was pointed as a possible concern [42]. On the other hand, when local anesthesia and rubber dam were used for infiltrating lesions in primary teeth, children reported higher levels of discomfort than when other non-invasive approaches were used [83]. Therefore, we consider that those techniques that cause less discomfort should be preferred and considered by clinicians. In addition, patient's and parents' satisfaction with treatments for initial caries lesions have not been evaluated. Staining caused by inactivation of caries lesions and/or using of SDF has not been systematically assessed. That is one of our concerns when testing the SDF as a possibility to treat initial caries [67]. Based on some preliminary findings, we believe this consequence of the mentioned treatment will not impact on patient's and parent's perceptions, especially due to the position of the surface, which hides the effect of SDF application (see Figure 23).

Finally, cost-efficacy of the mentioned treatment should be considered. More complex treatments as sealing or infiltrating caries lesions are more time-consuming [83], which will certainly lead to higher costs. Thus, even being equally effective, simpler procedures tend to

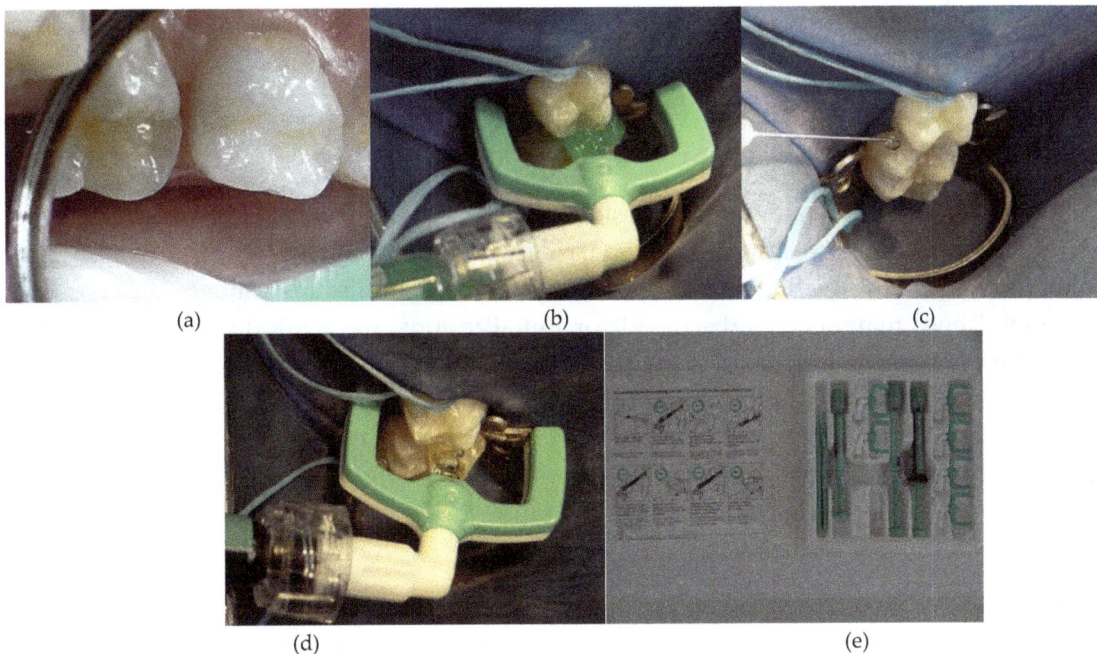

Figure 24. Resin infiltration of an initial caries lesion – (a) direct visual inspection after tooth separation - distal surface of element 54 presented a white spot lesion without any cavity. (b) After local anesthesia and adaptation of the rubber dam, 15%hydrochloric acid was applied on the lesion for 120s, followed by washing and air-drying. (c) Dehydration using 95% ethanol, followed by air-drying. (d) Resin infiltrant application on the lesion for 120s, followed by excess removal and light-curing for 40s. Further, resin is applied for more 30s and light-cured again. (e) All products used in resin infiltration are included in a specific kit commercialized for this purpose by the manufacturers (Icon® - Dental Milestones Guaranteed – DMG, Germany). *Note: For caries sealing, the steps A, B and D will be the same, but without the use of special applicators and using other materials (dental adhesives and resin sealants).*

be more cost-efficacious than complex ones. This is another point to be weighed in the decision-making process. Although our investigation is ongoing, we believe the SDF may be a more cost-efficacious/effective approach to be used in treating initial caries compared to other available treatments.

In summary, the scientific evidence regarding the effectiveness for treating initial caries on approximal surfaces in primary teeth is still scarce. However, some possible alternatives may be used until stronger evidences may be available. Additionally, it is important to consider the simplest techniques are cheaper and seem to be more accepted by children. Therefore, all these properties of the technique chosen for treating enamel caries on approximal surfaces in primary teeth should be considered conjointly.

7. Options to be used when cavitated

As discussed earlier, the greater susceptibility to caries experience of the approximal surface [1] linked to the faster progression rate for enamel to reach the dentin in primary teeth [19] results in a high prevalence of cavitated dentin caries lesions. These lesions need procedures that allow to arrest them and, especially, to reestablish the previous anatomy.

The treatments recommended to cavitated dentin lesion in approximal surfaces can be assigned according to depth and extent of the lesions.

Initially, when observed one cavitated lesion reaching outer dentin of approximal surface in primary teeth, without breaking the marginal ridge (see Figure 15), the utilization of infiltrating technique [82] or the sealing with adhesive system [42] or fissure sealants [77] has been proposed. These materials, as discussed for initial lesions, mechanically block the biofilm accumulation over the lesion. Previous studies have shown that both treatments seem to be good option to control caries progression in outer third of dentin [42, 82]. These previous studies included cavitated caries lesions clinically into enamel (despite their radiographic extension into dentin) [42, 82]. However, as few lesions with this severity were included in the samples, we could not draw definitive conclusions on the efficacy of these techniques or dental materials for cavitated lesions.

Sealing has been proved to be an option for small occlusal cavities exposing dentine [84]. Once more, the purpose of preventing the contact with cariogenic biofilm and enabling plaque removal from the surface instead is performing operative procedure care [84]. The same approach, if used on approximal surfaces, would avoid removal of sound enamel to access small lesions into dentine with preserved marginal bridge (Figure 25). A pilot study that compared the sealing to restoration for approximal cavitated dentin lesions showed almost 70% of sealed lesions have failed after 18 months compared to 11% of the restorations [85]. Besides, 54% of sealed lesions showed progression [85]. This finding seems to be linked with the technical difficulties in performing approximal caries sealing. Since the resin-based sealant is hydrophobic, there is a need to use rubber dam; however, sometimes there is a difficulty to maintain the work area without water (saliva, fluid) contamination [85]. Moreover, inserting both acid phosphoric and resin-based sealant into approximal cavities may have been a challenge which may justify the high proportion of observed failures [85]. Thus, although resin-based sealing represents the most conservative option to control cavitated dentin lesions, until the present moment, it is still not a satisfactory option to treat approximal cavitated caries lesions.

Depending on the size of the cavity and its location, it is also possible to improve the plaque removal from the cavity in order to promote caries lesions arrestment. This choice is especially interesting in areas in which restoration may be a greater challenge to deal than the mechanical control of the biofilm. Small approximal cavities in anterior primary teeth may be one indication for that, since restorations in these teeth may require sound tissue removal in order to access the cavity (Figure 26). Slicing has been also tested to approximal caries in posterior primary teeth [86]. Although, this technique seems to be a most conservative option for such cases, strongest evidences are necessary concerning it.

A recent systematic review showed that there is no difference concerning the choice of restorative material to treat occlusoproximal dentin cavities [87]. In this study, both conventional approaches as amalgam and composite resin were compared to Atraumatic Restorative

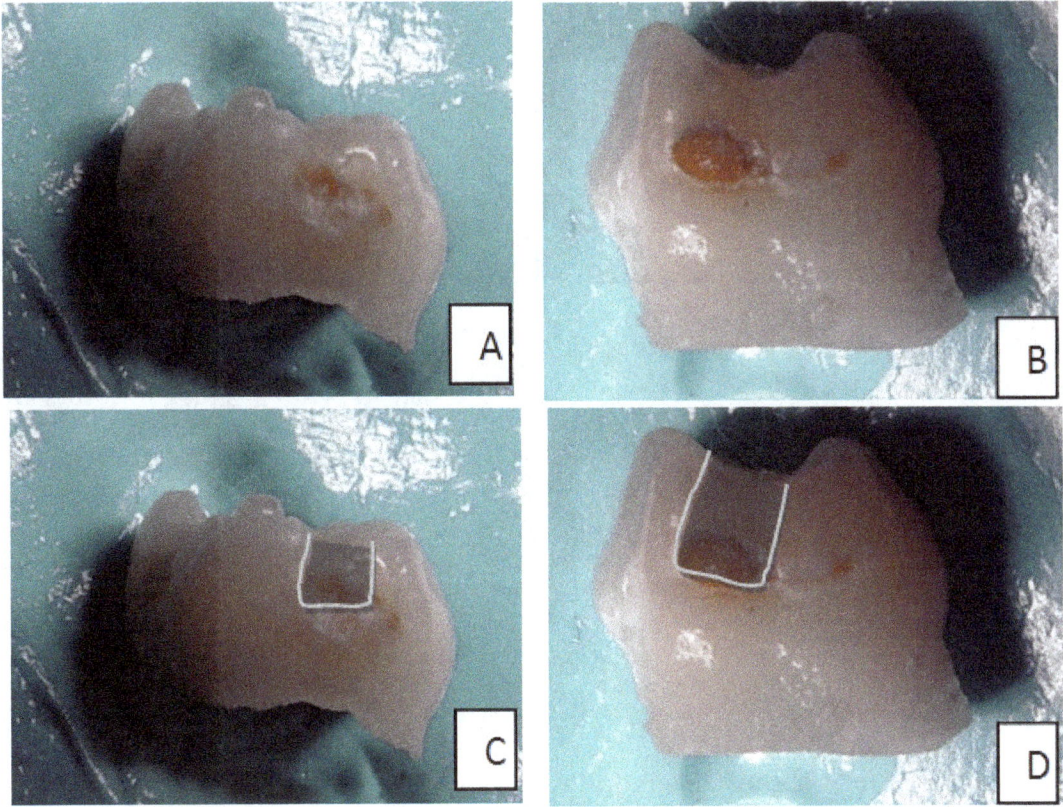

Figure 25. Cavitated dentine caries lesions (a-b). To restore these lesions, sound tissues should have to be removed, as schematically drawn (c-d).

Treatment (ART) performed with high-viscous glass ionomer cement (GIC), demonstrating similar results and satisfactory options to treating these lesions in primary teeth, until 3 years of follow up. However, when we think about the minimal intervention, which has the partial caries removal as one of its concepts, there is no reason to perform the amalgam restoration. Due to that, this procedure will not be discussed in this chapter.

Worldwide, the composite resin associated to adhesive system is, in approximately 25% of cases, the material of choice for restoring primary teeth [88-90]. This material shows satisfactory efficacy when used under local anesthesia and rubber dam, regardless of the brand of composite resin [91], demonstrating a success rate around 90% on occlusal and occlusal-proximal surface of primary teeth [92]. On the other hand, when it is considered the adhesive system, a systematic review reported that both three-step etch-and-rinse and two-step self-etching adhesive system present the best clinical performances [93]. However, this systematic review only considered the clinical trials performed in permanent teeth and these results should be interpreted with caution to primary teeth.

Some specific protocols to be applied in primary teeth in order to obtain similar results that observed to permanent teeth have been suggested. One of the proposals is shortening the etching time in dentin, for etch-and-rinse adhesive systems in order to increase the bond

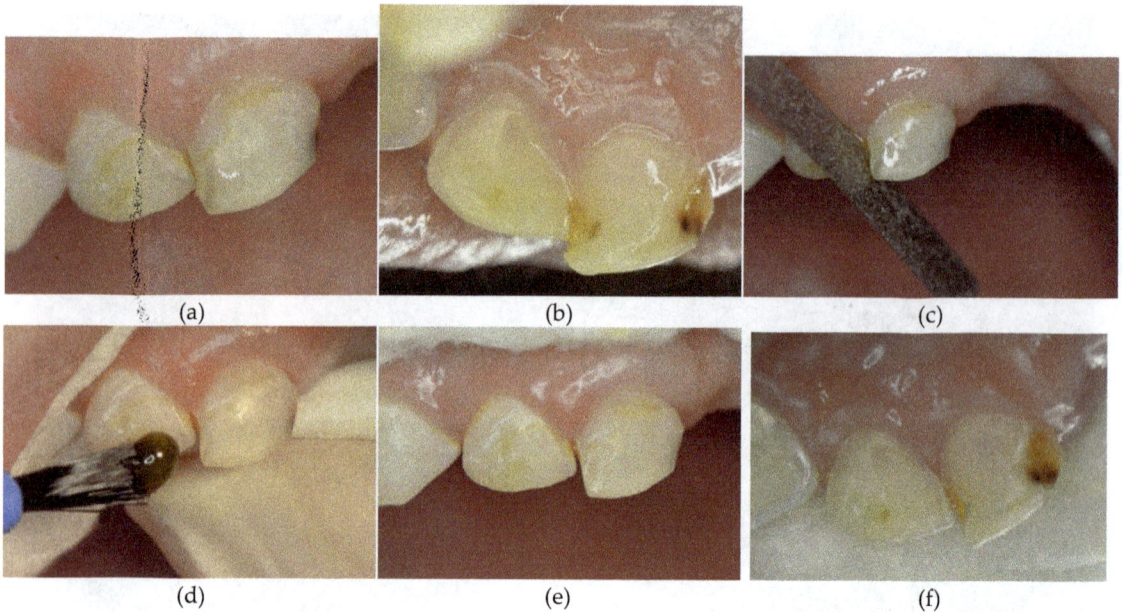

Figure 26. Small cavity on distal surface of upper primary central incisor – buccal (a) and palatal (b) view. Treatment: (c) access to the cavity to facilitate the mechanical removal of the biofilm; (d) application of fluoride varnish to enhance the remineralization. (e/f) follow-up after two weeks evidences the best control of the biofilm in the region.

stability of the restorations in primary teeth [94]. This protocol is based on previous studies that demonstrated the primary dentin is more reactive to acid etching [95, 96] and showed good results *in vitro* studies [94, 97]. Thus, the authors suggest the dentin etching of 35-37% acid phosphoric for 7 seconds before the adhesive system application [94]. Etching enamel remains in 15 seconds.

One important point to be pondered is that the main reason to failure of resin composite restorations is caries around restorations [92]. Due to that, other options of restorative materials may be considered. A previous study evidenced the effect of the resin-modified GIC restoration in prevention of secondary caries when compared to resin composite [98], probably due to fluoride release and uptake of the glass ionomer cements. The resin-modified GIC may be a good alternative, since presents a similar behavior of resin composite in clinical situation [91]. Its longevity is on average 5 years in occlusoproximal cavities [99]. However, this material contains resin monomers in its composition and may increase susceptibility to the presence of humidity compared to other ionomers. This characteristic associated to the need of a light source to polymerization of the material can be pointed as disadvantages of using resin-modified GIC.

On the other hand, similar trend regarding the protection of the margin of restorations can be observed with ART (Figure 26), since this treatment has high-viscous GIC as the material of choice. The GIC shows results such like the RMGIC in prevention of new caries lesion [100]. Moreover, studies have considered GIC as a viable alternative due to the similar survival rates compared to others restorative materials/techniques [87]. Other proprieties of GIC may also contribute to this choice, i.e., ability to chemically bond to enamel and dentine with insignificant heat formation or shrinkage, biocompatibility with the pulp and periodontal tissues and a similar coefficient of thermal expansion to tooth structure [101].

More recently, a new advantage related to GIC in occlusoproximal restoration has been addressed. Studies have claimed the contact with an approximal cavity offers a higher risk to the adjacent surfaces developing caries lesion [1]. In these cases, GIC restoration could prevent the new lesions and even to arrest the initial ones [102]. This hypothesis has been confirmed by a practice-based research, which showed that the progression rate of caries lesion on tooth surfaces adjacent to amalgam restorations was 30%, whilst to GIC restorations was only 16% [103]. These premises associated with no need of local anesthesia and rubber dam application have contributed for indicating GIC restoration associated to partial caries removal as the best option to treat cavitated lesions in children (Figure 27).

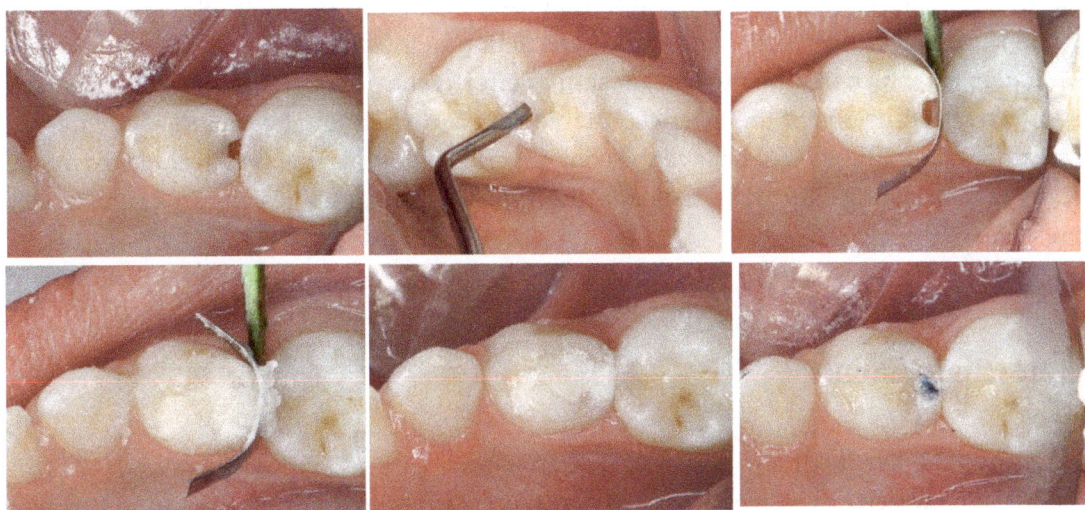

Figure 27. Step-by-step of an occlusoproximal restoration based on atraumatic restorative treatment, using partial caries removal and high-visous glass ionomer cement (GIC). (a) cavity into dentine; (b) accessing the cavity using a manual instrument; (c) preparing for restoration – to restore the contact point and avoid marginal excess; (d) after inserting the GIC and using finger pressure over the material; (e) final restoration; (f) checking the occlusal contacts. (images gently donated by Dr. Isabel Olegario)

8. Final considerations

It is evident, based on topics discussed in this paper, that approximal caries lesions are an actual challenge to dentists deal with. Indeed, the detection of caries lesion on these surfaces presents a duality. On one hand, the surfaces position in oral cavity makes the direct visual inspection almost impossible. On the other hand, if additional caries detection methods are used sequentially, they may lead to overtreatment in some situations (e.g. indiscriminate use of bitewings) or result in a greater doubt regarding options for treating those lesions (e.g. temporary tooth separation), since weak scientific evidences have been found for corroborating some available for clinical decision-making for approximal cavities clinically restricted to enamel.

Even if caries detection has been an overcome stage, treating approximal caries is not a simple task. Unfortunately, few strong evidences are available to support these treatments. Therefore, clinicians should try to use the best available evidences at the occasion. Based on that, we tried to contribute to clinical decision-making process joining the description of present evidences to a critical appraisal of them. We believe the critical judgment of the published evidences is crucial to guide the better clinicians' conduct to their patients.

Nowadays, the adoption of the minimal intervention philosophy has been a reality. Based on that, we have looked into evidences that may support our clinical decision-making not only based on effectiveness or efficacy of therapies used. We have also looked for manners of treating our children minimizing destruction/loss of healthy or reparable structures and guaranteeing higher levels of comfort and satisfaction to them. Due to that, we have insisted on situations in which treatments present similar effectiveness/efficacy, the simplest, the most cost-effective/efficacious or the most acceptable approaches should be preferable by dentists for treating their patients. We believe the conjoint critical appraisal of these requisites may be helpful when dealing with the challenge that approximal caries lesions in primary teeth represents.

Acknowledgements

Authors would like to thank the CNPq, Capes and Fapesp (Protocol 2012/50716-0 and 2014/00271-7), which have given financial support for investigations performed in this field. They were also very thankful to Dr. O´Such for English revision and to Dr. Olegario to donation of some images for illustrating this chapter.

Author details

Mariana Minatel Braga[1*], Isabela Floriano[1], Fernanda Rosche Ferreira[1], Juliana Mattos Silveira[1], Alessandra Reyes[1], Tamara Kerber Tedesco[1], Daniela Prócida Raggio[1], José Carlos Pettorossi Imparato[2] and Fausto Medeiros Mendes[1,2]

*Address all correspondence to: mmbraga@usp.br

1 Dental School, Department of Pediatric Dentistry, University of São Paulo, São Paulo, Brazil

2 University Camilo Castelo Branco, São Paulo, Brazil and CPO São Leopoldo Mandic, Campinas, Brazil

References

[1] Cagetti MG, Campus G, Sale S, Cocco F, Strohmenger L, Lingström P. Association between interdental plaque acidogenicity and caries risk at surface level: a cross sectional study in primary dentition. Int J Paediatr Dent. 2011 Mar;21(2):119-25. PubMed PMID: 20731733. eng.

[2] Seki M, Karakama F, Terajima T, Ichikawa Y, Ozaki T, Yoshida S, et al. Evaluation of mutans streptococci in plaque and saliva: correlation with caries development in preschool children. J Dent. 2003 May;31(4):283-90. PubMed PMID: 12735923. Epub 2003/05/09. eng.

[3] Choo A, Delac DM, Messer LB. Oral hygiene measures and promotion: review and considerations. Aust Dent J. 2001 Sep;46(3):166-73. PubMed PMID: 11695154. eng.

[4] Ashkenazi M, Bidoosi M, Levin L. Factors associated with reduced compliance of children to dental preventive measures. Odontology. 2011 Jun. PubMed PMID: 21698350. ENG.

[5] Longbottom CL, Huysmans MC, Pitts NB, Fontana M. Glossary of key terms. Monogr Oral Sci. 2009;21:209-16. PubMed PMID: 19494688. eng.

[6] Rao A, Malhotra N. The role of remineralizing agents in dentistry: a review. Compend Contin Educ Dent. 2011 2011 Jul-Aug;32(6):26-33; quiz 4, 6. PubMed PMID: 21894873. eng.

[7] Milsom KM, Tickle M, Humphris GM, Blinkhorn AS. The relationship between anxiety and dental treatment experience in 5-year-old children. Br Dent J. 2003 May; 194(9):503-6; discussion 495. PubMed PMID: 12835786. eng.

[8] Fejerskov O. Concepts of dental caries and their consequences for understanding the disease. Community Dent Oral Epidemiol. 1997 Feb;25(1):5-12. PubMed PMID: 9088687.

[9] Fejerskov O. Changing paradigms in concepts on dental caries: Consequences for oral health care. Caries research. 2004;38(3):182-91.

[10] Featherstone JD. The continuum of dental caries--evidence for a dynamic disease process. J Dent Res. 2004;83 Spec No C:C39-42. PubMed PMID: 15286120. eng.

[11] Bjørndal L, Mjör IA. Pulp-dentin biology in restorative dentistry. Part 4: Dental caries--characteristics of lesions and pulpal reactions. Quintessence Int. 2001 Oct;32(9): 717-36. PubMed PMID: 11695140. eng.

[12] Manji F, Fejerskov O, Nagelkerke NJ, Baelum V. A random effects model for some epidemiological features of dental caries. Community Dent Oral Epidemiol. 1991 Dec;19(6):324-8. PubMed PMID: 1764899. eng.

[13] Kidd EA, Fejerskov O. What constitutes dental caries? Histopathology of carious en-amel and dentin related to the action of cariogenic biofilms. Journal of dental re-search. 2004;83 Spec No C:C35-8. PubMed PMID: 15286119.

[14] Fejerskov O, Nyvad B, Kidd E. Pathology of Dental Caries. In: Fejerskov O, Kidd E, editors. Dental Caries: The Disease and Its Clinical Management. 2nd ed. Oxford: Wi-ley; 2008.

[15] Holmen L, Thylstrup A, Ogaard B, Kragh F. A scanning electron microscopic study of progressive stages of enamel caries in vivo. Caries Res. 1985;19(4):355-67. PubMed PMID: 3861258. eng.

[16] Cochrane NJ, Anderson P, Davis GR, Adams GG, Stacey MA, Reynolds EC. An X-ray microtomographic study of natural white-spot enamel lesions. Journal of dental re-search. 2012 Feb;91(2):185-91. PubMed PMID: 22095069.

[17] Holmen L, Thylstrup A, Artun J. Clinical and histological features observed during arrestment of active enamel carious lesions in vivo. Caries research. 1987;21(6): 546-54. PubMed PMID: 3479261.

[18] Bjørndal L, Thylstrup A. A structural analysis of approximal enamel caries lesions and subjacent dentin reactions. Eur J Oral Sci. 1995 Feb;103(1):25-31. PubMed PMID: 7600246. eng.

[19] Vanderas AP, Manetas C, Koulatzidou M, Papagiannoulis L. Progression of proximal caries in the mixed dentition: a 4-year prospective study. Pediatric dentistry. 2003 May-Jun;25(3):229-34. PubMed PMID: 12889698.

[20] Ekstrand KR, Ricketts DN, Kidd EA. Do occlusal carious lesions spread laterally at the enamel-dentin junction? A histolopathological study. Clin Oral Investig. 1998 Mar;2(1):15-20. PubMed PMID: 9667149. eng.

[21] Bjørndal L, Kidd EA. The treatment of deep dentine caries lesions. Dent Update. 2005 Sep;32(7):402-4, 7-10, 13. PubMed PMID: 16178284. eng.

[22] Bjørndal L. Buonocore Memorial Lecture. Dentin caries: progression and clinical management. Oper Dent. 2002 2002 May-Jun;27(3):211-7. PubMed PMID: 12022450. eng.

[23] Ratledge DK, Kidd EA, Beighton D. A clinical and microbiological study of approxi-mal carious lesions. Part 1: the relationship between cavitation, radiographic lesion depth, the site-specific gingival index and the level of infection of the dentine. Caries research. 2001 Jan-Feb;35(1):3-7. PubMed PMID: 11125189.

[24] Marshall GW, Marshall SJ, Kinney JH, Balooch M. The dentin substrate: structure and properties related to bonding. J Dent. 1997 Nov;25(6):441-58. PubMed PMID: 9604576. eng.

[25] Pitts NB, Rimmer PA. An in vivo comparison of radiographic and directly assessed clinical caries status of posterior approximal surfaces in primary and permanent teeth. Caries Res. 1992;26(2):146-52. PubMed PMID: 1521308. eng.

[26] González-Cabezas C. The chemistry of caries: remineralization and demineralization events with direct clinical relevance. Dent Clin North Am. 2010 Jul;54(3):469-78. PubMed PMID: 20630190. eng.

[27] Almahdy A, Downey FC, Sauro S, Cook RJ, Sherriff M, Richards D, et al. Microbio-chemical analysis of carious dentine using Raman and fluorescence spectroscopy. Caries Res. 2012;46(5):432-40. PubMed PMID: 22739587. eng.

[28] Banerjee A, Watson TF, Kidd EA. Dentine caries: take it or leave it? Dent Update. 2000 2000 Jul-Aug;27(6):272-6. PubMed PMID: 11218463. eng.

[29] Fusayama T. Two layers of carious dentin; diagnosis and treatment. Operative dentistry. 1979 Spring;4(2):63-70. PubMed PMID: 296808.

[30] Bjørndal L, Larsen T, Thylstrup A. A clinical and microbiological study of deep carious lesions during stepwise excavation using long treatment intervals. Caries Res. 1997;31(6):411-7. PubMed PMID: 9353579. eng.

[31] Schupbach P, Lutz F, Guggenheim B. Human root caries: histopathology of arrested lesions. Caries research. 1992;26(3):153-64. PubMed PMID: 1628289.

[32] Kidd EA. How 'clean' must a cavity be before restoration? Caries research. 2004 May-Jun;38(3):305-13. PubMed PMID: 15153704.

[33] Mejare I, Stenlund H, Zelezny-Holmlund C. Caries incidence and lesion progression from adolescence to young adulthood: a prospective 15-year cohort study in Sweden. Caries research. 2004 Mar-Apr;38(2):130-41. PubMed PMID: 14767170.

[34] Holmen L, Thylstrup A, Artun J. Surface changes during the arrest of active enamel carious lesions in vivo. A scanning electron microscope study. Acta odontologica Scandinavica. 1987 Dec;45(6):383-90. PubMed PMID: 3481156.

[35] Artun J, Thylstrup A. A 3-year clinical and SEM study of surface changes of carious enamel lesions after inactivation. American journal of orthodontics and dentofacial orthopedics : official publication of the American Association of Orthodontists, its constituent societies, and the American Board of Orthodontics. 1989 Apr;95(4):327-33. PubMed PMID: 2705413.

[36] Nyvad B, Fejerskov O. Assessing the stage of caries lesion activity on the basis of clinical and microbiological examination. Community Dent Oral Epidemiol. 1997 Feb;25(1):69-75. PubMed PMID: 9088694.

[37] Igarashi K, Lee IK, Schachtele CF. Comparison of in vivo human dental plaque pH changes within artificial fissures and at interproximal sites. Caries Res. 1989;23(6):417-22. PubMed PMID: 2598230. Epub 1989/01/01. eng.

[38] Novaes TF, Matos R, Celiberti P, Braga MM, Mendes FM. The influence of interdental spacing on the detection of proximal caries lesions in primary teeth. Brazilian oral research. 2012 Jul-Aug;26(4):293-9. PubMed PMID: 22790495.

[39] Martignon S, Ekstrand KR, Ellwood R. Efficacy of sealing proximal early active lesions: an 18-month clinical study evaluated by conventional and subtraction radiography. Caries Res. 2006;40(5):382-8. PubMed PMID: 16946605. Epub 2006/09/02. eng.

[40] Schüz B, Sniehotta FF, Wiedemann A, Seemann R. Adherence to a daily flossing regimen in university students: effects of planning when, where, how and what to do in the face of barriers. J Clin Periodontol. 2006 Sep;33(9):612-9. PubMed PMID: 16856896. eng.

[41] Hujoel PP, Cunha-Cruz J, Banting DW, Loesche WJ. Dental flossing and interproximal caries: a systematic review. Journal of dental research. 2006 Apr;85(4):298-305. PubMed PMID: 16567548. Epub 2006/03/29. eng.

[42] Martignon S, Tellez M, Santamaria RM, Gomez J, Ekstrand KR. Sealing distal proximal caries lesions in first primary molars: efficacy after 2.5 years. Caries research. 2010;44(6):562-70. PubMed PMID: 21088401.

[43] Guedes RS, Piovesan C, Ardenghi TM, Emmanuelli B, Braga MM, Ekstrand KR, et al. Validation of Visual Caries Activity Assessment: A 2-yr Cohort Study. J Dent Res. 2014 Apr;93(7 suppl):101S-7S. PubMed PMID: 24713370. ENG.

[44] Nyvad B, Machiulskiene V, Baelum V. Construct and predictive validity of clinical caries diagnostic criteria assessing lesion activity. Journal of dental research. 2003 Feb;82(2):117-22. PubMed PMID: 12562884.

[45] Peyron M, Matsson L, Birkhed D. Progression of approximal caries in primary molars and the effect of Duraphat treatment. Scandinavian journal of dental research. 1992 Dec;100(6):314-8. PubMed PMID: 1465563.

[46] Craig GG, Powell KR, Cooper MH. Caries progression in primary molars: 24-month results from a minimal treatment programme. Community dentistry and oral epidemiology. 1981 Dec;9(6):260-5. PubMed PMID: 6955124.

[47] Foster LV. Three year in vivo investigation to determine the progression of approximal primary carious lesions extending into dentine. British dental journal. 1998 Oct 10;185(7):353-7. PubMed PMID: 9807919.

[48] Sonju Clasen AB, Ogaard B, Duschner H, Ruben J, Arends J, Sonju T. Caries development in fluoridated and non-fluoridated deciduous and permanent enamel in situ examined by microradiography and confocal laser scanning microscopy. Adv Dent Res. 1997 Nov;11(4):442-7. PubMed PMID: 9470502.

[49] Novaes TF, Matos R, Raggio DP, Braga MM, Mendes FM. Children's discomfort in assessments using different methods for approximal caries detection. Brazilian oral research. 2012 Mar-Apr;26(2):93-9. PubMed PMID: 22473342.

[50] Abazov VM, Abbott B, Abolins M, Acharya BS, Adams M, Adams T, et al. Search for resonant pair production of neutral long-lived particles decaying to bb in pp collisions at square root(S)=1.96 TeV. Phys Rev Lett. 2009 Aug 14;103(7):071801. PubMed PMID: 19792632. Epub 2009/10/02. eng.

[51] Bader JD, Shugars DA, Bonito AJ. A systematic review of the performance of methods for identifying carious lesions. J Public Health Dent. 2002 Fall;62(4):201-13. PubMed PMID: 12474624.

[52] Espelid I, Mejare I, Weerheijm K, Eapd. EAPD guidelines for use of radiographs in children. European journal of paediatric dentistry : official journal of European Academy of Paediatric Dentistry. 2003 Mar;4(1):40-8. PubMed PMID: 12870988.

[53] Mendes FM, Novaes TF, Matos R, Bittar DG, Piovesan C, Gimenez T, et al. Radiographic and laser fluorescence methods have no benefits for detecting caries in primary teeth. Caries research. 2012;46(6):536-43. PubMed PMID: 22907166.

[54] Braga MM, Mendes FM, Ekstrand KR. Detection activity assessment and diagnosis of dental caries lesions. Dental clinics of North America. 2010 Jul;54(3):479-93. PubMed PMID: 20630191.

[55] Rimmer PA, Pitts NB. Temporary elective tooth separation as a diagnostic aid in general dental practice. British dental journal. 1990 Aug 11-25;169(3-4):87-92. PubMed PMID: 2206652.

[56] Mialhe FL, Pereira AC, Pardi V, de Castro Meneghim M. Comparison of three methods for detection of carious lesions in proximal surfaces versus direct visual examination after tooth separation. The Journal of clinical pediatric dentistry. 2003 Fall;28(1): 59-62. PubMed PMID: 14604144.

[57] Ridell K, Olsson H, Mejàre I. Unrestored dentin caries and deep dentin restorations in Swedish adolescents. Caries Res. 2008;42(3):164-70. PubMed PMID: 18446024. eng.

[58] Mendes FM, Braga MM. Caries detection in primary teeth is less challenging than in permanent teeth. Dental Hypotheses. 2013;4:17-20.

[59] Corby PM, Biesbrock A, Bartizek R, Corby AL, Monteverde R, Ceschin R, et al. Treatment outcomes of dental flossing in twins: molecular analysis of the interproximal microflora. J Periodontol. 2008 Aug;79(8):1426-33. PubMed PMID: 18672992. Epub 2008/08/05. eng.

[60] Merchant AT. Flossing for 2 weeks reduces microbes associated with oral disease. J Evid Based Dent Pract. 2009 Dec;9(4):223-4. PubMed PMID: 19913742. Epub 2009/11/17. eng.

[61] Schüz B, Wiedemann AU, Mallach N, Scholz U. Effects of a short behavioural intervention for dental flossing: randomized-controlled trial on planning when, where and how. J Clin Periodontol. 2009 Jun;36(6):498-505. PubMed PMID: 19453572. eng.

[62] Tellez M, Gomez J, Kaur S, Pretty IA, Ellwood R, Ismail AI. Non-surgical management methods of noncavitated carious lesions. Community dentistry and oral epidemiology. 2013 Feb;41(1):79-96. PubMed PMID: 23253076.

[63] Vanderas AP, Skamnakis J. Effectiveness of preventive treatment on approximal caries progression in posterior primary and permanent teeth: a review. European journal of paediatric dentistry : official journal of European Academy of Paediatric
Dentistry. 2003 Mar;4(1):9-15. PubMed PMID: 12870982.

[64] Jiang H, Bian Z, Tai BJ, Du MQ, Peng B. The effect of a bi-annual professional application of APF foam on dental caries increment in primary teeth: 24-month clinical trial. Journal of dental research. 2005 Mar;84(3):265-8. PubMed PMID: 15723868.

[65] Sarner B, Lingstrom P, Birkhed D. Fluoride release from NaF- and AmF-impregnated
toothpicks and dental flosses in vitro and in vivo. Acta odontologica Scandinavica.
2003 Oct;61(5):289-96. PubMed PMID: 14763781.

[66] Sarner B, Birkhed D, Huysmans MC, Ruben JL, Fidler V, Lingstrom P. Effect of fluoridated toothpicks and dental flosses on enamel and dentine and on plaque composition in situ. Caries research. 2005 Jan-Feb;39(1):52-9. PubMed PMID: 15591735.

[67] Mattos-Silveira J, Floriano I, Ferreira FR, Viganó ME, Frizzo MA, Reyes A, et al. New
proposal of silver diamine fluoride use in arresting approximal caries: study protocol
for a randomized controlled trial. Trials 2014 15:448.

[68] Braga MM, Mendes FM, De Benedetto MS, Imparato JC. Effect of silver diammine
fluoride on incipient caries lesions in erupting permanent first molars: a pilot study. J
Dent Child (Chic). 2009 Jan-Apr;76(1):28-33. PubMed PMID: 19341576. Epub
2009/04/04. eng.

[69] Chu CH, Lo EC, Lin HC. Effectiveness of silver diamine fluoride and sodium fluoride varnish in arresting dentin caries in Chinese pre-school children. Journal of dental research. 2002 Nov;81(11):767-70. PubMed PMID: 12407092. Epub 2002/10/31. eng.

[70] Rosenblatt A, Stamford TC, Niederman R. Silver diamine fluoride: a caries "silver-
fluoride bullet". J Dent Res. 2009 Feb;88(2):116-25. PubMed PMID: 19278981. eng.

[71] Beltrán-Aguilar ED. Silver diamine fluoride (SDF) may be better than fluoride varnish and no treatment in arresting and preventing cavitated carious lesions. J Evid
Based Dent Pract. 2010 Jun;10(2):122-4. PubMed PMID: 20466328. eng.

[72] Yamaga R, Nishino M, Yoshida S, Yokomizo I. Diammine silver fluoride and its clinical application. The Journal of Osaka University Dental School. 1972 Sep;12:1-20.
PubMed PMID: 4514730.

[73] Llodra JC, Rodriguez A, Ferrer B, Menardia V, Ramos T, Morato M. Efficacy of silver
diamine fluoride for caries reduction in primary teeth and first permanent molars of
schoolchildren: 36-month clinical trial. J Dent Res. 2005 Aug;84(8):721-4. PubMed
PMID: 16040729. Epub 2005/07/26. eng.

[74]   Ammari MM, Soviero VM, da Silva Fidalgo TK, Lenzi M, Ferreira DM, Mattos CT, et al. Is non-cavitated proximal lesion sealing an effective method for caries control in primary and permanent teeth? A systematic review and meta-analysis. Journal of dentistry. 2014 Oct;42(10):1217-27. PubMed PMID: 25066832.

[75]   Ahovuo-Saloranta A, Forss H, Walsh T, Hiiri A, Nordblad A, Makela M, et al. Sealants for preventing dental decay in the permanent teeth. The Cochrane database of systematic reviews. 2013;3:CD001830. PubMed PMID: 23543512.

[76]   Heller KE, Reed SG, Bruner FW, Eklund SA, Burt BA. Longitudinal evaluation of sealing molars with and without incipient dental caries in a public health program. J Public Health Dent. 1995 Summer;55(3):148-53. PubMed PMID: 7562727. Epub 1995/01/01. eng.

[77]   Gomez SS, Basili CP, Emilson CG. A 2-year clinical evaluation of sealed noncavitated approximal posterior carious lesions in adolescents. Clinical oral investigations. 2005 Dec;9(4):239-43. PubMed PMID: 16167153.

[78]   Phark JH, Duarte S, Jr., Meyer-Lueckel H, Paris S. Caries infiltration with resins: a novel treatment option for interproximal caries. Compend Contin Educ Dent. 2009 Oct;30 Spec No 3:13-7. PubMed PMID: 19891346. Epub 2009/11/07. eng.

[79]   Paris S, Hopfenmuller W, Meyer-Lueckel H. Resin infiltration of caries lesions: an efficacy randomized trial. Journal of dental research. 2010 Aug;89(8):823-6. PubMed PMID: 20505049. Epub 2010/05/28. eng.

[80]   Meyer-Lueckel H, Bitter K, Paris S. Randomized controlled clinical trial on proximal caries infiltration: three-year follow-up. Caries Res. 2012;46(6):544-8. PubMed PMID: 22922306. eng.

[81]   Martignon S, Ekstrand KR, Gomez J, Lara JS, Cortes A. Infiltrating/sealing proximal caries lesions: a 3-year randomized clinical trial. Journal of dental research. 2012 Mar; 91(3):288-92. PubMed PMID: 22257664. Epub 2012/01/20. eng.

[82]   Ekstrand KR, Bakhshandeh A, Martignon S. Treatment of proximal superficial caries lesions on primary molar teeth with resin infiltration and fluoride varnish versus fluoride varnish only: efficacy after 1 year. Caries research. 2010;44(1):41-6. PubMed PMID: 20090327. Epub 2010/01/22. eng.

[83]   Mattos-Silveira J, Floriano I, Ferreira FR, Vigano ME, Mendes FM, Braga MM. Children's discomfort may vary among different treatments for initial approximal caries lesions: preliminary findings of a randomized controlled clinical trial. Int J Paediatr Dent. 2014 Sep 17. PubMed PMID: 25229641.

[84]   Hesse D, Bonifacio CC, Mendes FM, Braga MM, Imparato JC, Raggio DP. Sealing versus partial caries removal in primary molars: a randomized clinical trial. BMC Oral Health. 2014;14:58. PubMed PMID: 24884684. Pubmed Central PMCID: 4045925.

[85] Celiberti P. Novas possibilidades de manejo e monitoramento de lesões de cárie em superfícies proximais.. São Paulo: Dental School, University of São Paulo; 2011.

[86] Hansen HV, Heidmann J, Nyvad B. Non-Operative Control of Cavitated Approximal Caries Lesions in Primary Molars Over 6–24 Months: A Practice-Based Approach. Caries Res 2014. p. 414.

[87] Raggio DP, Hesse D, Lenzi TL, C ABG, Braga MM. Is Atraumatic restorative treatment an option for restoring occlusoproximal caries lesions in primary teeth? A systematic review and meta-analysis. Int J Paediatr Dent. 2013 Nov;23(6):435-43. PubMed PMID: 23190278.

[88] Guelmann M, Mjor IA. Materials and techniques for restoration of primary molars by pediatric dentists in Florida. Pediatr Dent. 2002 Jul-Aug;24(4):326-31. PubMed PMID: 12212875.

[89] Pair RL, Udin RD, Tanbonliong T. Materials used to restore class II lesions in primary molars: a survey of California pediatric dentists. Pediatr Dent. 2004 Nov-Dec; 26(6):501-7. PubMed PMID: 15646912.

[90] Buerkle V, Kuehnisch J, Guelmann M, Hickel R. Restoration materials for primary molars-results from a European survey. Journal of dentistry. 2005 Apr;33(4):275-81. PubMed PMID: 15781135.

[91] Casagrande L, Dalpian DM, Ardenghi TM, Zanatta FB, Balbinot CE, Garcia-Godoy F, et al. Randomized clinical trial of adhesive restorations in primary molars. 18-month results. Am J Dent. 2013 Dec;26(6):351-5. PubMed PMID: 24640441.

[92] dos Santos MP, Passos M, Luiz RR, Maia LC. A randomized trial of resin-based restorations in class I and class II beveled preparations in primary molars: 24-month results. J Am Dent Assoc. 2009 Feb;140(2):156-66; quiz 247-8. PubMed PMID: 19188412.

[93] Peumans M, Kanumilli P, De Munck J, Van Landuyt K, Lambrechts P, Van Meerbeek B. Clinical effectiveness of contemporary adhesives: a systematic review of current clinical trials. Dent Mater. 2005 Sep;21(9):864-81. PubMed PMID: 16009415.

[94] Lenzi TL, Braga MM, Raggio DP. Shortening the etching time for etch-and-rinse adhesives increases the bond stability to simulated caries-affected primary dentin. J Adhes Dent. 2014 Jun;16(3):235-41. PubMed PMID: 24669366.

[95] Senawongse P, Harnirattisai C, Shimada Y, Tagami J. Effective bond strength of current adhesive systems on deciduous and permanent dentin. Oper Dent. 2004 Mar-Apr;29(2):196-202. PubMed PMID: 15088732.

[96] Nor JE, Feigal RJ, Dennison JB, Edwards CA. Dentin bonding: SEM comparison of the dentin surface in primary and permanent teeth. Pediatr Dent. 1997 May-Jun; 19(4):246-52. PubMed PMID: 9200195.

[97] Lenzi TL, Mendes FM, Rocha Rde O, Raggio DP. Effect of shortening the etching time on bonding to sound and caries-affected dentin of primary teeth. Pediatr Dent. 2013 Sep-Oct;35(5):E129-33. PubMed PMID: 24290541.

[98] Yengopal V, Mickenautsch S. Caries-preventive effect of resin-modified glass-ionomer cement (RM-GIC) versus composite resin: a quantitative systematic review. Eur Arch Paediatr Dent. 2011 Feb;12(1):5-14. PubMed PMID: 21299939.

[99] Qvist V, Laurberg L, Poulsen A, Teglers PT. Class II restorations in primary teeth: 7-year study on three resin-modified glass ionomer cements and a compomer. Eur J Oral Sci. 2004 Apr;112(2):188-96. PubMed PMID: 15056118.

[100] Mickenautsch S, Tyas MJ, Yengopal V, Oliveira LB, Bonecker M. Absence of carious lesions at margins of glass-ionomer cement (GIC) and resin-modified GIC restorations: a systematic review. Eur J Prosthodont Restor Dent. 2010 Sep;18(3):139-45. PubMed PMID: 21077424.

[101] Anusavice KJ. Phillips' Science of Dental Materials. 12.ed. ed. Philadelphia: Saunders; 2012.

[102] Guglielmi CA. Efeito de materiais restauradores em contato proximal com lesões de cárie em dentes decíduos São Paulo: Dental School, University of São Paulo, 2013.

[103] Qvist V, Laurberg L, Poulsen A, Teglers PT. Eight-year study on conventional glass ionomer and amalgam restorations in primary teeth. Acta odontologica Scandinavica. 2004 Feb;62(1):37-45. PubMed PMID: 15124781.

6

Factors Associated with the Presence of Teeth in the Adult and Elderly Xukuru Indigenous Population in Ororubá, 2010

Cecilia Santiago Araujo de Lima and
Rafael da Silveira Moreira

1. Introduction

Indigenous peoples in Brazil have particular configurations of customs, beliefs and language, forms of integration with the environment, history of interaction with the settlers and relationship with the Brazilian state. Thus insert the different ways in national society [1].

In Brazil, as in many other parts of the world, indigenous peoples are constitute as one of the most disadvantaged segments of the economic, housing, educational standpoint and health indicators, as revealed by the census and other surveys that measure conditions life of the population. In addition, for cultural or relationship with the environment reasons, require specific public policies [1].

The indigenous people Xukuru has the largest indigenous ethnic population group among the 10 ethnic groups of Pernambuco. Located in Pesqueira in the Sierra Ororubá, 216km from Recife (principal city of Pernambuco State) and has a population of approximately 10.000 indigenous [2].

The Xukuru suffered from the loss of traditional lands to allow their social and cultural reproduction and were the target of every source of discrimination, especially from the eighteenth century [3]. After the retaking of their lands the indigenous territory Xukuru now has 25 villages that are distributed in three environmentally bounded regions: the Ribeira, the Serra and the Agreste (Figure 1). The approval of the land in this population resulted in changes in the social context [4] that seems to have contributed in some way to changes in the mode of life of this population. These changes are called acculturation, which is perceived as a result of an exchange process in which two cultures mutually absorb their characteristics and customs generating a new reference.

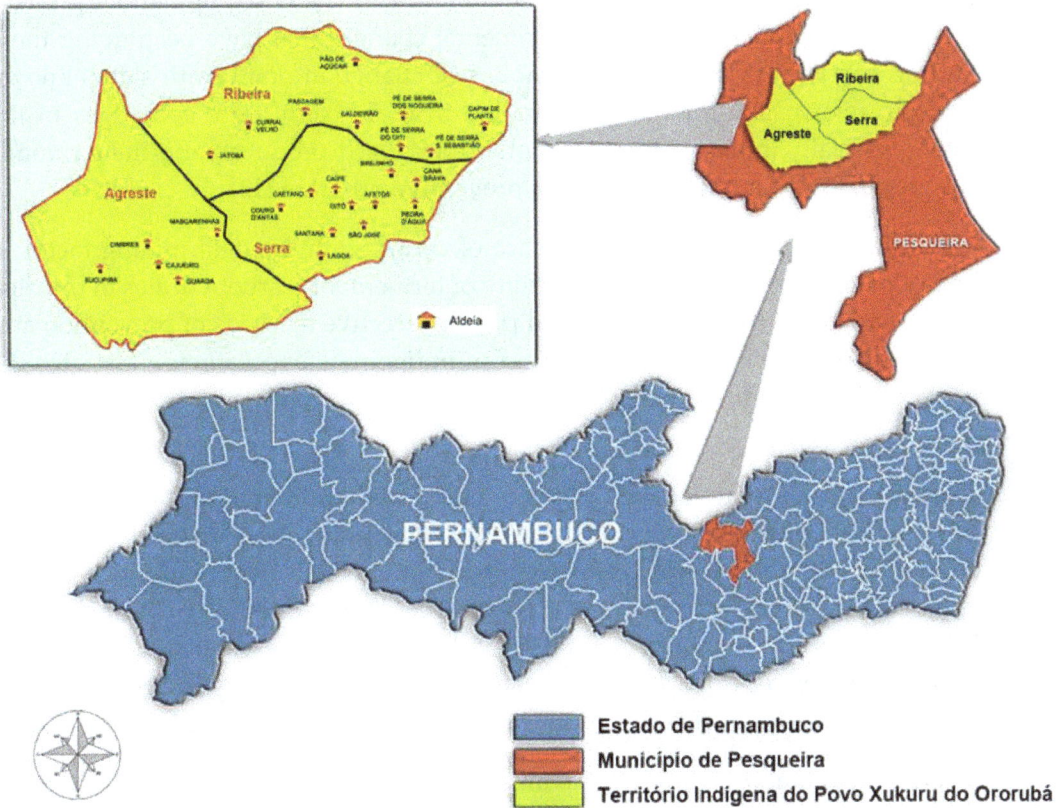

Figure 1. Geographical location of the Indian Territory Xukuru Ororubá and its division according to the socio-environmental regions and villages. Pesqueira, 2010 [5].

The health of indigenous peoples of Brazil presents complex and dynamic way. Is directly related to historical processes of social, economic and environmental changes, linked to the expansion and consolidation of demographic and economic fronts of society in various regions of the country [6].

The epidemiological profile of indigenous peoples is little known, which stems from the insufficiency of investigations, surveys and censuses, as well as the inaccessibility of information on morbidity and mortality systems. Any discussion of the health-disease process of indigenous peoples need to take into consideration, in addition to epidemiological and demographic dynamics, the enormous existing social diversity [7-11].

For proper understanding of the health-disease process on indigenous peoples it is necessary to appeal to the historical relations in which human societies are inserted [10]. Despite the fragmentation and lack of historical data on the history of contact between indigenous people and other population groups in Brazil records, it is known that the effects of this interaction on the profiles of illness and death were significant [12].

The epidemiology of oral health among indigenous peoples in Brazil is little known, which reflects a more general framework of ignorance about the health of these populations [7]. This perspective, intense socioeconomic and environmental changes that have been going these people, including subsistence and diet, are enablers of change in oral health status known aspects [10]. Main responsible for the deterioration in oral health are the changes in the traditional diet (especially intake of sugar and other processed products) and the economic system of this group, together with the lack of a preventive program [13].

From the 1960s, there was an increased incidence of caries, with the determining factor in changing dietary patterns and increased availability of fermentable carbohydrates in the diet. Although caries is a disease that has known and proven effective methods of prevention and control, precarious epidemiological profile found in indigenous populations illustrates the social exclusion of the latter from access to dental care groups and methods of oral health promotion [14].

Caries is the main cause of tooth loss. To a lesser degree are periodontal disease and dental injuries [15]. Tooth loss related to tooth extractions caused by preventable diseases, including, dental caries and periodontal diseases is very high and remains prevalent worldwide despite progress in prevention and early treatment of these diseases [16]. In addition to these diseases, tooth loss is due to attitudes of dental professionals and the public, accessibility and utilization of dental services, the type of financing of the health system and the way to provide dental care. Another primary cause or related of tooth extractions are the economic reasons [17-20].

Social conditions and dental practices hegemonic force the socioeconomically disadvantaged individuals to treat dental pain with extractions. Epidemiological data have shown significant increase of loss with age. In Brazil, the extraction mass begins at age 30 and is the most practical and economical solution for the accumulated oral health problems [16, 21].

The loss of teeth is the most common cause of impaired chewing, being related to the reduction of masticatory ability and perceptions of chewing ability. When associated with difficult access to prostheses result in functional and psychosocial disorders such as poor chewing, speech related problems, employment difficulties, dissatisfaction with appearance, among others. Little attention has been given to the impact that can cause tooth loss in chewing ability and changes in food thereon, which are determinants of nutritional status of these individuals as well as reduced self-esteem and social integration [21-25].

The variables related to tooth loss ranging from dental work (the increase in periodontal attachment loss, number of coronal and root surface caries, tooth mobility and fracture in restoration) to the individual level (the reporting dental pain, the need perceived dental treatment, frustration with dental care, preference for extraction instead of conservative treatment, older age group, black race and female) [26]. Early tooth loss should be considered a predictor of future tooth loss. There are significant correlations between early tooth loss and social variables, such as the human development index, ethnicity, education, income under the minimum wage, lack of fluoridated tap water and people living in cities with fewer than 10,000 inhabitants, which already were reported in other studies [27].

In Australia less than 2% of adults aged 35-54 years have complete tooth loss, but this increases to 36% for people aged 75 years or more [28]. The age distribution of edentulism for indigenous peoples is noticeably different from that of the total population. The level of edentulism is almost five times higher among people aged 35-54 years indigenous than among non-indigenous counterparts (7.6% compared with 1.6%). There is also a noticeable difference for those aged 55-74 years, 21% of indigenous peoples suffer from edentulism compared with 14% of non-Indians [29].

In general, lacking qualitative and quantitative information on the oral health status of indigenous peoples in Brazil, especially longitudinal studies to support an evolution of oral epidemiology. Particularly, in the northeast state of Pernambuco and the paucity of studies on the oral health status of indigenous peoples has become even more alarming which reflects the lack of information on the reality of these peoples and the consequent social exclusion which are submitted. This study aims to contribute to a better understanding of tooth loss in adults and elderly of this indigenous population, studying the factors associated with perma-nent teeth factors.

2. Methods

2.1. Location and study population

This study consists of a deepening of two studies entitled "Analysis of Living, Health and Vulnerability of Indigenous People Xukuru Ororubá as the tool for the Shares of Primary Health Care" [30] and "Health and Living Conditions of the Indigenous People Xukuru Ororubá of Pesqueira - PE "[31] that were developed in Pesqueira, Northeast Region of Brazil. The field work was developed with the participation of indigenous population only in the period January to March 2010.

2.2. Sampling plan

Due to the larger study have sought to analyze various health situations, the sample size was based on the condition of lower prevalence being studied which was equivalent to a third of the universe. This sampling strategy ensured the representativeness of the smaller study group, with the lowest prevalence being estimated. Consequently allowed the representation of the other study groups. It was found that the population of the ethnic group Xukuru is formed by 7,225 people, 1,896 households dwelling and socio-environmental distributed in 3 regions and 25 villages. From these census data, the sample consisted of 632 households (equivalent to a third of the universe).

The selection of households for the sample is given in a systematic random manner, ensuring all members of the population the same chance of being chosen. To systematize the sample, the following calculation was used: k = N (population) / n (sample). Then, the initial sampling unit was selected by lottery between 1 and k, ie, between the numbers one, two and three. With number three drawn, broke for the selection of households starting at home in 1001, ie, the first home of the village of number one. From there followed the systematization where every three households, the third was selected. This sampling was continued until the last possible home the last village. At the end, 632 households were randomly selected and all the inhabitants of these households who are aged 35-44 years and 60 years and older were included in the sample.

Those who were excluded during the visit had some temporary impossibility (as being hospitalized or sick) or a disability that prevented the completion of the oral clinical examination.

2.3. Instrument for data collection

The instruments for data collection were based on records proposed for the Project SB Brasil 2003 [32] and SB Brasil 2010[33]. The codes and criteria adopted are those proposed by the World Health Organization (WHO) publication *Oral health surveys: basic methods*, fourth edition [34].

Data collection was made up of eight teams formed by a dentist (examiner) and a annotator. Standardization was done as the criteria and approaches used to test intra-examiner and inter-examiner before and during the process of data collection. And were reexamined 5% of the sample that aimed to estimate the agreement of the main study findings.

The local and the organization of the examination areas were defined according to the availability of the site, with natural lighting, ventilation and proximity to a water source needed. The examiner, the annotator and the examined person sat for the exam. The tests were conducted using a combination of a dental mirror with handle, and a specific probe, developed by WHO, known as "CPI probe."

2.4. Description of variables

The dependent variable is being studied to tooth loss that represents the count of missing teeth (varying 0-32 teeth), is due to decay or other reasons.

The independent variables were collected through the questionnaire administered by a health survey and also by the census Xukuru be classified into three categories: Characterization of sociodemographic and socioeconomic profile (place of residence, income, age, sex, attends school, can read and write), Characterization of access to oral health care (dental visits, time of last dental appointment, place of last dental visit, reason for last dental visit) and characterization of self-perception and impact on oral health (dental appointment last assessment services, satisfaction with teeth / mouth, OIDP).

2.5. Processing of data

The data collected were criticized to correct fill failures and processed at the National School of Public Health - ENSP / FIOCRUZ, a partner institution of the Center Aggeu Magalhães - CPqAM / FIOCRUZ this health survey.

Before to the analysis, the database went through a cleansing process in which the entered data were compared with the information provided in the questionnaires. In case they found differences, the database was corrected.

2.6. Data analysis

The data were tabulated in EpiData (version 3.1). Data analysis was initially performed using the statistical package SPSS 13.0® with the distribution of frequencies and description of the measures of central tendency and dispersion. The analyzes were presented in tables.

Association analyzes/dependence were performed by means of parametric or non-parametric tests, depending on the type of distribution and the nature of the variables under study. Effect measures were calculated, emphasizing reason means (RM) and odds ratio (OR) simple and adjusted for confounding variables. For both, negative binomial regression models with inflated zero were adopted in order to check the direction and strength of the effect of independent variables on the outcome analyzed. This model is used when the variable is discrete with quantitative absence of normal distribution and when there is overdispersion of the data distribution [35]. Due to the large number of zeros present in the dependent variable (many adults and especially seniors had missing teeth, or teeth zero), it was recommended the use of this regression model. This model presents two regression coefficients, one for the non inflated zeros (whose measure of effect is the RM and is associated with increased number of teeth) and other coefficients for the part inflated zeros (whose measure is the OR and will be associated with the presence of teeth zero, ie the edentulous). The influence of the factors under study on tooth loss followed the hierarchical model proposed by Victora et al. [36] showed in the Figure 2.

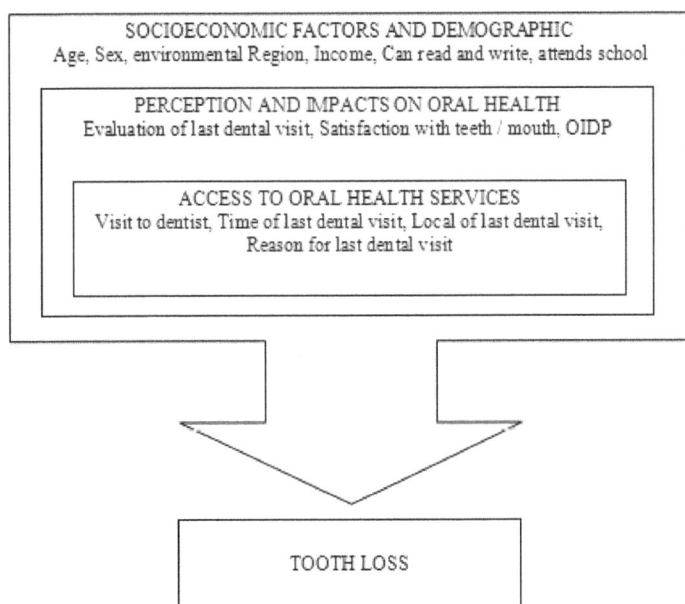

Figure 2. Theoretical Hierarchial Model of variables associated with the presence of permanent teeth. Pesqueira, 2010.

2.7. Ethical aspects

This study was based on "Health and Living Conditions of the Indigenous People Xukuru Ororubá the Pesqueira-PE" which was approved by the Ethics in Research-CEP (CPqAM / Fiocruz) and the National Committee for Research Ethics - CONEP / National Board of Health / Ministry of Health, through Opinion nº 34/2011. The study "Analysis of Living, Health and Vulnerability of Indigenous People Xukuru Ororubá as the tool for the Shares of Primary Health Care" that contains the census Xukuru also obtained approval of the CEP by Opinion nº 604/2009.

The project also received permission from FUNASA for this work, as well as the letter of consent from the ethnic Xukuru Ororubá signed by Cacique Marcos de Araújo Luidson after approval of the Local Council of Indigenous Health Xukuru was obtained and the Consent and Informed (IC) of the political leaders of each village existing in Indian Territory.

3. Results

A sample of the Survey of Health Xukuru the Ororubá constituted 632 selected households. Among these, 27 households were considered lost due to the absence of its residents in the three visits by field staff. Thus, the final sample consisted of 605 households.

The average of the presence of permanent teeth tooth was 10.43 (± 9.79). Table 1 shows the composition of the sample and the average of permanent teeth according to the independent variables. It was observed that 39.0% of individuals residing in the Agreste region of the Indigenous Territory and about 50.7% had an income between R$ 216,00 - 465,00.

The socio-demographic structure of the population studied was 45.6% of adults and 54.4% of elderly, composed mostly of males (50.7%). Among adults with an average age of 39.2 years and among older average age was 70.3 years. It was observed that 58.2% can not read and write and 56.1% have attended school.

Variable		N (%)	Average	±DP	CI 95%	Median	p-value *
Age group	Adults	195 (45,6%)	17,91	7,90	16,80-19,03	19,00	<0,001
	Elderly	233 (54,4%)	4,16	6,15	3,37-4,96	1,00	<0,001
Sex	Male	217 (50,7%)	11,49	9,97	10,15-12,82	10,00	0,010
	Female	211 (49,3%)	9,34	9,50	8,05-10,63	7,00	0,010
Enviromental region	Ribeira	131 (30,6%)	9,90	9,30	8,29-11,52	9,00	0,531
	Serra	130 (30,4%)	10,24	10,13	8,48-12,0	7,50	0,531
	Agreste	167 (39,0%)	11,16	9,95	9,61-12,72	11,00	0,531

	Variable	N (%)	Average	±DP	CI 95%	Median	p-value *
Income	Tertile 1 (R$ 0 - 215,00 reais)	140 (32,7%)	16,68	7,96	15,35-18,01	18,00	<0,001
	Tertile 2 (R$ 216,00 - 465,00)	217 (50,7%)	6,58	8,52	5,44-7,73	3,00	<0,001
	Tertile 3 (R$ 466,00 -1500,00)	62 (14,5%)	8,77	9,76	6,29-11,25	4,00	<0,001
	Missing	9 (2,1%)					
Can read and write	Yes	173 (40,4%)	13,47	9,89	11,98-14,95	13,00	<0,001
	No	249 (58,2%)	8,39	9,19	7,23-9,54	5,00	<0,001
	Missing	6 (1,4%)					
Attends school	Yes	25 (5,8%)	17,56	9,18	13,76-21,35	19,00	<0,001
	No, already attended	240 (56,1%)	11,76	9,74	10,52-13,0	11,00	<0,001
	No, never attended	154 (36,0%)	7,36	8,97	5,93-8,79	4,00	<0,001
	Missing	9 (2,1%)					
Satisfaction with teeth/mouth	Satisfied	235 (54,9%)	7,42	8,70	6,18-8,67	4,0	<0,001
	Neither satisfied nor dissatisfied	31 (7,2%)	12,28	8,35	9,04-15-52	11,50	<0,001
	Dissatisfied	158 (36,9%)	15,48	9,08	13,92-17,03	17,00	<0,001
	Missing	4 (0,9%)					
Review of last visit	Good	345 (80,6%)	10,58	9,66	9,51-11,65	9,00	0,424
	Regular	22 (5,1%)	12,94	8,82	8,69-17,19	14,00	0,424
	Bad	24 (5,6%)	10,81	9,60	6,55-15,07	9,00	0,424
	Missing	37 (8,6%)					
OIDP	No impact	155 (36,2%)	7,85	9,48	6,34-9,35	4,00	<0,001
	One or more impact	233 (54,4%)	13,07	9,40	11,85-14,28	13,00	<0,001
	Missing	40 (9,3%)					
Visit to dentist	Yes	397 (92,8%)	10,11	9,61	9,16-11,06	8,00	0,004
	No	28 (6,5%)	15,92	10,93	11,68-20,16	17,00	0,004
	Missing	3 (0,7%)					
Time of last visit	Less than 1 year	81 (18,9%)	15,37	8,40	13,51-17,22	17,00	<0,001
	1 to 2 years	84 (19,6%)	15,17	8,04	13,43-16,92	16,50	<0,001
	3 years and more	228 (53,3%)	6,62	8,90	5,44-7,79	2,00	<0,001
	Missing	35 (8,2%)					

Variable		N (%)	Average	±DP	CI 95%	Median	p-value *
Local of last visit	Public	241 (56,3%)	12,30	9,54	11,09-13,51	12,00	<0,001
	Particular, health plan, covenants	151 (35,3%)	7,02	8,79	5,58-8,45	3,00	<0,001
	Missing	36 (8,4%)					
Reason for last visit	Review, prevention, treatment and other	71 (16,6%)	13,91	10,42	11,44-16,38	16,00	<0,001
	Pain	47 (11,0%)	12,82	9,25	10,11-15,54	14,00	<0,001
	Extraction	278 (65,0%)	8,71	9,12	7,64-9,79	6,00	<0,001
	Missing	32 (7,5%)					
Total		428 (100%)	10,43	9,79		9,0	

*P-value from Mann-Whitney e Kruskall Wallis test.

Table 1. Description of average indigenous Xukuru permanent teeth in adults and the elderly. Pesqueira, 2010.

Regarding the perception and impact on oral health, 235 individuals (54.9%) say they are satisfied with their teeth / mouth, 80.6% rated the last query as good and 54.4% reported one or more impacts on oral health in daily life. Regarding access to dental services, 28 individuals (6.5%) had never been to the dentist, 53.3% had a dental appointment last three years and over and 56.3% held in the public service. The main reason for consultation to 65.0% of the subjects was to perform extraction.

Table 2 shows the results of a single regression model. The average ratio (RM) presented considers the variance present in each level and shown as a measure of effect corrected to factors associated presence of teeth.

Individuals of adult age group showed less tooth loss and RM 2.29. But women showed greater chance of tooth loss (OR = 1.99). Regarding environmental region and income were not significant for tooth loss. Reading and writing (RM = 1.27) is negatively associated to tooth loss as well as those attending (RM = 1.55) or have attended school at some time in life (RM = 1.26).

With regard to the variables of block 2, who says satisfied with teeth / mouth has greater tooth loss (RM = 0.74) and those with a greater number of teeth present in the mouth has more impact on oral health (RM = 1.23). Regarding the last consultation, evaluation dictates how fair and poor is related to having more teeth.

Among the variables in block 3 is important to note that anyone who has ever been to the dentist in life has more chance of not having teeth, or going to the dentist increases by 160% tooth loss than those who have never been. For people who performed the last visit for more than three years average of teeth present was lower (RM = 0.68). Having performed consulting in public service decreased the chance of tooth loss (OR = 0.36) and who was motivated to consultation with the purpose of extracting has fewer teeth (RM = 0.67).

Demographic variables Block 1		Not inflated			Inflated		
		RM	CI 95%	p-value	OR	CI 95%	p-value
Age group	Adults	2,29	2,02-2,59	<0,001	0,05	0,02-0,11	<0,001
	Elderly	1,00			1,00		
Sex	Male	1,00			1,00		
	Female	0,99	0,85-1,15	0.902	1,99	1,29-3,06	0,002
Can read and write	Yes	1,27	1,09-1,47	0,001	0,40	0,25-0,65	<0,001
	No	1,00			1,00		
Attends school	Yes	1,55	1,16-2,07	0,003	0,27	0,02-0,58	0,008
	No, already attended.	1,26	1,08-1,49	0,004	0,48	0,31-0,75	0.001
	No, never attended.	1,00			1,00		
Perception variables Block 2		Not inflated			Inflated		
		RM	CI 95%	p-value	OR	CI 95%	p-value
Satisfaction with teeth/mouth	Satisfied	0,74	0,63-0,86	<0,001	5,73	3,25-10,09	<0,001
	Neither satisfied nor dissatisfied	0,84	0,64-1,11	0,24	2,28	0,84-6,17	0,103
	Dissatisfied	1,00			1,00		
Review of last visit	Good	1,00			1,00		
	Regular	1,02	0,75-1,39	0,878	0,48	0,15-1,49	0,207
	Bad	0,86	0,64-1,17	0,348	0,42	0,13-1,33	0,143
OIDP	No impact	1,00			1,00		
	One or more impact	1,23	1,05-1,44	0,009	0,33	0,21-0,54	<0,001
Acess variables Block 3		Not inflated			Inflated		
		RM	CI 95%	p-value	OR	CI 95%	p-value
Visit to dentist	Yes	0,77	0,59-1,01	0,066	2,60	0,86-7,84	0,088
	No	1,00			1,00		
Time of last visit	Less than 1 year	1,00			1,00		
	1 to 2 years	0,92	0,75-1,12	0,421	0,37	0,10-1,39	0.143
	3 years and more	0,68	0,56-0,82	<0,001	6,78	3,17-14,47	<0,001
Local of last visit	Public	1,29	1,09-1,53	0,002	0,36	0,23-0,57	<0,001
	Particular, health plan, covenants	1,00			1,00		

Demographic variables Block 1		Not inflated			Inflated		
		RM	CI 95%	p-value	OR	CI 95%	p-value
Reason for last visit	Review, prevention, treatment and other	1,00			1,00		
	Pain	0,85	0,65-1,11	0,251	0,73	0,30-1,77	0,49
	Extraction	0,67	0,55-0,81	<0,001	1,29	0,72-2,32	0,38

RM: Ratio of average

OR: Odds Ratio

CI 95%: confidence interval of 95%

Table 2. Average Ratio (RM) and odds ratio (OR) of teeth present estimates of the simple model of zero-inflated negative binomial regression. Pesqueira, 2010.

Table 3 presents the results of multiple hierarchical model, according to the theoretical model presented in Figure 2. Was observed that among the variables in block 1 only age and sex were statistically significant. Being female is an increased likelihood of tooth loss (OR = 2.68). In block 2 only satisfaction variable in the final model and their effects were controlled for block 1.

In block 3 variables time of last visit and reason for last visit remained the final model. A higher probability of not having teeth was related to having made the last visit for more than 3 years (OR = 2.65).

Demographic variables Block 1		Not inflated			Inflated		
		RM	CI 95%	p-value	OR	CI 95%	p-value
Age Group	Adults	2,29	2,02-2,59	<0,001	0,04	0,02-0,09	<0,001
	Elderly	1,00			1,00		
Sex	Male				1,00		
	Female				2,68	1,63-4,43	<0,001
Perception variables Block 2		Not inflated			Inflated		
		RM	CI 95%	p-value	OR	CI 95%	p-value
Satisfaction with teeth/mouth	Satisfied	0,88	0,78-1,00	0,05	3,40	1,81-6,36	<0,001
	Neither satisfied nor dissatisfied	0,95	0,76-1,19	0,69	1,83	0,59-5,63	0,287
	Dissatisfied	1,00			1,00		
Acess variables Block 3		Not inflated			Inflated		

Demographic variables Block 1		Not inflated			Inflated		
		RM	CI 95%	p-value	OR	CI 95%	p-value
		RM	CI 95%	p-value	OR	CI 95%	p-value
Time of last visit	Less than 1 year				1,00		
	1 to 2 years				0,33	0,08-1,33	0,118
	3 years and more				2,65	1,05-6,70	0,038
Reason for last visit	Review, prevention, treatment and other	1,00			1,00		
	Pain	0,92	0,75-1,12	0,424	0,19	0,05-0,70	0,012
	Extraction	0,79	0,68-0,92	0,003	0,36	0,15-0,85	0,020

* Adjusted for variables in block 1.

* Adjusted for variables in block 1 and 2.

* Adjusted for variables in block 1, 2 and 3.

RM: Ratio of average

OR: Odds Ratio

CI 95%: confidence interval of 95%

Table 3. Average Ratio (RM) and Odds Ratio (OR) of teeth according to estimates from multiple hierarchical multilevel model of zero-inflated negative binomial regression. Pesqueira, 2010.

4. Discussion

The average number of permanent teeth found in this study was lower than that found by [37]. Adults in this study had an average of 17.91 permanent teeth (± 7.90) and older had an average of 4.16 permanent teeth (± 6.15). Early tooth loss is considered a predictor of future tooth loss and grows with increasing age. In studies carried out by [37-39] confirmed an increase in the loss of teeth with increasing age.

The increase in edentulism with age seems to be a universal trend, creating the social imaginary figure of the old toothless elderly and the acceptance of tooth loss as a natural evolution of the human dentition, more or less in the sense of "we are born without teeth and die without teeth" [40].

Females had increased likelihood of tooth loss. This finding corroborates the results found in the study done by Indians of the Guarani tribe [39] and in studies of the general population [21, 41, 42]. A possible explanation would be the increased use of dental services by women, resulting in overtreatment would cause the loss of the tooth.

According to [43], increased tooth loss in women reveals some phenomena related to gender differences in health. Among these phenomena, we have the longest life expectancy of women who would be prolonging exposure to determinants of edentulism or the greatest care that the woman spends with their health.

Although the social and environmental areas of study have been insignificant to tooth loss, studies are needed to better understand the influence of acculturation on tooth loss among indigenous.

Although in distinct and involving other human, social, economic and environmental factors timescale, contemporary indigenous groups, once in contact with national societies also experience socio-economic and ecological changes with strong potential to change oral health conditions [10, 44].

When related tooth loss and income observed insignificance, but the study shows that those who have a higher income have less teeth in the mouth. This is due to the elderly who have a higher income than adults and they have fewer teeth than adults. In our study, those who can read and write and who attends or has attended school any time in life, proved to be less chances of tooth loss. These conditions influence the pattern and type of use of oral health services. This model is reaffirmed by [39], where low education is strongly associated with greater tooth loss.

There are significant correlations between early tooth loss and social variables, such as the human development index, ethnicity, education, income under the minimum wage, lack of fluoridation of city water and living in cities with fewer than 10,000 inhabitants, which have already been reported in other studies [27].

However, it is difficult to compare studies of tooth loss among Indians and the general population because of the few relevant studies, different methodologies and different age groups.

Individuals who said they were satisfied with their oral health have fewer teeth. This result is related to the elderly, given the absence of teeth does not seem to impact on daily life. The adults in the study expressed dissatisfaction with oral health, but reported no problems related to functional activity and/or social.

Regarding the visit to the dentist was possible to observe an increased risk of tooth loss. According to[45], considering that the only way to experience tooth loss is to enter the dental care system (with the small exception of the self-extraction), since having access people have increased risk of tooth loss.

The main reason for the last visit was extraction. There are two hypotheses for [26]: firstly, those first decide to remove a tooth due to a specific problem and will extract it to the dentist or, on the other hand, decide to see a dentist first because of a problem specific and go to the dentist to see what can be done. In the first case, the specific symptoms and problems determine the loss of teeth. In the second case, the dental care determines tooth loss and problems and symptoms would have a direct effect on the use of dental services and indirect about losing teeth.

This latter fact reveals the importance of the function of the dentist in maintaining oral health, yet there to highlight all the influence of hegemonic paradigms and dominant ideology contained in the dental practice of a particular historical moment [40]. This is one of the reasons why teeth are extracted could be recovered, since this alternative is considered the most convenient and also the most economical [18, 46].

In the daily routine of the people, the alterations produced by the loss of teeth should be the object of concern of the dental profession [47]. However, the approach of professionals, most often only considers the biological and restorative perspectives, ie, the restoration of teeth should be done according to the best principles of the technique, neglecting the effects of tooth loss in quality of life patients [48, 49].

Considering the results in multilevel analysis, it was possible to contemplate some of the complexity inherent in the health-disease process. This possibility ensured the simultaneous approach of contextual and individual factors in the analysis.

5. Conclusion

This study showed that: the average permanent teeth decreases considerably with advancing age, male sex is what has more teeth, self-perception is a satisfactory condition when there is tooth loss and oral health impacts are mainly perceived on who has more teeth. Access to services reveals a high proportion of the population that has already been to the dentist in public service for over three years and the reason for the visit was tooth extraction.

The differences between the oral health status of indigenous and non-indigenous constitute a framework of inequality between these two populations. It is necessary to rethink the routine visits to the dentist, since the factors associated with the presence of teeth are different for both individuals of the same age group, as different age groups. As well as the services of dental care does not have adequate infrastructure is sufficient to absorb the demand of the indigenous population, especially in adult and elderly.

Considering the epidemiological profile of the indigenous ethnic groups is important to highlight that are developed and put into public policies, in order to seek intervention strategies in oral health care.

Aknowledgements

Aknowledgements to facepe and CNPQ for the financial support.

Author details

Cecilia Santiago Araujo de Lima and Rafael da Silveira Moreira[*]

*Address all correspondence to: moreirars@cpqam.fiocruz.br

Department of Public Health. Oswaldo Cruz Foundation. Aggeu Magalhães Research Center. Recife. Pernambuco, Brazil

References

[1] Instituto Brasileiro de Geografia e Estatística. Censo Demográfico 2010. Características Gerais dos Indígenas. Resultados do Universo. Rio de Janeiro, p. 1-245, 2010. ftp://ftp.ibge.gov.br/Censos/Censo_Demografico_2010/Caracteristicas_Gerais_dos_Indigenas/pdf/Publicacao_completa.pdf (Acesso 26 fev. 2013).

[2] Fundação Nacional de Saúde. Sistema de Informação da Atenção à Saúde Indígena de Pernambuco. Distrito Sanitário Especial Indígena de Pernambuco. Dados demográficos dos índios de Pernambuco. Recife, 2008.

[3] Souza LC. "Doença que rezador cura" e "doença que médico cura": modelo etiológico Xukuru a partir de seus especialistas de cura. [Dissertação de Mestrado em Antropologia]. Recife: Universidade Federal de Pernambuco, 2004.

[4] Fundação Nacional do Índio. Atualização do levantamento fundiário do TI Xukuru: relatório GT PP nº 374. Brasília, DF, 2007.

[5] Mauricio, H.A. A Saúde Bucal do Povo Indígena Xukuru do Ororubá na Faixa Etária de 10 a 14 anos. [Dissertação Mestrado em Saúde Pública]. Recife: Centro de Pesquisas Aggeu Magalhães, Fundação Oswaldo Cruz, 2012.

[6] Leite MS. Transformações e persistência: antropologia da alimentação e nutrição em uma sociedade indígena amazônica. Rio de Janeiro: Editora Fiocruz, 2007.

[7] Coimbra Jr CEA, Santos RV. Saúde, minorias e desigualdade: Algumas teias de inter-relações, com ênfase nos povos indígenas no Brasil. Ciência & Saúde Coletiva, 2000; 5:125-132.

[8] Coimbra Jr CEA, Flowers NM, Santos RV, Salzano FM. The Xavánte in Transition: Health, Ecology, and Bioanthropology in Central Brazil. Ann Arbor: University of Michigan Press; 2002.

[9] Fundação Nacional de Saúde. Política Nacional de Atenção à Saúde dos Povos Indígenas, 2a Edição, Brasília:FUNASA/Ministério da Saúde; 2002.

[10] Santos RV, Coimbra Jr CEA. Saúde e Povos Indígenas. Rio de Janeiro: Editora Fiocruz; 1994. p. 545-566.

[11] Santos RV, Escobar AL. (eds.), 2001. Saúde dos povos indígenas no Brasil: Perspectivas atuais. Cadernos de Saúde Pública, 17(2) (número temático).

[12] Basta PC, Orellana, JDY. Arantes R. Perfil epidemiológico dos povos indígenas no Brasil: notas sobre agravos selecionados.In: Garnelo L, Pontes AL. Saúde Indígena: uma introdução ao tema. Brasília: MEC-SECADI, 280 p., 2012.

[13] Arantes R. Saúde oral de uma comunidade indígena Xavante do Brasil central: uma abordagem epidemiológica e bioantropológica. Dissertação (Mestrado em Saúde Pública) - Escola Nacional de Saúde Pública. Rio de Janeiro, 1998.

[14] Arantes R. Saúde bucal dos povos indígenas no Brasil: panorama atual e perspectivas. In: Coimbra Jr CEA, Santos RV, Escobar AL (organizadores). Epidemiologia e saúde dos povos indígenas do Brasil. Rio de Janeiro: Abrasco/Fiocruz; 2003. p. 49-72.

[15] Jovino-Silveira RC, Caldas Jr. AF, Souza EH, Gusmão ES. Primary reason for tooth extraction in a Brazilian adult population. Oral Health Prev Dent 2005; 3:151-7.

[16] Pinto VG. Epidemiologia das doenças bucais no Brasil. In: Kriger L. (Org.) Promoção da saúde bucal. São Paulo: Artes Médicas-Aboprev; 1997.

[17] Burt BA, Eklund AS. Dentistry, dental practice and the community. 4th Ed. Philadelphia: W.B. Saunders Company; 1992.

[18] Pinto VG. Saúde bucal coletiva. 4a Ed. São Paulo: Editora Santos; 2000.

[19] Barros AJD, Bertoldi AD. Desigualdades na utilização e no acesso a serviços odontológicos: uma avaliação em nível nacional. Ciência Saúde Coletiva 2002; 7:709-17.

[20] Cabral ED, Caldas Jr. AF, Cabral HA. Influence of the patient's race on the dentist's decision to extract or retain a decayed tooth. Community Dent Oral Epidemiol 2005; 33:461-6.

[21] Barbato PR, Nagano HCM, Zanchet FM, Boing AF, Peres MA. Perdas dentárias e fatores sociais demográficos e de serviços associados em adultos brasileiros: uma análise dos dados do Estudo Epidemiológico Nacional (Projeto SB Brasil 2002-2003). Cad Saúde Pública. 2007; 23(8):1803-14.

[22] Moyniham P. Bradbury J. Compromised Dental Function and Nutricion. Nutricion, United States, 2001 feb; 17(2): 177-178.

[23] N'Gom PI, Woda A. Influence of impaired mastication on nutricion. J. Prosthet Dent, United States, 2002 feb; 87(6): 667-673.

[24] Marcenes W, Steele JG, Sheiham A, Walls AWG. The relationship between dental status, food selection, nutrient intake, nutricional status, and body mass index in older people. Cad Saúde Pública, Rio de Janeiro, 2003 mai-jun; 19: 809-816.

[25] Musacchio E, Perissinotto E, Binotto P, Sartori L, Silva-Netto F, Zambon S, et al. Tooth loss in the elderly and its association with nutritional status, socio-economic and lifestyle factors. Acta Odontol Scand 2007; 65:78-86.

[26] Gilbert GH, Miller MK., Duncan RP, Ringelberg ML, Dolan TA, Foerster U. Tooth-specific and person level predictors of 24-month tooth loss among older adults. Community Dent Oral Epidemiol 1999; 27:372-85.

[27] Frazão P, Antunes JLF, Narvai PC. Perda dentária precoce em adulto de 35 a 44 anos de idade. Estado de São Paulo, Brasil, 1998. Rev Bras Epidemiol. 2003; 6(1): 49-57.

[28] Slade GD, Spencer AJ, Roberts-Thomson KF. Australia's dental generations: the national survey of adult oral health 2004-06. Canberra: Australian Institute of Health and Welfare 2007.

[29] Williams S, Jamieson L, MacRae A, Gray C. Review of Indigenous oral health. 2011. http://www.healthinfonet.ecu.edu.au/oral_review (Acesso 20 jan. 2013).

[30] Costa AM et al. Projeto de pesquisa: Análise das condições de vida, saúde e vulnerabilidade do povo indígena Xukuru do Ororubá como ferramenta para as ações de atenção primária de saúde. Projeto submetido ao edital FACEPE 09/2008 - Pesquisa para o SUS: Gestão compartilhada em saúde PPSUS – Pernambuco MS/CNPQ/FACEPE/SES. Recife: CPqAM/FIOCRUZ, 2009.

[31] Costa AM et al. Projeto de pesquisa: Saúde e condições de vida do povo indígena Xukuru do Ororubá, Pesqueira – PE. Projeto submetido ao Edital CNPq – Chamada: Edital MCT/CNPq Nº 014/2008 – Universal. Recife: CPqAM/FIOCRUZ, 2009.

[32] Brasil. Ministério da Saúde. Projeto SB Brasil 2003: Condições de saúde bucal da população brasileira 2002-2003: resultados principais. Brasília: Ministério da Saúde; 2004.

[33] Brasil. Ministério da Saúde. Projeto SB Brasil 2010 – Manual da Equipe de Campo. Brasília – DF: 2009. www.saude.gov.br/bucal (Acesso 15 jan. 2013).

[34] World Health Organization. Oral health surveys: basic methods. 4 ed. Geneva; 1997.

[35] Gschlößl S, Czado C. Modelling count data with overdispersion and spatial effects. Statistical papers, 2008; 49(3): 531-532.

[36] Victora CG, Huttly SR, Fuchs SC, Olinto MT. The role of conceptual frameworks in epidemiological analysis: a hierarchical approach. Int J Epidemiol 1997; 26: 224–227.

[37] Ulhôa Netto, E.; Ferreira, T. F. L.; Drummond, M. M.; Sanchez, H. F.; Tooth loss and need of denture in Pataxó Natives. Rev Gaúcha Odontol., 2012 abr./jun; 60(2): 195-201.

[38] Arantes R, Santos RV, Coimbra Jr CEA. Saúde bucal na população indígena Xavante de Pimentel Barbosa, Mato Grossso, Brasil. Cad. Saúde Pública, 2001 mar.-abr; 17(2): 375-384.

[39] Alves Filho P, Santos RV, Vettore M V. Saúde bucal dos índios Guarani no Estado do Rio de Janeiro, Brasil. Cad. Saúde Pública, 2009 jan; 25(1): 37-46.

[40] Moreira RS, Nico LS, Tomita NE. O risco espacial e fatores associados ao edentulismo em idosos em município do Sudeste do Brasil. Cad. Saúde Pública, 2011 out; 27(10): 2041-2053.

[41] Susin C, Oppermann RV, Haugejorden O, Albandar JM. Tooth loss and associated risk indicators in an adult urban population from south Brazil. Acta Odontol Scand 2005; 63:85-93.

[42] Silva DD, Rihs LB. Sousa M LR. Fatores associados à presença de dentes em adultos de São Paulo, Brasil. Cad. Saúde Pública, Rio de Janeiro, 2009 nov; 25(11): 2407-2418.

[43] Moreira RS. Perda dentária em adultos e idosos no Brasil: a influência de aspectos individuais, contextuais e geográficos. [Tese Mestrado Acadêmico em Saúde Pública]. São Paulo: Faculdade de Saúde Pública, Universidade de São Paulo, 2009.

[44] Wirsing R. The health of traditional societies and effects of acculturation. Current Anthropology 1985; 26: 303-322.

[45] Gilbert GH, Duncan RP, Shelton BJ. Social determinants of tooth loss. Health Service Research 2003; 38: 1843-1862.

[46] Guimarães MM, Marcus B. Expectativa de perda de dente em diferentes classes sociais. REVCROMG 1996; 2(1): 16-20.

[47] Chianca TK, Deus MR, Dourado AS, Leão AT, Vianna RBC. El impacto de la salud bucal en calidad de vida. Rev Fola/oral 1999; 16: 96-102.

[48] Wolf SMR. O significado da perda dos dentes em sujeitos adultos. Rev Assoc Paul Cir Dent. 1998; 52(4): 307-315.

[49] Vargas AMD, Paixão HH. Perda dentária e seu significado na qualidade de via de adultos usuários de serviço público de saúde bucal do Centro de Boa Vista, em Belo Horizonte. Cien Saude Colet 2005; 10(4): 1015-1024.

Pain Evaluation Between Stainless Steel and Nickel Titanium Arches in Orthodontic Treatment

M. Larrea, N. Zamora, R. Cibrian, J.L. Gandia and
V. Paredes

1. Introduction

The pain has traditionally been one of the most common side effects in orthodontic treatment. Orthodontic movement causes an inflammatory reaction in the periodontium and the pulp, which stimulates the production of biochemical mediators that cause the sensation of pain [1].

Different factors such as gender, personality and previous experience with other dental treatments may influence the concrete experience that each patient experiences with a particular orthodontic treatment [2].

It has been described by several authors [3-10] that pain begins at 4 hours after application of the force, after 24 hours, it descends, maintaining a plateau of lower intensity for two or three days, to continue descending from the fifth and sixth day until it disappears.

In the beginning, the pain was evaluated in a subjective manner, though in recent decades, numerous studies [11-12] have focused on the composition of crevicular fluid and changes that occur in it during orthodontic treatment as a more objective assessment of pain.

The application of mechanical forces moves the tooth and induces an inflammatory reaction by compression of the periodontal ligament. As a result, a variety of mediators are produced within the periodontal space, spread out at the crevicular fluid and reflecting the biological processes taking place. Several in vivo studies have used crevicular fluid analysis to monitor changes.

Crevicular fluid analysis is a noninvasive study of the cellular responses of the periodontal ligament during orthodontic treatment [13]. There are a variety of substances involved in the bone remodeling, produced in the cells of the periodontal ligament, that are spread out in the crevicular fluid [14].

Three substances, interleuquin 1β (IL-1β), prostaglandin E2 (PG-E2) and substance P (SP) were independently associated with pain [15-17], and are expressed during initial tooth movement in sufficient amounts to be detected in the crevicular fluid [18].

2. Problem statement

95% patients perceive pain during orthodontic treatment [6, 19], this pain being an important factor in rejecting treatment [20] or in interrupting it [21]. The pain involved has been described by various authors [3-10], there being different factors that modify it; gender, personality and previous experience with other dental treatments [2].

Ogura *et al.* [22] found a relationship between the magnitude of the force applied on the tooth and pain response, although other authors did not [23-25]. Additionally, the type of force (continuous or non-continuous) is also important. High and non-continuous forces [11,26,27] tend to significantly reduce the levels of IL1β at 168 hours from applying the force, which suggests the need for reactivation in order to maintain a sufficient production of IL1β. These types of forces not only increase the risk of radicular resorption on raising the hyalinization of the periodontal tissue [28,29], but also induce very sharp peaks of rises and falls in cytokine levels of which lead to undesirable results on the tissular level and the need for reactivating the forces. Light and continuous forces, however, tend to maintain high levels of IL1β so the need for reactivation is diminished [30-32]. These forces keep cytokine levels, which are necessary for continuous periodontal remodelling, high for a longer time.

The efficiency of orthodontic forces with different intensity and different duration has long been a major problem in the orthodontic clinic. In this study, to evaluate the efficacy and duration of each type of orthodontic force inducing initial tissue reaction two potent mediators of pain and bone resorption were measured; Prostaglandin E2 (PGE2) and substance P (SP).

Lastly, the material of the archwires that are fitted in the mouths of patients stailess-steel (SS) and nickel-titanium (Ni-Ti) exercise the force that may have an influence on pain, although there is controversy on this point [33]. There are few studies that compare pain depending on the type of archwire employed.

The aims of this work were, therefore:

- To compare pain during the initial stages of orthodontic treatment depending on the type of archwire employed; stainless steel (SS) or nickel-titanium (Ni-Ti).

- To determine a mathematical equation for predicting the level of pain depending on the time elapsed from fitting the archwire and that, therefore, would allow us to obtain the moment of peak of pain and to establish the moment when pain begins and ends depending on the type of archwire.

• To determine the difference in pain between time intervals.

• To analyse the crevicular fluid samples taken from patients to whom it has been performed the subjective study of pain.

3. Application area

A comparative, prospective clinical study was carried out at the Orthodontics Teaching Unit of the University of Valencia, Spain from January to April 2010. The study had previously been approved by the Ethics Committee of the University of Valencia. Rights have been protected by an appropriate Institutional Review Board and written informed consent was granted from all subjects. The Helsinki declaration was considered and its guidelines were followed in our investigation. All patients agreed to participate in the study, even though the diagnosis material was gathered as part of their treatment protocol.

4. Material and methods

4.1. Sample

A total of 150 patients who presented themselves at the Master in Orthodontics in order to receive Orthodontic treatment were selected.

The following inclusion criteria were established:

Patients who were to undergo a fitted Orthodontic treatment without dental extractions.

The presence of bracket cementing throughout the upper and/or lower arch.

The presence of good oral and periodontal health.

Whereas the exclusion criteria were:

The taking of any drug during the study.

The presence of active two band dental appliances during the treatment that would cause additional pain.

The presence of extra-oral appliances during the treatment that would cause additional pain.

On applying all these criteria, we obtained a total of 112 patients with a mean age of 19.8 years, ranging from between 9.5 and 64 years old. The sample comprised 37 males and 75 females.

The sample was divided according to the type of archwire that each of the patients wear: 49 patients with stainless-steel (SS) archwires and 63 patients with nickel-titanium (Ni-Ti) archwires. Of the 49 patients with SS archwires, 31 were females and 18 males and of the 63 patients with Ni-Ti archwires, 44 were females and 19 males.

Table 1 shows the distribution of the sample depending on age, gender, archwire type and according to where their archwires were fitted (upper, lower or both arches).

Archwire type	Female	Male	Arch upper	Arch lower	Both arches	Age (mean)
Ni-Ti Archwire (N =63)	44	19	38	25	4	22.6
Stainless-Steel Archwire (N=49)	31	18	31	18	2	17.2

Table 1. Sample distribution according to gender, the arch on which the archwire was fitted, age and archwire type used.

4.2. Method

After completing the appropriate orthodontic diagnosis, bracket bonding, which was carried out by 8 previously trained students of the Master of Orthodontics, Faculty of Medicine and Dentistry, University of Valencia, was scheduled.

Once the bonding of the brackets was performed, a 0.12"(diameter) Ni-Ti or SS arches were placed ramdomly in the patients enrolled in the study in order to compare the difference between groups in relationship with pain. In order to standardize the protocol, o elastomeric ligatures were used in all patients to hold the arches into the bracket system. The placement of the selected type of archwires did not alter the treatment of each patient.

5. Subjective assessment of pain — Patient questionnaire

First of all, a questionnaire was designed in order to assess the subjective level of pain. Having fitted the orthodontic appliance and the different archwires (SS and Ni-Ti), the patients filled in a pain questionnaire especially designed for this study, specifying the amount of pain (0=No pain; 1=discomfort; 2=slight pain; 3=intense pain) they experienced each day (from day 1 to day 14) and the time of day (morning, afternoon and night) they felt it. They were instructed to stop filling in this questionnaire after two consecutive days with an absence of pain. By doing so, the subjective values were obtained on an arbitrary scale. The appraisal of the questionnaire allowed us to assess both the subjective level of pain at each moment after the archwire was fitted and the total pain level experienced during the entire process of adapting to the archwire, obtained as the sum of the reported pain.

6. Objective assessment of pain — Crevicular fluid analysis

Secondly, an objective evaluation of pain was performed by analyzing the biochemical pain mediators in the crevicular fluid, in the laboratory.

The crevicular fluid samples were taken at the following stages of orthodontic treatment:

Before bracket bonding.

After 24 hours of placement of the archwire (Stainless Steel or Nickel Titanium).

A week after the archwire and bracket placement.

One month after the positioning of the initial archwire.

Crevicular fluid, using sterile paper strips (Periopaper Strip®. Proflow Incorporated. New York), was collected. Each sample was collected according to the technique described by Offenbacher et al. [34] and later modified by Uematsu et al. [11], without removing the plaque of the tooth in order to not alter the outcome of the study. However, efforts were made to collect the sample in the absence of plaque. The collection of all the crevicular fluid samples was taken by the same observer.

The technique used for sample collection was made by: firstly, drying of the mouth with suction; after that, isolating the area with cotton rolls;thirdly, looking for drying places where the paper strip is placed; and then, taking the sample of crevicular fluid by placing the Periopaper ® in the binding groove between the tooth and gum. The paper strip is kept in this position within 30 seconds; and finally, the samples are placed between the sensors of the Periotron® 8000 (Proflow Incorporated. New York. USA) in order to obtain the crevicular fluid collection in Periotron units (Figures 1 and 2).

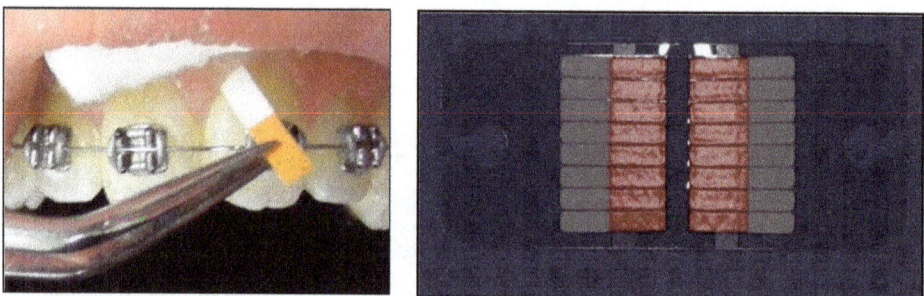

Figure 1. Sample collection of crevicular fluid with Periopaper®.

The extracted samples obtained were measured by ELISA immunofluorescence technique. To quantify the levels of substance P and PGE2, all samples were measured in duplicate. In our case, kits of high purity of the R & D Systems (Inc Minneapolis brand, USA) were used.

The spectrophotometer UV.vis shown in Figure 3 was used for the sample analysis. The spectrometer is an instrument used in biochemical analysis that measures, as a function of

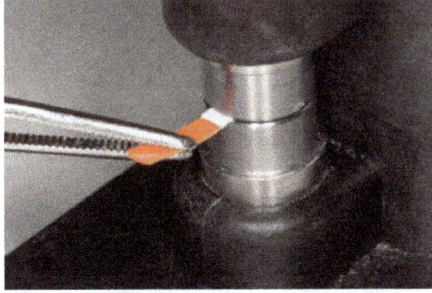

Figure 2. Crevicular fluid sample placement between Periotron® sensors.

wavelength, the relationship between the values of the same photometric magnitude related to two beams of radiation and the concentration and chemical reactions that are measured in a sample.

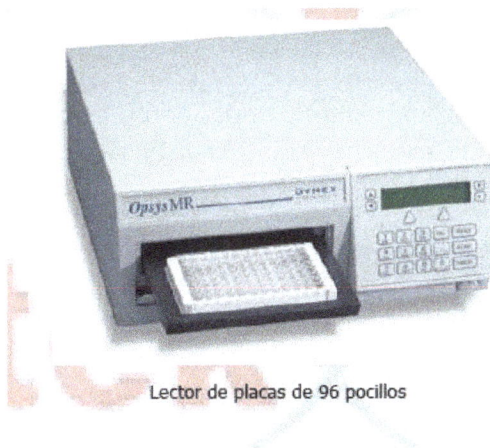

Lector de placas de 96 pocillos

Figure 3. Spectrophotometer UV. vis

The Periotron® (Figure 4), must be properly calibrated before its use. It consists in a device for measuring the volume of the gingival crevicular fluid, collected by the paper strips (Periopaper®). Usually, a number, defined as Periotron unit, appears on the screen; constructing calibration graphs is required to obtain microliters, by using known amounts of fluid.

Once the device is switched on, it should be heated for 10 minutes. Then, it should be set to zero. After that, a dry paper strip must to be placed inside and the dial has to be adjusted until the zero value appears on the digital screen. A Hamilton microsyringe is then used (maximum volume 2µl, with 0'02µl gradations) to dispense known volumes of calibration liquid (human serum, being similar to the gingival crevicular fluid viscosity and composition) in the paper strips.

In our study, the paper strips were transferred to the Periotron® sensors (2-3 seconds) quickly to avoid evaporation errors. These paper strips were positioned in a standardized way, with the orange tips off the sensors.

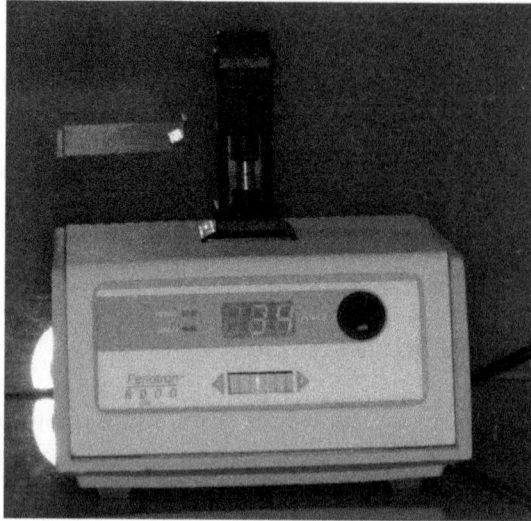

Figure 4. Periotron® machine.

After about 16 seconds, the Periotron Unit of each of the samples analysed was obtained. This occurred when the screen went from position I to position II in the frontal side of the device. Using moistened gauze with alcohol, the Periotron® sensors were cleaned between each sample.

Each volume was measured at least three times and the machine was set after each sample to zero.

In this way two variables were obtained:

1.   The volume (in µl) of serum dispensed with Hamilton microsyringe (Figure 5).

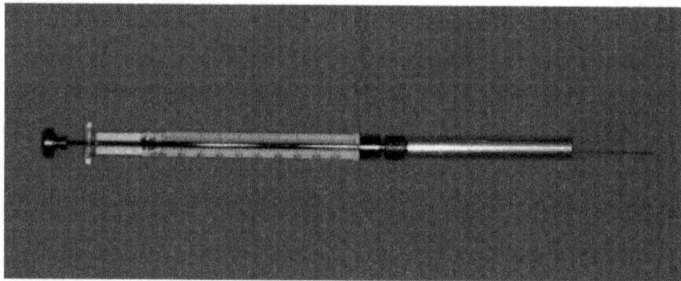

Figure 5. Hamilton Microjsyringe.

2.   The Periotron Unit values of each of the parameters of the sample (average of the measurements made three times).

With these measurements, a linear regression curve was performed, obtaining a formula of the type y=ax+b, where "a" is the slope of the curve, "b" the intersection of the axis, and "x" in the crevicular fluid in Periotron Units.

6.1. Statistical method

The normality of the total pain (TP) distribution experienced by the patients throughout the treatment was checked using the Kolmogorov-Smirnovtest, which allows us to compare the means of independent samples using Student's t-test.

A two-factor (time and archwire type) ANOVA was applied with the Scheffé test for multiple comparisons.

The χ^2 test was used to analyse factor dependence.

Non-linear regression was used for the variables, PL: pain level and T: time elapsed from fitting the dental archwire, with an estimation of best-fit parameters and quality assessment of the same through R^2, which indicates the percentage of variation of one variable that can be explained by the variation of the other.

7. Results

The total pain (TP) experienced throughout treatment, the pain level (PL) associated with each time section (morning, afternoon, night) and, therefore, the time elapsed from the beginning of treatment and the peak of maximum pain experienced have all been analysed.

7.1. Subjective study of pain

7.1.1. Total pain associated with treatment

From the data provided by the patients in the questionnaire, the total subjective pain (TP) reported by each patient throughout the study was determined as the sum of pain level at each time of the day.

With both types of archwires, there was no case of pain after the tenth day onwards so, in the study that follows, we are only going to consider the data up until that moment, which amounts to 232 hours following the fitting of the initial archwires. With these considerations, the maximum TP possible would be 90 points, even though the maximum value suffered was 48 points for the SS archwires and 36 points for Ni-Ti archwires.

TP data distribution for each type of archwire (Ni-Ti and SS) corresponded to a normal distribution with p>0.850 and p>0.150, respectively. Data on level, mean, standard deviation and percentiles of 25% and 75% for each type of archwire and for the total of the sample are presented in Table 2.

It could then be confirmed that the mean pain value for SS archwires was greater than for Ni-Ti archwires with p<0.007.

Using the percentile values of the total group, the pain suffered throughout the treatment can be classified as: "slight" for under 10 points; "moderate" for between 10 to 20 points; and

Treatment	mean	SD	Minimum	Maximum	Percentile 25%	Percentile 75%
Ni-Ti	14.6	7.2	0	36	10	19
SS	19.8	11.5	3	48	11	29
TOTAL	16.8	9.5	0	48	10	21

Table 2. Total pain (TP) over the 10 days following the beginning of treatment with Ni-Ti or SS archwires regardless of the archwire used. Mean and standard deviation (SD), minimum and maximum values and the percentiles of 25 and 75% were also presented.

"intense" for over 21 points. Applying this criterion, figure 6 shows the percentage of TP suffered using the two types of archwire in the study.

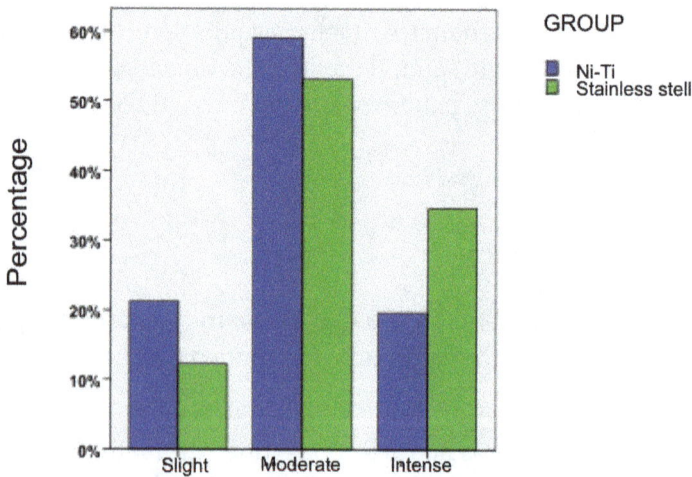

Figure 6. Percentage of total pain, slight (less than 10 points), moderate (between 10 and 20 points) and intense (over 20 points) for the two types of archwire studied (SS and Ni-Ti).

Dependence between the pain level and type of archwire was found to be $p < 0.006$. It can be observed that the percentage of cases with intense pain in the SS group, 34.7%, is greater than in that of the Ni-Ti group, 19.7%, whereas in the case of slight pain, the percentage is the other way around being greater in that of the Ni-Ti group with 21.2% than the 12.2% of the SS group, although, in this case, without statistically significant difference.

Furthermore, the mean of the days that the patients experienced pain was 4.84 days in general, with 4.5 of mean for patients with Ni-Ti archwires as opposed to 5.4 days of mean for the group with SS archwires, with a statistically significant difference of $p < 0.04$.

7.1.2. Pain level depending on the time elapsed from beginning of treatment

The subjective pain level (PL) for each time period was analysed according to the pain experienced during those same periods. As has been indicated in Material and Methods section, the possible evaluation in this case ranges from 0-3 points. The experimental results for each type of archwire are shown in figure 7.

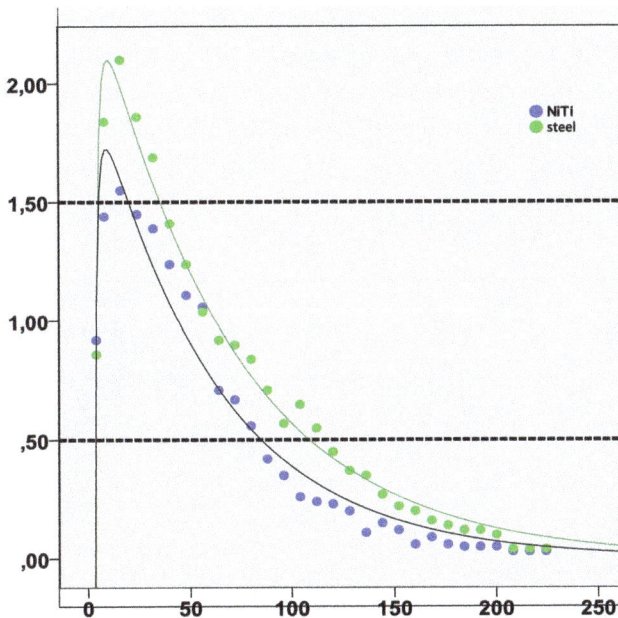

Figure 7. Experimental results and fit to the proposed curve PL=a* T^{-3}+c * exp (-b*T) for the two types of archwires studied. PL values have been categorized as slight: less than 0.5; moderate from 0.5 to 1.5; and high: greater than 1.5.

It can be observed that, in general, the shape of the curve is similar for both types of archwires, pain appearing after a few hours and decreasing gradually. This similarity in pain behaviour encouraged us to look for a mathematical function that would fit the points of the curve in order to evaluate pain depending on time and that, therefore, would provide a predictive study of the pain associated with the archwire or with the physiological characteristics of the process them self.

Given that the representation of pain level (PL) with the time period, regardless of the archwire used, also had a similar shape to that shown in figure 7, we then analysed this situation, as here the number of cases was higher and the fitting of the mathematical function would have more statistical validity and offer information on the evolution of pain in general. The points were fitted using non-linear regression curves of different types, the maximum fit being found to be a curve of the form: PL=a* T^{-3}+c * exp (-b*T), where PL, is pain level, T is the time elapsed in hours and the values "a", "b" and "c" correspond to the best-fit parameters that could differ or not depending on the type of archwire. The curve chosen for fitting consists of two terms: a decreasing exponential in which the parameters "b" and "c" are related, respectively, to the fall in the exponential and to PL in each time period, and a potential term that becomes insignificant for long times, but which modulates the growth of the exponential for low times, being responsible for the height that the peak of the curve reaches and is characterized by the "a" parameter. In this way, the first term of the equation and, therefore, the "a" coefficient is important in the first hours following the fitting of the archwire and represents the higher or lower PL corresponding to the "peak". The "b" parameter indicates the greater or lesser speed in the reduction of pain and value "c" represents the higher or lower PL throughout the treatment.

The parameters of fit for the 3 cases considered (pain in general regardless of the type of archwire, pain due to Ni-Ti archwire and pain due to SS archwire) are shown in Table 3. The goodness of fit for the three cases analysed is provided by the correlation coefficient R^2, which is very high, 0.983, 0.964 and 0.987, for the total group, the SS archwires group and the Ni-Ti group respectively.

| | Parameter | Estimation | Typical error | IC 95% | | |
				Lower limit	Upper limit	R^2 value
Total	a	-83.1	6.4	-96.2	-70.0	
	b	0.016	0.001	0.015	0.017	0.983
	c	2.31	0.07	2.17	2.45	
SS archwires	a	-70.4	8.8	-88.5	-52.4	
	b	0.017	0.001	0.015	0.019	0.964
	c	2.12	0.09	1.93	2.32	
Ni-Ti archwires	a	-100.8	6.1	-113.3	-88.2	
	b	0.015	4.8 E-4	0.014	0.016	0.987
	c	2.56	0.06	2.43	2.68	

Table 3. Values of parameters (a,b,c) and IC95% of the same corresponding to the non-linear fit of pain level (ND) depending on time in hours (T) elapsed since the beginning of treatment for the two types of archwires used and for the set of all cases. The non-linear fit corresponds to the expression PL=a* T^{-3}+c * exp (-b*T)

The values of the best-fit parameters indicate that: patients with SS archwires have a higher pain level at first than Ni-Ti patients (statistically significant difference in parameter a); a parallel reduction in pain level takes place (statistical equality in parameter b); but during the entire treatment patients with SS archwires experience more pain (statistically significant difference in parameter c).

Figure 7 also shows that after the tenth day no patient reported any pain, which is why our study ended at that point, 232 hours from the fitting of the archwire. The moment of the pain disappearing was practically the same for the two types of archwires, but it is interesting to calculate the average time that pain may be considered as high, moderate or slight. To do so, the PL experienced during the treatment was categorized on these three levels. The criterion was established that under 0.5 points (approximately 30% of the maximum PL experienced) pain could be considered as slight, between 0.5 and 1.5 as moderate, and above 1.5 (approximately 70% of the maximum PL experienced) as high. These stratification values are shown in figure 7. Using this categorization we can consider that the Ni-Ti archwires cease to hurt from 85h (3.5 days) from beginning of treatment as opposed to 109 hours (4.5 days) for SS archwires.

7.1.3. Peak of maximum pain

It is interesting to analyse the moment at which the peak of maximum pain intensity is reached. In our experimental data, the maximum pain is reached in the morning of the day after fitting the archwires, both for Ni-Ti and SS archwires. More specifically, if we observe the fits made (figure 7), maximum pain arrives at between 10 to 12 hours after fitting either of the types of archwire. However, if we consider the peak of the pain when the PL$\geq$ 1.5, as we commented earlier, we can see that that the peak takes place between 8-36 hours in SS and 8-20 hours in Ni-Ti, being, therefore, longer in patients with SS archwires.

7.1.4. Comparison of pain between time periods

Figure 8 represents the average PL for each time period and it can be observed that there are no "pain peaks" associated with night time, although in the first 5 days, during the night time period a slight increase in pain or a lower decrease than that which would correspond to the 8 hours elapsed from the previous afternoon is noted. This has no statistical significance as the increase or decrease in pain is associated more with the number of hours elapsed since fitting the appliance. Indeed, the AVOVA carried out on the PL values for morning, afternoon and night, the results of which can be seen in Table 4, shows that there is no difference between the mean values with p>0.999, although a very slightly higher mean value of PL can be appreciated for the night period.

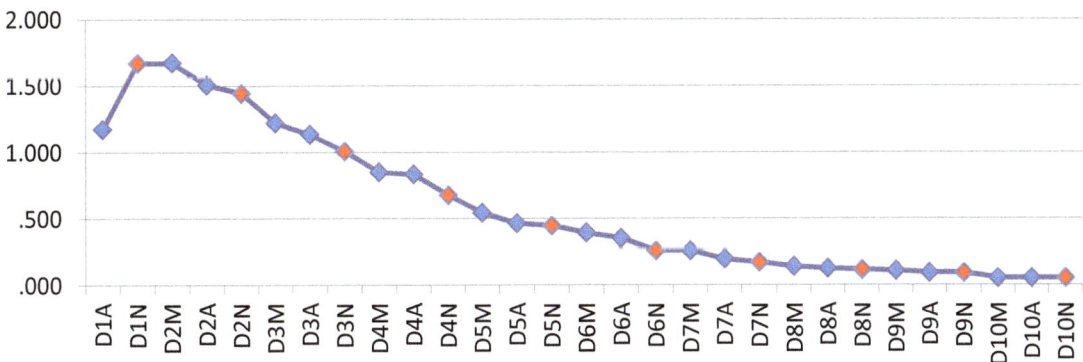

Figure 8. Pain level (PL) for each time period, regardless of the archwire used. The points in red correspond to the PL of night time periods.

	Mean PL	SD	IC95%	Minimum	Maximum
Morning	.58	.56	0.15 - 1.01	.06	1.67
Afternoon	.59	.53	0.27 - 0.97	.06	1.51
Night	.60	.59	0.17 - 1.02	.06	1.67

Table 4. Mean values and standard deviation (SD) of pain level (PL), confidence interval for the mean of PL at 95% (IC95%) and minimum and maximum values of each time period (morning, afternoon and night), regardless of the type of archwire used.

7.2. Subjective study of pain

7.2.1. Biochemical mediators analysis

To complete the study of pain, an objective assessment was performed. Two biochemical mediators of pain (Prostaglandin E2 (PGE2) and Substance P (SP)) were determined for each patient during treatment in four time intervals: prior to bracket bonding, 24 hours after bonding, a week and a month after bonding. In all cases, direct measurements were not considered but the proportion to the amount of crevicular fluid collected.

It was analyzed the possible correlations between the subjective pain reported by the patient with the levels of these mediators in the crevicular fluid for all the times studied.

7.2.2. Prostaglandin E2 (PGE2).

Correlations have been found between the concentration of PGE2 (PC) in the 4 times in which the determinations of this mediator were taken (PCT1: start, PCT2: 24 hours, PCT3: 7 days and PCT4: 30 days) and the subjective pain level of each individual in each interval analyzed, taking into account the 10 days in which there was existence of subjective pain. The results are shown in Table 5.

		D6N	D7M	D7T	D7N	D8M	D8T
P_Ct1	r-Pearson	0,102	0,274*	,280*	0,288*	,303**	0,140
	Sig. (bilateral)	0,386	0,017	,015	0,012	0,008	0,231
P_Ct2	r-Pearson	-0,032	0,053	,064	0,020	0,029	0,001
	Sig. (bilateral)	0,787	0,650	,583	0,862	0,803	0,993
P_Ct3	r-Pearson	0,010	0,161	,122	0,139	0,273*	0,173
	Sig. (bilateral)	0,931	0,167	,296	0,234	0,018	0,137
P_Ct4	r-Pearson	0,242*	0,326**	0,420**	0,442**	0,252*	0,295*
	Sig. (bilateral)	0,037	0,004	0,000	0,000	0,029	0,010

Table 5. Study of the correlation between the level of concentration of PGE2 (PC) in the 4 time times analyzed (PCT1 correspond to the time prior to bracket bonding, PCT2 to 24 hours after, PCT3 a week after and PCT4 a month after) and the level of pain reported by each patient. Values with * correspond to the times when correlation was found between the two measures of pain.

It can be seen that, in general, individuals with initially high values of PC mediator have a correlation with higher levels of pain one week after the archwire placement. This situation is also shown with PCT3 values and with those of PCT4, with no significant correlation with PCT1.

If the correlation of this mediator is analysed, not with the level of pain but with the total pain experienced by the subjects during the first 10 days, we find that high values of PC are correlated with subjects having more total level of pain throughout the treatment (Table 6). This finding does not happen with this marker in the other periods of time.

		P_Ct1	P_Ct2	P_Ct3	P_Ct4
Total Pain	r- Pearson	0,229*	0,059	0,025	0,166
	Sig. (bilateral)	0,048	0,616	0,831	0,156

Table 6. Study of the correlation between the level of PGE2 concentration (PC) and total pain level.

Furthermore, we analyzed whether there was correlation between the values of PGE2 in the four times studied. The results are shown in Table 7 and confirm that initially high values of this mediator are correlated to high values along the entire treatment.

		Total Sum	P_Ct1	P_Ct2	P_Ct3	P_Ct4
P_Ct1	CP	-0,042	1	0,484**	0,352*	0,365*
	SG	0,797		0,002	0,026	0,021
	N	40	40	40	40	40
P_Ct2	CP	-0,037	0,484**	1	0,120	0,297
	SG	0,821	0,002		0,462	0,063
	N	40	40	40	40	40
P_Ct3	CP	-0,268	0,352*	0,120	1	0,318*
	SG	0,094	0,026	0,462		0,046
	N	40	40	40	40	40
P_Ct4	CP	-0,004	0,365*	0,297	0,318*	1
	SG	0,978	0,021	0,063	0,046	
	N		40	40	40	40

Table 7. Study of the correlation between the values of prostaglandin PGE2 in the four times tested. CP (Pearson Correlation) and SG (Sig. Bilateral) ** significant correlation at the 0.01 level and * at the 0.05 level (bilateral).

7.2.3. Substance P (SP)

In orther to analyse this biochemical mediator, 86 cases were taken into account. The mean values of SP in the four times analysed of the study are shown in Table 8 and Figure 9.

Factor 1	Mean	Error	IC 95%	
			Lower limit	Upper limit
SPC1	173,165	21,470	130,469	215,860
SPC2	139,728	20,928	98,111	181,345
SPC3	190,621	26,825	137,278	243,965
SPC4	230,510	45,338	140,351	320,670

Table 8. Mean values of SP for each of the times studied.

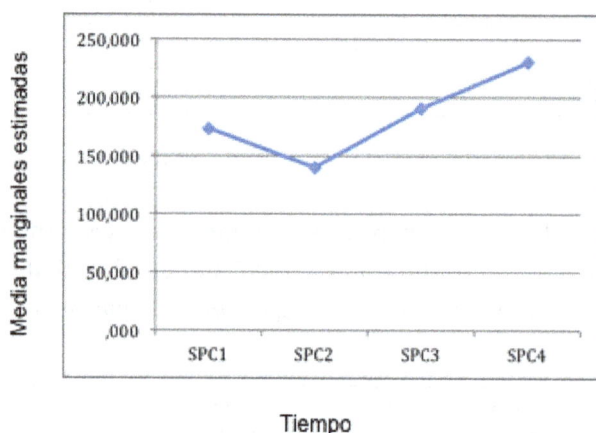

Figure 9. SP concentration at each time for each of the times studied.

According to these data, no statistical difference was found between the objective pain (SP crevicular fluid analysis) with the SS or Ni-Ti archwires, and the total subjective pain experienced according to the questionnaire.

8. Further research

In the literature, we have found few studies that compare pain depending on the type of archwire used [5, 32, 35] and none that introduces a mathematical equation for predicting pain level or peak of pain.

8.1. Subjective study of pain

8.1.1. Pain level

Our results coincide with those of Lee *et al.* [32] in stating that there is less pain in the group of patients treated with Ni-Ti archwires than in the group treated with SS archwires. However, neither our results nor the previously mentioned ones coincide with those of Jones and Chan

[5], who did not find differences in the pain experienced by patients between Ni-Ti archwires or SS archwires. Moreover, despite being a quite different study, Fernandes et al. [35] also did not find any difference on comparing conventional Ni-Ti archwires with super elastic Ni-Ti archwires.

In our results, pain receded at 4.5 days in cases treated with SS archwires, whereas it receded one day earlier (at 3.5 days) in those cases treated with Ni-Ti archwires. Moreover, the pain level was lower in the group with Ni-Ti archwires than in those with SS archwires.

If we analyse the results of the subjective study of pain recorded by the patients, we observe how 38.2% of patients felt discomfort and 43.1% felt slight pain, whereas only 18.6% experienced intense pain. These results do not coincide with those of Kaneko et al. [36], where only 10.3% felt discomfort and the great majority (72.4%) felt only slight pain. However, their results are in line with ours in stating that 17.2% experienced intense pain.

8.1.2. Peak of maximum pain

If we analyse when the peak of maximum pain takes place, the results of our study show that the peak occurs 15 hours after fitting the archwires into the mouth of the patient, both in the Ni-Ti group and the SS archwire group, results that are similar but not identical to those of other authors [1, 3, 6,18, 25, 37] who observed a maximum peak of pain 24 hours after fitting the archwire in the patient's mouth.

In contrast, our results and those mentioned above do not coincide with the results of the work of Jones and Chan [5] who found the maximum peak of pain to be on the same morning when fitting the archwire in the mouth, or the results of Jones and Richmond [38] who found the maximum peak of pain in the afternoon or night of the same day that the archwire was fitted.

8.1.3. Duration of pain

On studying how long pain lasts, the results of our study show that pain ceased at 3.5 days in the Ni-Ti group, whereas, in the SS group, it ceased at 4.5 days, the decrease in pain taking place earlier in the Ni-Ti group than in the SS group. These results do not coincide with those of Jones and Richmond [38], Jones and Chan [5], Ngan et al. [4] or Scheurer et al. [6] in whose studies, the pain caused by the fitting of the archwires was observed to last for approximately 5 days.

Our results show how both groups of patients, both the patients fitted with SS archwires and those fitted with Ni-Ti archwires, began to experience pain at 4 hours, results similar to those of Jones and Richmond [38] with the same intensity of pain.

However, SS and Ni-Ti metals do not have the same stress deformation curve and it can be observed that in order to achieve the same deformation, the stress that has to be applied in the case of steel is greater than in the case of Ni-Ti, which would account for the greater initial pain of the patient in cases treated with SS archwires. Nevertheless, as the teeth adapt to the forces applied and, therefore, the stress applied on the archwire material diminishes, these two materials behave differently, SS maintains a residual deformation, whereas Ni-Ti returns to practically its original dimensions, meaning that its effect on the tooth is more continuous and produces a sensation of pain over a longer time, so evening out the total time of pain duration for both types of archwire.

8.1.4. Comparison of pain between time periods

In our study, we did not find pain peaks associated with night time, unlike those shown in the results of Kaneko et al. [36] but that the increase or decrease of pain was similar in the morning or afternoon and was only associated with the number of hours following the fitting of the appliance. These results coincide with those of Scheurer et al. [6] who found that pain increased as the day elapsed.

8.2. Objective study of pain

Authors like Erdinic and Dincer [8] or Awawdeh et al. [39] have observed that the perception of pain during orthodontic movement is related to substance P. Substance P is involved in the nervous system signals required to perceive pain [40] also influencing the concentration of other pain mediators associated with dental pain like the metalloproteinase 8 [41], and in the secretion of IL-1β from the monocytes. These three substances (IL-1β, PG-E2 and SP) were independently associated with pain [15-17] and are expressed during initial tooth movement in sufficient amounts to be detected in the crevicular fluid [18].

Then we will discuss some variables affecting the collection of this sample.

8.2.1. Sources of error in the collection of the crevicular fluid

Before taking the samples, one have to keep in mind that the most frequent sources of contamination of the crevicular fluid samples are blood, saliva and plaque. Respect to the presence of plaque, its presence in the paper strips used for collecting the sample has a considerable effect on the volume of the sample, thus being a source of bias [42-44].These considerations have been supported also by other authors, who demonstrate that the non-removal of the plaque has a bad effect on the determination of the volume [43,45].

In order to avoid these problems of contamination prior to bracket bonding, scaling was performed to all patients of the study, thus reducing the possibility of bleeding and contamination by plaque.

Also, in our study, in order to reduce saliva contamination, a good insulation protocol was carried out by placing the aspiration system and cotton rolls in each patient. Saliva contamination is a problem when the sample is collected with paper strips, as it can alter the volume of the sample collected [46].

8.2.2. Sample recording time

The first authors who described the use of Periotron® [43] recommended a sample recording time of five seconds. However, to increase the volume of the sample in order to subsequently analyze it sometimes it is necessary to increase the sample time.

Therefore, in our work, a sample time of 30 seconds was established following the recommen-dations from other authors [32, 47-50]. For the analysis of the crevicular fluid, the collection should be made in such way that minimum groove environment deterioration occurs in the shortest time possible. By doing so, correct protein concentrations are maintained and also sufficient time is achieved to collect the required sample volume.

8.2.3. Methods of collection of crevicular fluid

There are many ways to collect the crevicular fluid; gingival washing, micropipettes and paper strips. Gingival washing method is suitable for obtaining cells of the gingival groove. It is a complex method and has limited applications since it can only be used in the maxillary arch due to the complexity of the technique. On the other hand, samples cannot be analyzed later in the laboratory and all the fluid cannot be recovered during aspiration and re-aspiration.

With micropipettes is difficult to collect a necessary amount of fluid in a short period of time unless there is gingival inflammation, resulting in more volume of crevicular fluid. It can cost up to 30 minutes to collect the amount of fluid necessary and this makes this technique traumatic [51].

The crevicular fluid analysis it is a useful and advantageous method, especially for in vivo studies, it is not invasive, and the sample can be split as many times as necessary. This allows the perfect monitor development in a given area for a certain period of time. Therefore and because of the complications mentioned above with the two methods described, in our work we decided to take the sample by this method, using paper strips, like other authors [32, 47-50] because it is a simple, rapid and non-traumatic method and can be applied to isolated areas.

Crevicular fluid samples of each patient who also had filled the subjective pain questionnaire were collected, in order to later compare the subjective data of pain with the objective values obtained from the analysis of the biochemical mediators.

8.3. Biochemical mediators analysis

8.3.1. Prostaglandin E2 (PGE2)

In our study, PGE2 production reached its maximum peak at 24 hours, coinciding with the results found by Bergius et al. [37], Giannopoulou et al. [18] and Grieve et al. [52]. In another study by Lee et al. [32], initial measurements of IL-1 β and PGE2 showed little variation, however, once force is applied, the individual variation became large enough to estimate the overall response.

Lee et al. [32] observed an increase in the levels of interleukins in patients during the third week, even without the revive forces, causing an increase in the average concentration but without statistical significance. Iwasaki et al. [30] found that IL-1β levels fluctuate with a period of 28 days when a force is applied continuously.

Interestingly, when a discontinuous force (equivalent to steel arches) is reactivated after a week, a significant increase in the levels of IL-1β, 24 hours after reactivation was found, compared with the results found 24 hours after the initial activation. This finding implies that timely reactivating discontinuous forces might be more effectively in the regulation of IL-1β than the continuous application of forces. Instead, they did not found any increased after a second reactivation. This could be due to a refractory period or excessive applied pressure. Since excessive pressure causes a large area of hyalinization in the pressure side and a wide acellular area, which produces impairment in cytokine secretion and its spread to the periodontal space. These results suggest that the application of a suitable pressure force intermittent and timely recovery may be effective to promote secretion of IL-1 β. However, authors like Yamaguchi et al. [26], Tian et al. [27] or Uematsu et al. [11], argue that the intense and discontinuous forces tend to significantly reduce levels of IL1β suggesting the need for reactivation to maintain sufficient production of IL1β. Such forces not only increase the risk of root resorption but also increase the hyalinization of periodontal tissue [28,29] which also induce very pronounced rise and fall peaks in the levels of cytokines, leading to undesirable tissue level and the need for the reactivation of the forces.

On the contrary, continuous light forces [30-32] tend to maintain high levels of IL1β so the need for reactivation is reduced. These forces maintain, high longer, cytokine levels, which are necessary for continuous periodontal remodeling.

The efficiency on the recovery is shown in a series of experiments in rats done by King et al. [53] where the reactivation during the end of the cycle stimulates bone resorbing osteoclasts and reduce root resorption.

In the study by Lee et al. [32], changes in the levels of PGE2 to mechanical stress and the interactions between the IL-1β and PGE2 in vivo were investigated. The mechanical loads applied to the periodontal ligament cells are known to induce the expression of cyclooxygenase-2 (COX-2), which facilitates the formation PGE2 [54]. In the study of Saito et al. [55], a significant increase in PGE2 was observed when IL-1β was applied to periodontal ligament cells alone or in combination with mechanical stress. The synergistic action of IL-1β and mechanical stress on the production of PGE prove the hypothesis that mechanical stress provides more substrate for cyclooxygenase by activation of phospholipase A2, while IL-1β formation increases cyclooxygenase.

PGE2 levels in this initial study showed significant peaks at 24 hours (T2) of the application of force, compared to the control site. This appears to be a direct effect of mechanical stress. By applying continuous force, high levels of PGE2 was observed only temporarily, compared to the control site, even though the average concentration is maintained at a high level during the experiment. With discontinuous forces, significantly higher levels of PGE2 for 1 week were observed. This regulation is an example of the synergistic effect of the mechanical stresses sustained and secreted IL-1β.

In this study we found that, if the total pain recorded by the subjects is determined and their correlation is sought with the values of this mediator, patients with high values of PC1 have more total level of pain during the treatment. Furthermore, PC3 high values are related with high values one week after the archwire placement. We did not find association between patients who had elevated levels of PC4 with high levels of pain between the 6th and 8th day.

These results cannot be compared with other authors as there are no studies reported in the literature.

8.3.2. Substance P (SP)

The results of the substance P values were inconsistent with what would be expected of a biochemical mediator of pain as, in the initial time of the study, when no level of pain exists (and therefore this substance should have a baseline), we found higher values, both overall levels and concentrations, than in the rest of study for 56 of the 86 patients analyzed.

The apparently anomalous behavior of this marker with a decrease at 24 hours and a later increased tendency to grow up is not statistically significant because, due to the high variability of the data. However, other authors as Giannopoulou et al. [18], found more predictable values in the levels of these biochemical mediators after insertion of ligatures.

The experience of pain has its peak 1 day after starting treatment and is reduced to normal levels at 7 days. The IL-1β, SP, PGE2 mediators are expressed during initial tooth movement. The initial perception of pain (1h) is related to the levels of PGE2, the IL-1β is related to pain at 24 hours and the SP has its peak at 24 hours. This is possible because of the relationship that has with PGE2 as an indicator of periodontal inflammation [56].

On the other hand, Yao et al. [57], did not find relationship between pain intensity and PGE2 at 12, 24 and 72 hours of the beginning of tooth movement. Another authors, though [26], found no relationship between IL-1β and substance P. Indirectly, this finding also has an association between IL-1β and pain.

9. Conclusions

This paper has analyzed the pain associated with the placement of the first archwire in the beginning of the orthodontic treatment, analyzing the influence that several variables have (such as the type of wire used) on pain.

A questionnaire for the subjective assessment of pain has been designed, registering the pain indicated by the patient at each time interval (morning, afternoon and evening), from the time of placing the archwire for the first time until it disappears. Furthermore, the objective assessment of pain has been determined in the crevicular fluid through the different biochemical mediators of pain, such as prostaglandin 2 (PGE2) and substance P (SP).

- Total pain (TP) and the maximum level of pain (PL) are lower in the group of patients fitted with Ni-Ti archwires than in the group fitted with SS archwires, although pain for both groups recedes at the same time.

- Pain level (PL) is determined by the mathematical equation:

$PL = a * T^{-3} + c * \exp(-b*T)$ where parameters a, b and c represent: "a" coefficient represents the higher or lower PL corresponding to the "peak". The "b" parameter indicates the greater or lesser speed in the reduction of pain and value "c" represents the higher or lower PL throughout the treatment.

- Both the patients with SS archwires and those with Ni-Ti archwires began to feel pain after 4 hours of the placement of the archwires. The maximum peak of pain is established generally within the first hours of the placement of the archwire (10 hours) and lasts for about 20 hours. The pain becomes moderate and mild, respectively, about one and a half (30 hours) and 4 days (100 hours) after the beginning of the treatment. Pain disappears generally before 10 days after the placement of the archwire. There is no difference in the time when pain is greatest for both types of archwire, being situated at between 15 and 20 hours following the fitting of the archwire in the mouth.

- Biochemical mediators (prostaglandin E2 (PGE2) and substance P (SP)) have not reported generally good correlation with the subjective pain reported by the patient. Only it should be noted that high values of PGE2 before treatment (PCT1), correlate with higher levels of subjective pain a week after the archwire is placed. This situation is also shown in the values determined after one week (PCT3) and after a month (PCT4).

Author details

M. Larrea[1], N. Zamora[1*], R. Cibrian[2], J.L. Gandia[1] and V. Paredes[1]

*Address all correspondence to: natalia.zamora@uv.es

1 Department of Orthodontics. Faculty of Medicine and Dentistry, University of Valencia, Spain

2 Department of Physiology. Faculty of Medicine and Dentistry, University of Valencia, Spain

References

[1] Krishnan V. Orthodontic pain: from causes to management-a review. European Journal of Orthodontics. 2007; 29:170–9.

[2] Williams JM, Murray JJ, Lund CA, De Franco A. Anxiety in the child dental clinic. Journal of Child Psychology and Psychiatry. 1985; 26:305-10.

[3] Ngan P, Kess B, Wilson S 1989. Perception of discomfort by patients undergoing orthodontic treatment. American Journal of Orthodontics and DentofacialOrthopedics 96:47-53.

[4] Ngan P, Wilson S, Shanfeld J, Amini H 1994 The effect of ibuprofen on the level of discomfort in patients undergoing orthodontic treatment. American Journal of Orthodontics and DentofacialOrthopedics106: 88-95

[5] Jones M, Chan C 1992 The pain and discomfort experienced during orthodontic treatment. A randomized controlled clinical trial of two initial aligning arch wires. American Journal of Orthodontics and DentofacialOrthopedics 102: 373-381.

[6] Scheurer PA, Firestone AR, Burgin WB 1996 Perception of pain as a result of Orthodontic treatment with fixed appliances. European Journal of Orthodontics 18:349-357

[7] Firestone A R, Scheurer P A, Bürgin W B 1999 Patient's anticipation of pain and pain-related side effects, and their perception of pain as a result of orthodontic treatment with fixed appliances. European Journal of Orthodontics 21: 387-396

[8] Erdinç A M E, Dinçer B 2004 Perception of pain during orthodontic treatment with fixed appliances. European Journal of Orthodontics 26:79-85

[9] Polat O, Karaman A 2005 Pain control during fixed appliance therapy. Angle Orthodontist 75: 214-219

[10] Jones ML 1984 An investigation into the initial discomfort caused by placement of an archwire. European Journal of Orthodontics 6:48-54.

[11] Uematsu S, Mogi M, Deguchi T 1996 Interleukin (IL)-1 beta, IL-6, tumor necrosis factor-alpha, epidermal growth factor, and beta 2-microglobulin levels are elevated in gingival crevicular fluid during human orthodontic tooth movement. Journalof Dental Research75: 562-567

[12] Hofbauer LC, Lacey DL, Dunstan CR, Spelsperg TC, Riggs BL, Khosla S. (1999) Interleukin-1beta and tumor necrosis factoralpha, but not interleukin-6 stimulate osteoprotegerin ligand gene expression in human osteoblastic cells. Bone. 25: 255-259.

[13] Ren Y, Maltha JC, Van't Hof MA, Von den Hoff JW, Kuijpers-Jagtman AM, Zhang D. (2002) Cytokine levels in crevicular fluid are less responsive to orthodontic force in adults than in juveniles. J Clin Periodontol. 29:757-762.

[14] Kavadia-Tsatala S, Kaklamanos E, Tsalikis L. (2002) Effects of orthodontic treatment on gingival crevicular fluid flow rate and composition: Clinical implications and applications. Int J Adult Orthod Orthog Surg. 17;191-205.

[15] Hori T, Oka T, Hosoi M, Aou S. (1998) Pain modulatory actions of cytokines and prostaglandin E2 in the brain. Ann NY Acad Sci. 840:269-281.

[16] Lundy FT, Linden GJ. (2004) Neuropeptides and neurogenic mechanisms in oral and periodontal inflammation. Crit Rev Oral Biol Med. 15;82-98.

[17] Sommer C, Kress M. (2004) Recent findings of how proinflammatory cytokines cause pain: peripheral mechanisms in inflammatory and neuropathic hyperalgesia. Neurosci Lett. 361:184-187.

[18] Giannopoulou C, Dudic A, Kiliaridis S 2006 Pain discomfort and crevicular fluid changes induced by Orthodontic elastic separators in children. Journal of Pain7: 367-76

[19] Kvam E, Gjerdet N, Bondevik O 1987 Traumatic ulcers and pain during orthodontic treatment. Community Dentistry and Oral Epidemiology 15:104-110

[20] Oliver R G, Knapman Y M 1985 Attitudes to Orthodontic treatment. BritishJournal of Orthodontics 12: 179-188

[21] Patel V 1992 Non-completion of active orthodontic treatment. British Journal of Orthodontics 19: 47-54

[22] Ogura M,Kamimura H, Al-KalalyA, Nagayama K, Taira K, Nagata J, MiyawakiS2009 Pain intensity during the first 7 days following the application of light and heavy continuous forces. European Journal of Orthodontics 31: 314-319

[23] Dubner R 1968 Neurophysiology of pain. Dental Clinics of North America 22: 11-30

[24] Brown D F, Moerenhout R G 1991 The pain experience and psychological adjustments to orthodontics treatment of preadolescents, adolescents and adults. American Journal of Orthodontics and DentofacialOrthopedics 100: 349-356

[25] Bergius M, Kiliardis S, Berggren U 2000 Pain in orthodontics: a review and discussion of the literature. Journal of OrofacialOrthopedics 61:125-137

[26] Yamaguchi M, Yoshii M, Kasai K 2006 Relationship between substance P and interleukin-1beta in gingival crevicular fluid during orthodontic tooth movement in adults. European Journal of Orthodontics 28: 241-246

[27] Tian YL, Xie JC, Zhao ZJ, Zhang Y 2006 Changes of interlukin-1beta and tumor necrosis factor-alpha levels in gingival crevicular fluid during orthodontic tooth movement.Hua Xi Kou Qiang Yi XueZaZhi 24: 243-245

[28] Maltha JC, Van Leeuwen EJ, Dijkman GE, Kuijpers-Jagtman AM 2004 Incidence and severity of root resorption in orthodontically moved premolars in dogs. Orthodontics and Craniofacial Research 7:115-121

[29] Von Bohl M, Maltha JC, Von Den Hoff JW, Kuijpers-Jagtman AM 1986 Focal hyalinization during experimental tooth. American Journal of Orthodontics and DentofacialOrthopedics 125:615-623

[30] Iwasaki LR, Haack JE, Nickel JC, Reinhardt RA, Petro TM 2001 Human interleukin-1 beta and interleukin-1 receptor antagonist secretion and velocity of tooth movement. Archives of Oral Biology46: 185-189

[31] Iwasaki LR, Crouch LD, Tutor A, Gibson S, Hukmani N, Marx DB, Nickel JC 2005 Tooth movement and cytokines in gingival crevicular fluid and whole blood in growing and adult subjects. American Journal of Orthodontics and DentofacialOrthopedics128: 483-491

[32] Lee KJ, Park YC, Yu HS, Choi SH, Yoo YJ 2004 Effects of continuous and interrupted orthodontic force on interleukin-1beta and prostaglandin E2 production in gingival

crevicular fluid. American Journal of Orthodontics and DentofacialOrthopedics 125:168-177

[33] Fuck LM, Drescher D2006 Force systems in the initial phase of orthodontic treatment-a comparison of different leveling arch wires.Journal of OrofacialOrthopedics 67(1): 6-18

[34] Offenbacher S, Farr DH, Goodson JM. (1981) Measurement of prostaglandin E in crevicular fluid. J Clin Periodontol. 8:359-367.

[35] Fernandes LM, Ogaard B, Skoglund L 1998 Pain and discomfort experienced after placement of a conventional or a super-elastic NiTi aligning archwire. Journal of OrofacialOrthopedics 59:331-339

[36] Kaneko K, Kawai S, Tokuda T, Kamogashira K, Kawagoe H, Itoh T, Matasumoto M 1990 On the pain experience of the tooth caused by placement of initial archwire. Fukuoka ShikaDaigakuGakkaiZasshi17(1): 22-27

[37] Bergius M, Berggren U, Kiliaridis S 2002 Experience of pain during an orthodontic procedure. European Journal of Oral Sciences 110: 92-98

[38] Jones M, Richmond S 1985 Initial tooth movement: force application and pain. A relationship? American Journal of Orthodontics 88: 111-116

[39] Awawdeh LA, Lundy FT, Linden GJ, Shaw C, Kennedy JG, Lamey PJ. (2002) Quantitative analysis of substance P, neurokinin A and calcitonin gene–related peptide in gingival crevicular fluid associated with painful human teeth. Eur J Oral Sci. 110:185-191.

[40] Cerveró F. (1998) El papel de la sustancia P en el dolor. Rev SocEsp Dolor. 5, N.º 4, Julio-Agosto.

[41] Avellán NL, Sorsa T, Tervahartiala T, Forster C, Kemppainen P.(2008) Experimental tooth pain elevates substance P and matrix metalloproteinase-8 levels in human gingival crevice fluid. Acta Odontol Scand.66:18-22.

[42] Stoller NH, Karras DC, Johnson LR. (1990) Reliability of crevicular fluid measurements taken in the presence of supragingival plaque. J Periodontol. 61:670-673.

[43] Griffiths GS, Wilton JM, Curtis MA. (1992) Contamination of human gingival crevicular fluid by plaque and saliva. Arch Oral Biol. 37:559-564.

[44] Hanschke M, Splieth C, Kramer A. (1999) Activities of lysozyme and salivary peroxidase in unstimulated whole saliva in relation to plaque and gingivitis scores in healthy young males. Clin Oral Investig. 3:133-137.

[45] Martin P, D'Aoust P, Landry RG, Valois M. (1994) The reliability of the Periotron 6000 in the presence of plaque. J Can Dent Assoc. 60: 895-898.

[46] Nakashima K, Demeurisse C, Cimasoni G. (1994) The recovery efficiency of various materials for sampling enzymes and polymorphonuclear leukocytes from gingival crevices. J Clin Periodontol. 21:479-483.

[47] Reinhardt RA, Masada MP, Kaldahl WB, DuBois IM, Kornman KS, Choi JI, Kalkwarf KL, Allison AC. (1993) Gingival fluid IL-1, and IL-6 levels in refractory periodontitis. J Clin Periodontol. 20:225-231.

[48] Rossomando EF, Kennedy JE, Hadjimichael J. (1990) Tumor necrosis factor alpha in gingival crevicular fluid as a possible indicator of periodontal disease in humans. Arch Oral Biol.35:431-434.

[49] Atilla G, Kütükçüler N. (1998) Crevicular fluid interleukin-β tumor necrosis factor-α and interleukin-6 levels in renal transplant patients receiving cyclosporine. Am J Periodontol. 69:784-790.

[50] Ataoglu H, Alptekin NÖ, Haliloglu S, Gürsel M, Ataoglu T, Serpek B, Durmus E. (2002) Interleukin-1β tumor necrosis factor-α levels and neutrophil elastase activity in peri-implant crevicular fluid. Clin Oral Implants Res.13:470-476.

[51] Sueda T, Bang J, Cimasoni G. (1969) Collection of gingival fluid for quantitative analysis. J Dent Res.48: 159.

[52] Grieve III WG, Johnson GK, Moore RN, Reinhardt RA, DuBois LM. (1994) Prostaglandin E (PGE) and interleukin-1 beta (IL-1β) levels in gingival crevicular fluid during human orthodontic tooth movement. Am J Orthod Dentofacial Orthop.105: 369-374.

[53] King GJ, Archer L, Zhou D. (1998) Later orthodontic appliance reacti-vation stimulates immediate appearance of osteoclasts and linear tooth movement. Am J Orthod Dentofacial Orthop. 114; 692-697.

[54] Kanzaki H, Chiba M, Shimizu Y, Mitani H. (2002) Periodontal ligament cells under mechanical stress induce osteoclastogenesis by re-ceptor activator of nuclear factor kB ligand up-regulation via prostaglandin E2 synthesis. J Bone Miner Res. 17; 210-220.

[55] Saito S, Ngan P, Saito MJ, Lanese R, Shanfeld J, Davidovitch Z. (1990) Interactive effects between cytokines on PGE production by human periodontal ligament fibroblasts in vitro. J Dent Res. 69:1456-1462.

[56] Hanioka T, Takaya K, Matsumori Y, Matsuse R, Shizukusihi S. (2000) Relationship of the substance P to indicators of host response in human gingival crevicular fluid. J Clin Periodontol. 27: 262-266.

[57] Yao YL, Feng XP, Jing XZ. (2003) The correlation between tooth pain and bioactivators changes in gingival crevicular fluid after applying orthodontic stress. Shanghai Kou Qiang Yi Xue. 12: 331-333.

Advances in Radiographic Techniques Used in Dentistry

Zühre Zafersoy Akarslan and Ilkay Peker

1. Introduction

Conventional radiographic techniques have been used in dental radiography since the discovery of the x-rays. With the revolution in electronic systems, equipment's have been produced to achieve a radiographic image in a digital format. Digital images are in numeric format and differ from conventional radiographs in terms of pixels, and the different shades of gray given to these pixels [1].

A digital image is produced by analog-to-digital conversion (ADC). First, the small ranges of voltage values in the signal are grouped together as a single value. Second, every sampled signal is assigned a value and stored in the computer. Last, the computer organizes the pixels in their proper locations and displays a shade of gray corresponding the number assigned and the image becomes visible on the computer screen [1].

Two dimensional and three dimensional digital imaging modalities have been developed for dentomaxillofacial diagnosis, treatment planning and several clinical applications. These modalities consist of digital intraoral imaging, digital panoramic and cephalometric imaging and cone-beam computed tomography.

The knowledge of advances regarding radiographic techniques and proper use of them gives the opportunity to the practitioner for improvement in diagnostic tasks and treatment planning. Therefore, the aim of this chapter is to focus on the requirements, applications, advantages and disadvantages and artifacts of the currently available digital imaging techniques according to the literature.

2. Two dimensional digital imaging in dentistry

Two dimensional imaging is an adjunct of clinical examination in dentistry. It has an important role in the diagnosis of dental pathologies and treatment planning.

Two dimensional imaging could be broadly categorized as intraoral and extraoral imaging. Intraoral imaging includes periapical, bitewing and occlusal projections, while extraoral imaging includes panoramic and cephalometric projections. These both were acquired with conventional radiography; which is a technique using films, cassettes and wet film processing for long time, but nowadays with the introduction of digital systems they could be achieved with digital imaging.

Two dimensional digital imaging systems have been considerably improved since their initial introduction. This improvement in type, size, shape, radiation effective dose, and resolution of the sensors made them to be adopted in routine use in dental clinics [2,3]. The diagnostic performance of two dimensional digital imaging systems was found to be comparable with conventional radiography. Studies reported the usefulness of digital imaging in caries diagnosis [4-6], periodontal bone defects [7-9], endodontic applications and diagnosis of periapical lesions [10,11], root fractures [12] and root resorption [13,14].

2.1. Digital intraoral imaging

Digital intraoral imaging could be achieved by periapical, bitewing and occlusal projections. Periapical images show the crown and root of the investigated tooth/teeth and some of the surrounding structures. It is useful in dentistry as it shows the entire image of tooth/teeth, periapical region and some of the surrounding structures. Bitewing images show only the crown of the tooth/teeth and part of the root(s), but allow the visualization of both the maxillary and mandibular teeth crowns and alveolar crest in one image. Occlusal images show the palate and the floor of the oral cavity and a larger area of teeth and surrounding structures compared to periapical and bitewing projections. Assessment of bucco-lingual direction of interested regions is also possible with the cross-sectional occlusal technique. It is useful for the examination of the palate and floor of mouth and for the anterior teeth when patients are unable to open their mouth wide enough for the placement of receptors in periapical projections. Although two dimensional intraoral digital imaging is useful and has several advantages, the superimposition of unwanted structures is the main problem in capable of decision-making for correct diagnosis and treatment planning [15].

Intraoral digital imaging could be achieved with indirect, semi-direct and direct digital intraoral techniques. The dentists should have knowledge about the requirements, advantages and disadvantages of these systems in detail to maximize benefits and safe use of the systems.

Indirect Digital Intraoral Imaging: In this method, conventional radiographs (analog images) are transferred to digital medium with the aid of a flatbed scanner with a transparency adapter, a slide scanner and a digital camera. It is a simple way to obtain a digital image and it is less expensive compared to semi-direct and direct digital systems. This technique was used more commonly at the beginning of digital image acquisition. With the improvement and widespread of other digital techniques, it has lost its popularity nowadays [16].

Semi-Direct Digital Intraoral Imaging: Semi-direct digital intraoral imaging is possible with a system using photo-stimulable phosphor coated plates (PSP) (Figure 1). These plates are placed in the mouth of the patient and exposed to x-rays. After the exposure, they are scanned with a special laser scanner system and the latent image becomes visible on the computer monitor [17]. The latent image is erased by exposing the plates with bright light prior to a new x-ray exposure after the plates are scanned [18,19].

The plates should not be exposed to light because this will release some of the energy captured by the plate before it is scanned and degrade the quality of the radiographic image. Hence, the plates exposed to x-ray should be kept in subdued light environment prior to scanning. [18]

Different types of scanners are present. Some of the scanners scan only one plate in each step, and other are capable of scanning more than one at each scan. [19] Scanning time also differ among modalities from 4 seconds to several minutes and according to the spatial and contrast resolution of the image.

Similar to films used in conventional radiography there are different sizes of plates, including child size, adult size, adult bitewing size and occlusal size and they can be used with the film holders used in conventional radiography [20].

Semi-direct digital imaging is a more comfortable technique for patients' compared to direct digital intraoral imaging as the plates' are flexible to some extent and the size, shape and thickness are similar to films used in conventional radiography [21].

Direct Digital Intraoral Imaging: Direct digital intraoral images could be achieved with solid-state sensors. There are two types of solid state-sensors; charged-coupled device (CCD) and complementary metal oxide semiconductor (CMOS).

CCD sensors: A solid state silicon chip is used to record the image in this technology. Silicon crystals convert absorbed radiation to light and the electrons constitutes the latent image according to the light intensity. This signal is sent to the computer with a cable connecting the sensor and the computer, and the image becomes visible on the screen (Figure 2) [1,19].

CMOS sensors: This technology was adapted to intraoral digital imaging after the CCD sensors were invented. These sensors have a similar working principle with CCD, only the chip design differ in terms of integration of the control circuitry directly into the sensor [16]. CMOS sensors are less expensive than CCD's [1]. Initial CMOS systems had a cable connected to the sensor and computer, but nowadays cable-free type is also produced. In cable-free type, the radiographic data stored in the chip are transferred to the computer in radio-waves with the aid of a stationary radio-wave receiver connected to the computer. The manufactures instruction recommends the distance between the sensor and this receiver should not be more than 180cm, but in a study it was reported that this distance could be more than this, but should not exceed 350cm [22].

2.2. Digital extraoral imaging

The revolution in digital extraoral radiography includes digital panoramic imaging and digital cephalometric imaging. Digital extraoral and panoramic systems have not been widely adopted since their first introduction in the dental market (Figure 3). This was due to their very high costs. Sometime after their invention, relatively cost effective systems with improved computer settings (computer speed, data storage capacities) have been manufactured and they

(a)   (b)

(c)

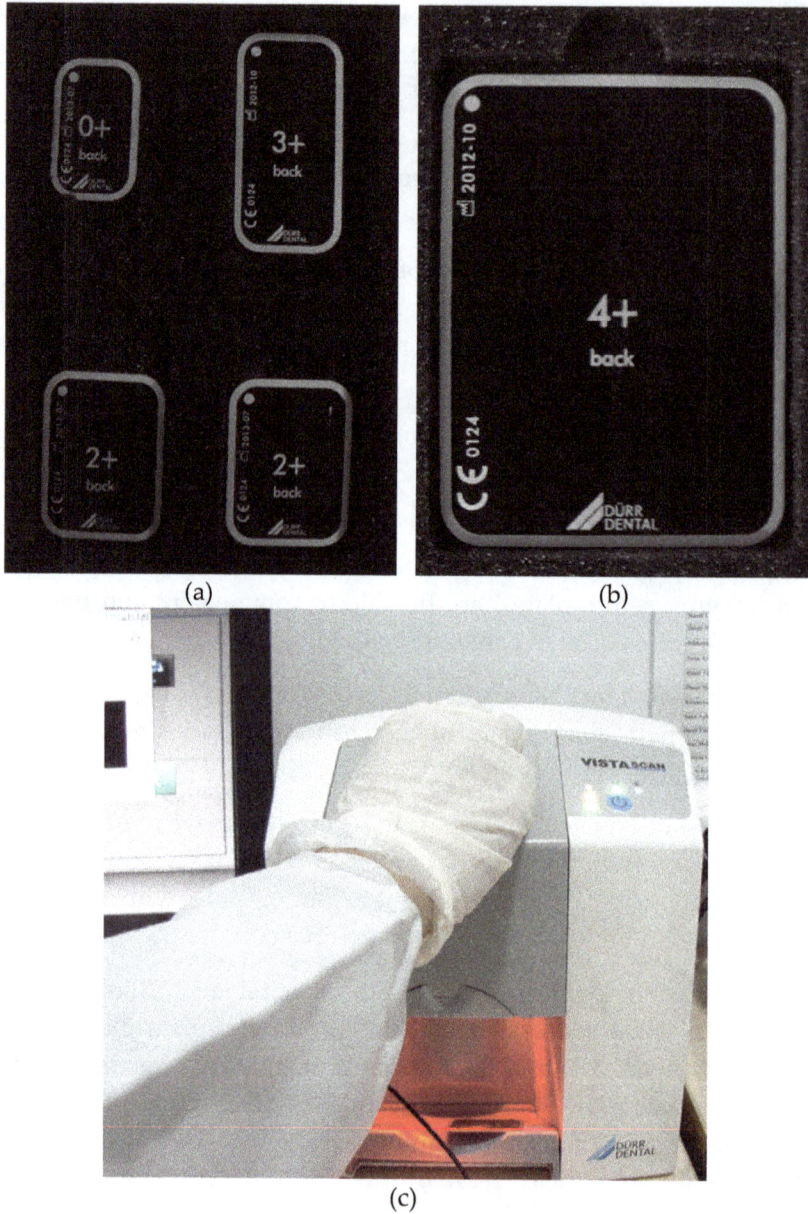

Figure 1. PSP plates (a,b) and plate scanning system (c)

have been started to be adopted in dental practice [23]. The image quality of direct digital panoramic images has been reported to be equal to conventional panoramic radiographs [24].

Panoramic radiography has been one of the most common imaging method among dentists. This technique provides facial structures that includes both maxillary and mandibular teeth and their supporting structures to be imaged on a single film with a single exposure. It is simple and could be applied in cases when mouth opening is not enough to place an intraoral receptor, and an extreme gag reflex (Figure 4) [25].

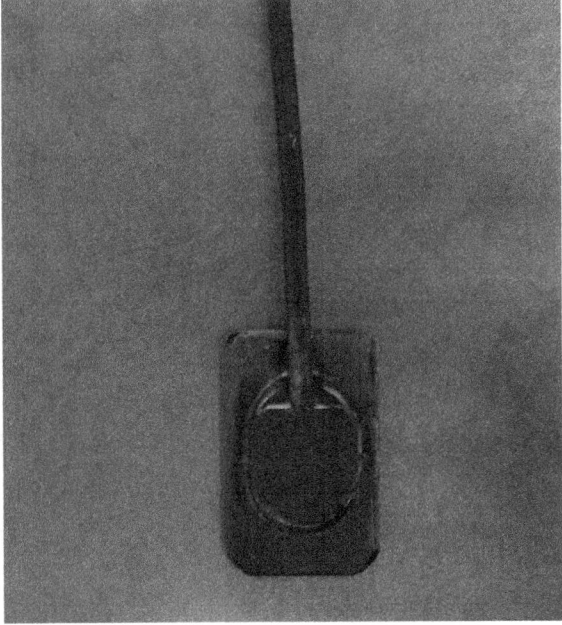

Figure 2. Cabled CCD sensor

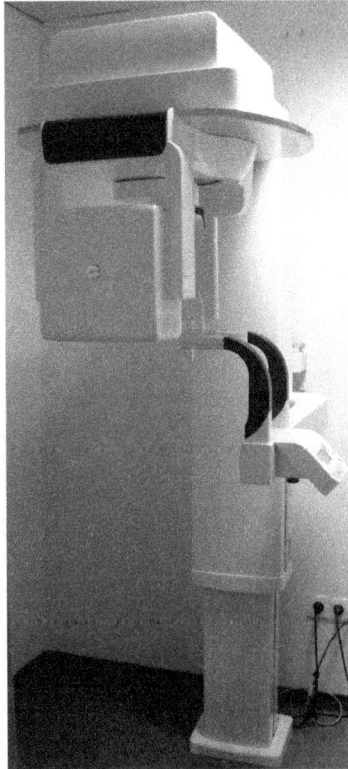

Figure 3. A digital panoramic unit

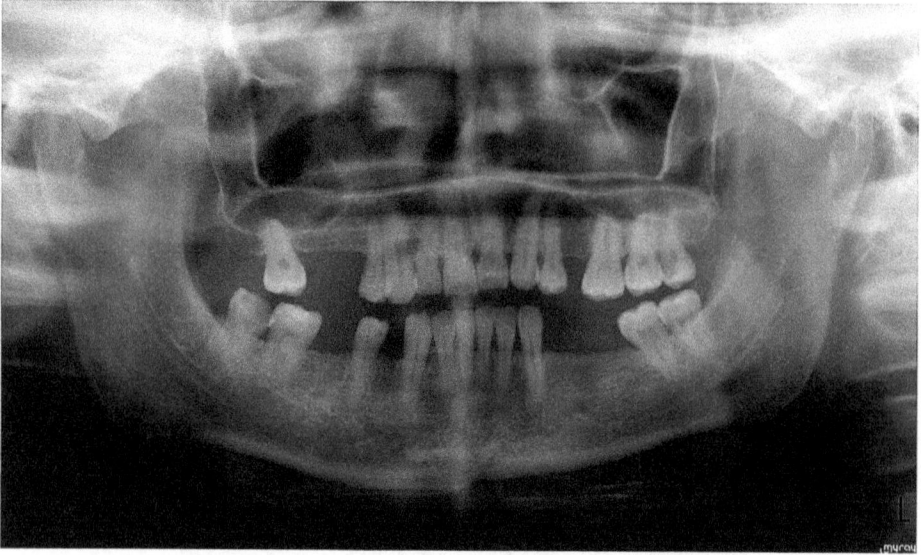

Figure 4. An example of digital panoramic image

Similar to panoramic imaging the same revolution took place in cephalometric radiography. Cephalometric radiography is a technique providing the image of the head in lateral and posterioanterior view (Figure 5). It is frequently used by orthodontists as a treatment planning tool. Some manufacturers made special digital units with a cephalometric attachment to allow exposure of standardized skull views. Digital cephalometric images make it possible to perform cephalometric analysis and superimposition on chair side computer, enhancement of the images for further aid in diagnosis, ease of storage and data transmission [26].

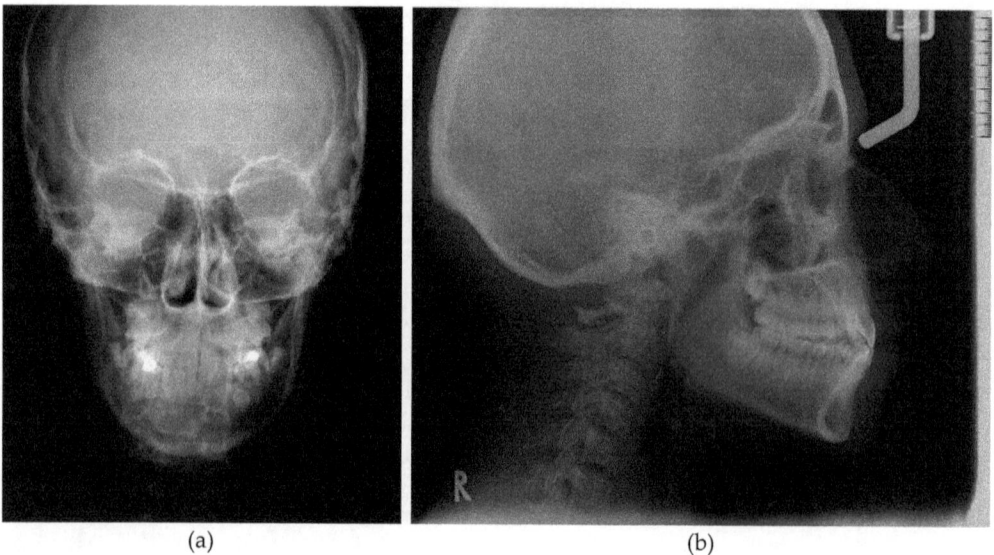

(a)   (b)

Figure 5. Digital posterioanterior (a) and lateral cephalometric image (b)

CCD sensor and PSP plate technology have been used in panoramic and cephalometric devices to capture the image. Compared with digital intraoral sensors, CCD's used in extraoral imaging contains more quantity of pixels to make the image wide and long compared with intraoral imaging. In panoramic units, the CCD is placed opposite to the x-ray source and the long axis of the array is oriented to the x-ray beam. The mechanics used for digital panoramic machine is similar to conventional technique however, it differs for cephalometric imaging. A CCD receptor in a size which could completely take the image of the skull simultaneously is very expensive; therefore to reduce the cost a different mechanic was constructed. In this system, a linear CCD array and a slit shaped x-ray beam with a scanning motion is present and this provides scanning of the skull in short time. The disadvantage of this mechanic is the increased possibility of patient movement artifacts during scanning [1].

2.3. Advantages and disadvantages of two dimensional digital imaging in comparison with conventional radiography

Digital intraoral and extraoral systems have some advantages and disadvantages compared with conventional radiographic techniques. Recently, with the routine use of these systems some aspects which were stated to be advantages initially have been started to be questioned also.

Image enhancement: Image enhancement is the improvement of the original image to make the image visually more appealing. This could be both applied to digital intraoral and extraoral images. Image enhancement could be made by adjusting the contrast and brightness, applying various filters to reduce unsharpness and noise and zooming the image [27].

Radiographic contrast describes the range of densities on a radiograph. It is defined as the differences in densities between light and dark regions [15]. First generation digital sensors performed suboptimal images in terms of contrast and spatial resolution. This has been improved with the new detector technology [2]. The resultant image of an underexposed or overexposed digital detector could be corrected in terms of density and contrast. This especially helps to prevent the retakes due to improper contrast and density [28]. It was reported that contrast enhancement was useful for the detection of low contrast objects both in solid-state and PSP systems [29] and contrast and brightness-enhanced digital images enabled better signal detection and showed a comparable performance with film for detection of artificially induced recurrent caries [30].

There are various filters in each system which could be applied to the digital images for image enhancement. In general, there are filters which sharpen, smooth and emboss the image [31] Filters that smooth the image remove high frequency noise. Filters that sharpen the images either remove low frequency noise or enhance boundaries between regions with different intensities. (edge enhancement) [1]. Filters that emboss the image make it appear as an image with depth. This is named as "3D" in some software's as the resultant image resembles a three dimensional image. It was reported that filtration of a digital panoramic image with the emboss filter may have a value in detecting approximal caries especially in the mandibular molar region [31] and the sharpen filter may be useful for detecting subtle approximal caries [32].

However, controversial results were reported also. Digitally enhanced images with sharpness, zoom and pseudocolour were found not to be effective for the detection of occlusal caries [33].

Image processing is task dependent. Filters should be applied in special cases and they should be used properly and carefully by the clinicians. An edge enhancement filter could be useful for marginal bone height measurements around implants [29] while, it may not improve the level of accuracy for cephalometric points detection [34].

A study demonstrated digital image magnification at X3, X6 and X12 had a significant influence on observer performance in the detection of approximal caries but magnification over these values reduced the diagnostic accuracy [35]. In another study, it was reported that three digital magnifications; 1 : 1, 2 : 1, and 1 : 2 did not affect the detection of root fractures [36].

The operator should be very careful during image enhancement, because inaccurate application of these functions may lead to inaccurate diagnosis of pathology! [1]

Image analysis: Image analysis functions help to obtain diagnostically relevant information from the image. Linear, curved and angle measurements, area calculation, densitometric analysis, complex tools and procedures are present in this extent. Simple linear, curved and angle measurements, area calculation and densitometric analysis functions are generally present in the software of digital imaging devices, but complex tools and procedures require special software [1].

Measurements can be performed with a special digital ruler and are expressed as pixels and in millimeters or inches in digital images. The operator could measure something with the aid of the electronic ruler by drawing lines or curves with the cursor. If the measurement is going to be expressed as pixels the detector should be exposed with an object with known dimensions for the conversation of the pixels into real length [19]. It was reported that radiographic measurements of bone height around implants in images obtained from a PSP system was accurate and precise as much as conventional radiographs [29].

Computer aided cephalometric analysis is faster in data acquisition and analysis than conventional radiographic techniques. Special programs have been developed to perform computer aided cephalometric analysis directly on the screen displayed images. This could reduce the potential errors occurring form digitizing of the radiographs and the need of hardcopies. [37, 38] The reliability of landmark identification and linear and angular measurements in conventional and digital lateral cephalometry was found to be comparable with each other, but all landmarks were not accurately identified in both techniques [39]. A software developed for quantitative analysis of cervical vertebrae maturation was found to be useful [40].

Decrease in radiographic working time: CCD and CMOS sensors provide an important decrease in radiographic working time, especially for radiographic evaluation during endodontic treatment or surgical procedures. Reduction in radiographic working time differs among sensors and plates. Images with sensors are obtained simultaneously after the exposure on the screen, but the PSP plates require an additional scanning procedure after exposure and this increases working time. Working time differ between cable-free and cabled sensors. Cable-free sensors require less time compared with cabled sensors [20,22,41].

Ease in archiving and electronically transmission of the images: Images can be easily archived in digital medium and can be electronically transferred to other clinics or for consultation without any impairment in the image quality by web or CD, flash disk etc. in a very short time and little effort. In addition, other operators have the chance to enhance the image when required [1, 26].

Elimination of film processing step and hazardous wastes: One of the important advantages of digital systems is the elimination of a dark room, film processing equipment's and hazardous wastes such as processing chemicals, lead foil present in the film package and rare earth products in extraoral film cassettes [1,26,27].

In direct digital panoramic and cephalometric imaging the step of inserting and removing a film in cassette in a dark room is eliminated. Besides, the elimination of film processing step puts away the artifacts due to improper processing which could be a reason for retakes of radiographs both in digital intraoral and extraoral radiology [1].

Radiation dose: It was suggested that direct digital intraoral systems [1,26,42,43,44] and direct digital cephalometric systems require less radiation dose to obtain an image compared with conventional film in the first presentation of the systems [45,46].

The radiation dose required for CCD and CMOS sensors for a single exposure is lower compared to that of films. PSP plates require less radiation exposure than conventional film while, they require higher radiation dose compared with CCD and CMOS sensors [1].

The active imaging area of CCD and CMOS sensors are smaller than films thus, they do not show the same number of teeth or area [20]. According to a study additional retakes of images due to placement errors compared with films were higher in these sensors as they have a smaller active imaging area [47]. Therefore the number of images required for the radiographic examination of the same region increases. Due to these factors the effect in radiation dose decrease in sensor systems may be speculated [20].

The dynamic range of the sensors is lower from the PSP plates. This means that, the quality of the image decrease in systems using sensors when overexposed, however, the quality remains unchanged even at overexposure of the PSP plates. This could be an advantage for decreasing the retakes, but a disadvantage which may result in unnecessary high patient radiation dose [48].

Disadvantages

Cost: The cost of shifting from film based systems to digital intraoral and extraoral systems is very expensive [1,26]. This leads to a decrease in the popularity of these systems especially in countries having low income rates.

Lack in cross infection control: Compared with films, the sensors and plates used in digital imaging are not disposable and could not be sterilized thus; special attention is required for infection control. The sensors and plates could be covered with a special film protecting cover, traditional plastic sheaths or latex finger cots. The traditional plastic sheath covering the sensor during exposure was found to leak in some cases [49] and although latex finger cot stretched over the sensor resulted in less contamination it did not fully eliminate the risk [50]. Therefore, authors suggested the use of both a plastic sheath and a latex finger cot especially during invasive procedures [20,49,50].

Wiping the plates covered with a special plastic cover with soap or alcohol before placing in the scanner was reported as a useful method in disinfection control [21,51].

Structures of sensors and plates: CCD and CMOS sensors are thicker and stiff than conventional films and the patients feel more uncomfortable during the radiographic process compared with film. Besides, the cable attached to the sensor makes sensor placement in the oral cavity difficult [1,22,52].

PSP plates are similar to films in terms of dimension and thickness. Reports indicated that PSP plates were more tolerable by both adult [21] and pediatric patients than sensors [53] Although PSP plates are similar to films some kinds of plastic envelopes used for covering the plates have sharp edges, and their corners could not be bent. This leads to difficulty during placement of the plates in the oral cavity and the patients may feel uncomfortable [20].

Physical damage could occur if the patient bites the cable of the CCD and CMOS sensors and PSP plates. In addition PSP plates are prone to damage if they are dropped to floor, bended, and scratched. Mechanical wear and trauma influences the life span of the plates and sensors. This affects the cost-effectiveness of these systems compared with conventional radiography [20].

It is not possible to distinguish images from plates that have been exposed backward in most PSP systems [1,26]. One manufacturer has developed a PSP system with a metal disk present on the hard cover which protects the plates. In the case of opposite insertion of the plate, this object becomes visible on the radiographic image.

Ability of manipulation of the images for fraudulent purposes: Digital technology also brings the capability of manipulation of the original image. This is an important issue for legal purposes. Manufacturers are developing systems which keep the original of the image obtained subsequently after x-ray exposure. With this security key if anyone alters the contrast, density and other characteristics of the image, it is possible to acquire the original data. Thus if one could show the source of the original data these images are considered to be reliable [19,54].

2.4. Artifacts in two dimensional digital imaging

The term artifact describes any distortion or error in the image that is unrelated to the subject being studied [55]. Image artifacts decrease the rate of accurate diagnosis and treatment planning. Additionally, radiographic retakes cause unnecessary radiation dose exposure to patients, clinicians, radiology staff and the environment, as well as the loss of time and money [56]. These are going to be presented as artifacts in intraoral digital imaging and digital panoramic imaging in this section.

2.4.1. Artifacts in digital intraoral imaging

Although image artifacts in film-based radiography are well-known, digital radiography, like any emerging technology, produces new and different challenges. Thus, knowing the reasons of image artifacts is very important for the clinicians [57]. The artifacts of digital imaging can be categorized in three parts: **I)** Operator artifacts during exposed image receptors **II)** Image processing artifacts: and **III)** Defective sensor artifacts

I) Operator artifacts during exposed image receptors

Cone-cut image: It is resulted from improper alignment of the position-indicating device; partial image occurs.

Distorted images: These artifacts occur because bending of phosphor plates during intraoral placement [1].

Double images: It appears due to incomplete erasure of previous image in PSP plates.

Underexposed images: This could be related with i) placement of the opposite side of the PSP plate facing the x-ray tube, ii) noisy images and iii) overlapped sensor plate images.

Opposite side of the sensor plate wrongly placed facing the x ray tube: This is a significant problem for most phosphor plate systems due to backward placement of the phosphor plate in the mouth cannot be distinguished from correct placement. The images have little x-ray attenuation from the polyester base when exposed backward [1]. On the other hand, very few manufacturers had placed a metal disc back of the sensor plates to distinguish by the clinician.

The sensor plate wrongly placed in protector envelope.

Noisy images: It appears as a result of excessive exposure to ambient light between image acquisition and scanning [1].

Overlapped sensor plate images: It appears when plates are overlapped before scanning.

II) Image processing artifacts: This type of artifacts can be corrected thorough rescanning by another scanner without the need to retakes [57].

a. Incorrect usage of image processing tools: This type of artifact occurs form incorrect use of filters [1].

b. The artifacts resulting from image scanning resolution: Scanning under the 300 dpi causes lack of detail [1].

c. Undefined image artifacts [57].

The image of a horizontal white line after scanning

Brightness of images although scanning with optimal conditions and procedures

Half images after scanning

Reduction of the image size

Overlapped images after scanning of two different intraoral sensor plates in two different slots.

III) Defective sensor artifacts [1].

The image artifact resulting from scratching or biting mark.

The image artifact resulting from partial peeling of the coating of the intraoral sensor plate.

The image artifact resulting from surface contamination by glove powder smudging.

Geometric image artifacts resulting from mishandling of CCD sensors.

Examples of intraoral image artifacts are presented in Figure 6-13.

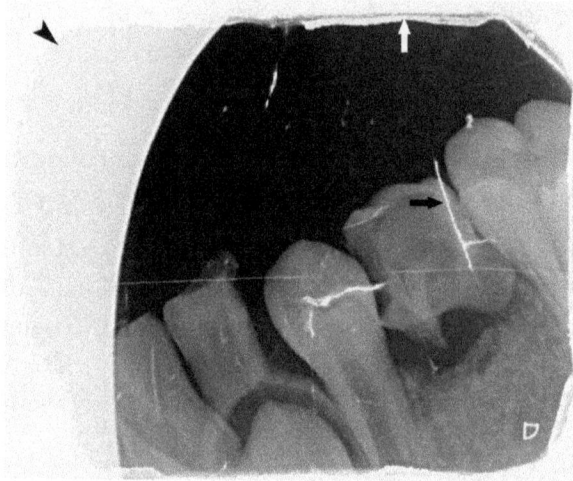

Figure 6. Cone-cut image (black arrowhead), the image artifact resulting from excessive bending of the plate within the mouth (black arrow) and image artifact resulting from partial peeling of the coating of the plate (white arrow).

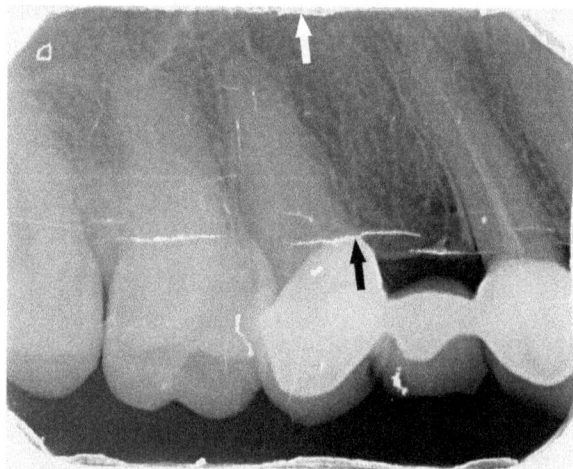

Figure 7. The image artifact resulting from excessive bending of the plate within the mouth (black arrow) and image artifact resulting from partial peeling of the coating of the plate (white arrow).

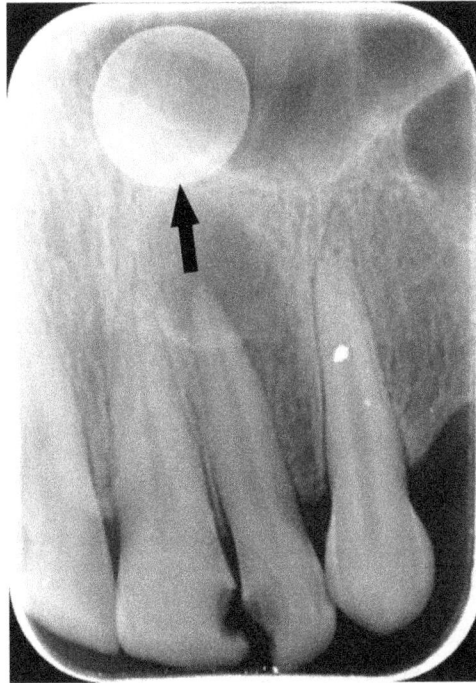

Figure 8. The image of metal disc resulting from opposite insertion of the plate facing the x ray tube (black arrow).

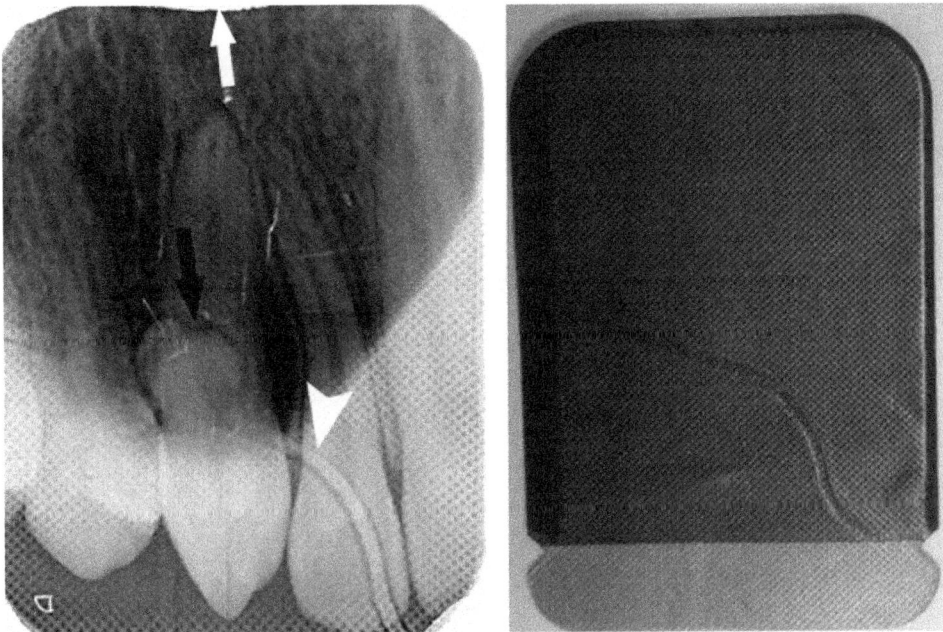

Figure 9. The image artifact resulting from opposite insertion of the plate in protector envelope (white arrowhead) and partial peeling of the coating of the plate (white arrow). Also overlapped sensor plate image is seen. Note the odontoma in the canine region (black arrow).

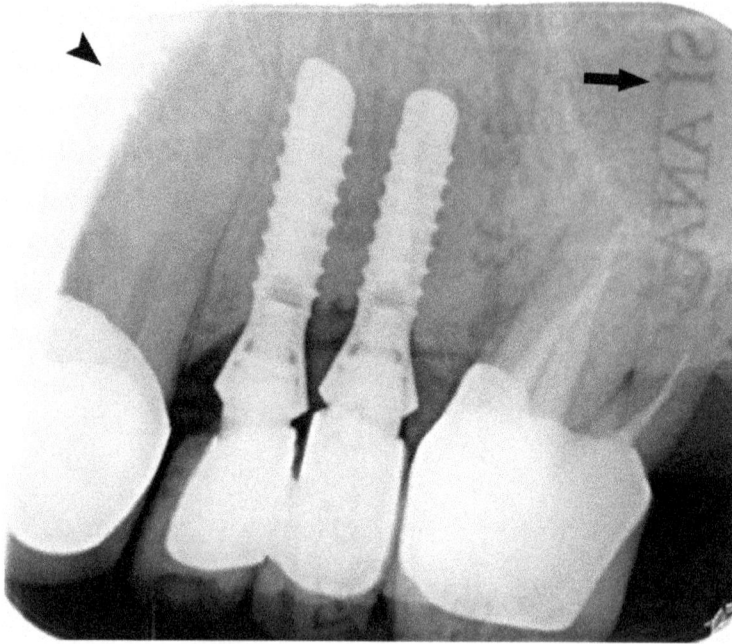

Figure 10. The image artifact resulting from cone-cut (black arrowhead) and image of letters due to contact of plate and letters before scanning (black arrow).

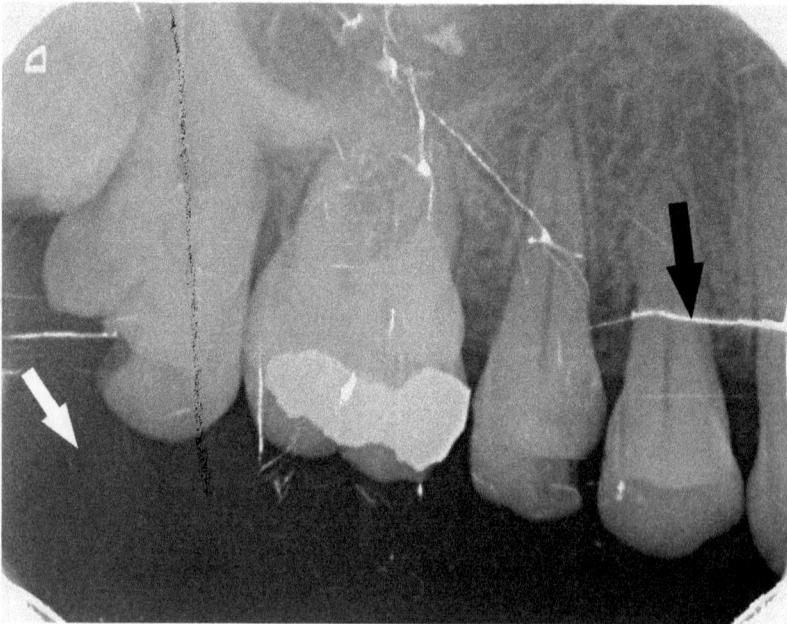

Figure 11. The bright image artifact resulting from non-uniform image density (white arrow), the image artifact resulting from excessive bending of the plate within the mouth (black arrow).

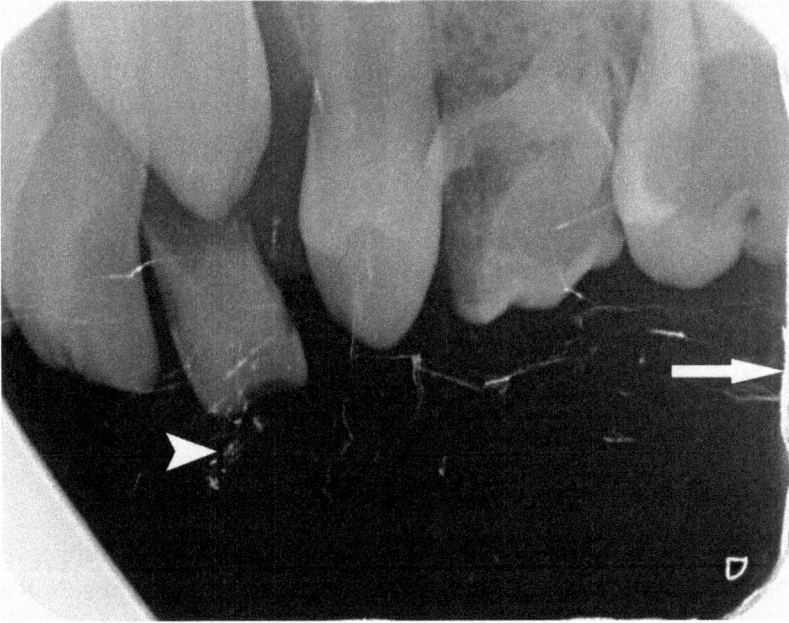

Figure 12. The image artifact resulting from scratching or biting mark the image artifact resulting from excessive bending of the plate within the mouth (white arrowhead) and generalized brightness of the image

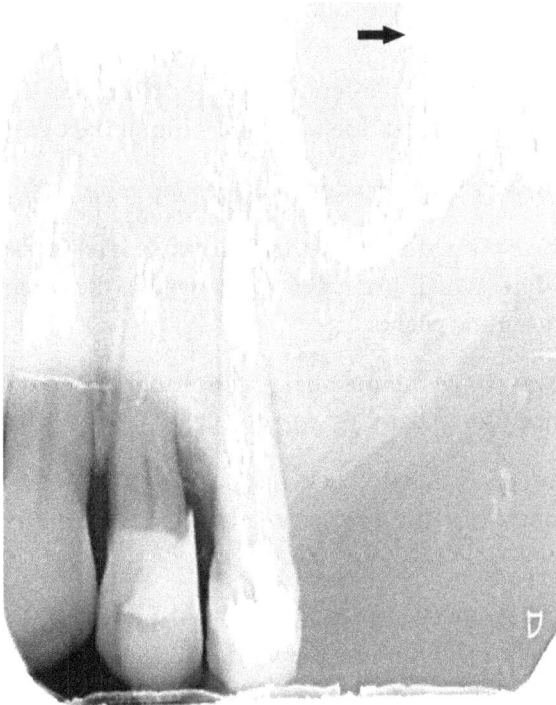

Figure 13. The image artifact resulting from surface contamination by glove powder smudging (black arrow) and image artifact resulting from partial peeling of the coating of the plate (white arrow).

2.4.2. Artifacts in digital panoramic imaging

Artifacts in digital panoramic imaging are similar to the errors occurring in conventional panoramic radiography. One of the advantages of digital panoramic imaging is that errors associated with film radiographs; such as static electricity and image processing are not present as in this technique.

Artifacts could occur due to I)technical errors, II)improper patient positioning and III)during x-ray exposure in digital panoramic imaging [58-60].

i.   **Artifacts due to technical errors**

   1.   Radiopaque artifacts (earrings, necklace, prosthesis, lead apron, spectacles, apron/thyroid shield etc.)

ii.   **Artifacts due to improper patient positioning**

   1.   Occlusal plane rotated downwards, the condyles approaching the upper edge of the image or are cut-off by its upper edge due to chin tipped too low.

   2.   Occlusal plane rotated upwards, the condyles approach the lateral edges of the image or are projected off its edges symmetrically and bilaterally due to chin raised too high.

   3.   Overlapped or unclear appearance of the anterior teeth because of patient not biting on the bite-block

   4.   Narrowed or blurring anterior teeth, superimposition of the spine on the condyles or rami caused due to patients biting the bite-block too far forward.

   5.   Widening of anterior teeth due to the patient biting the bite-block too far back.

   6.   Asymmetrical placement of teeth, the condyle is enlarged and is above the contra lateral condyle, which is smaller and lower in the image due to the rotation of the head in sagittal plane.

   7.   Radiolucency above the maxillary teeth roots due to the patient not raising the tongue against the palate.

   8.   The patient's neck is stretched forward on a slant, vertebral column causing extreme lightness in the anterior region as a result of the superimposed shadow of the spine.

   9.   Superimposition of the hyoid bone with the body of the mandible according to the patient's Frankfurt plane not being parallel to the floor

iii.   **Artifacts occurring during x-ray interpretation**

   1.   Missing or doubled objects or abrupt shifting of image vertically due to the horizontal or vertical movement of the patient during exposure.

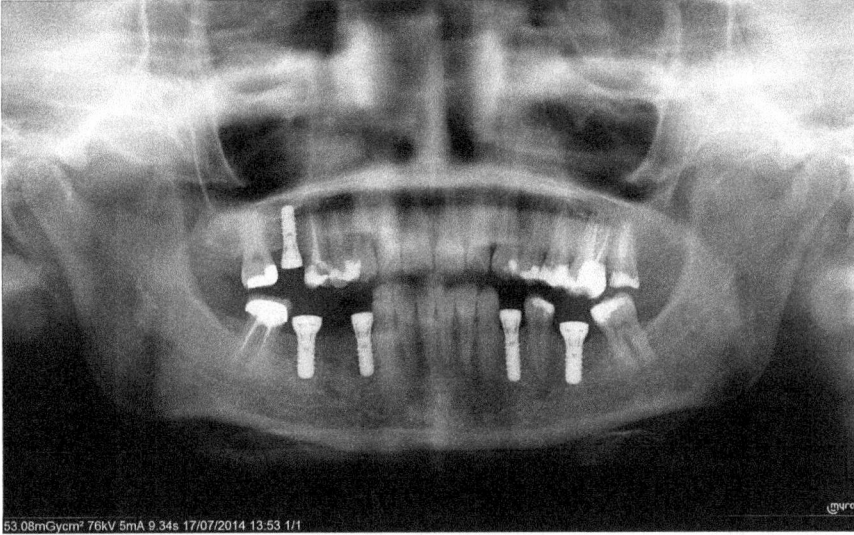

Figure 14. Digital panoramic image demonstrating occlusal plane rotated downwards, the condyles approach the upper edge of the image superimposition of the hyoid bone with the body of the mandible according to the patient's Frankfurt plane not being parallel to the floor.

It was reported that artifacts of digital panoramic images differed between patients with mixed dentition and permanent dentition and more artifacts were seen in permanent dentition. Positioning the patient too forward was seen more common in the mixed dentition. Slumped position and improper chin position were more commonly seen in the permanent dentition. Blurred or shortened upper incisors were more prevalent in the mixed dentition [61]. Training of dental personnel and a discussion of technical measures to be taken if errors occur are essential to maximize the quality of panoramic radiographs [59].

Examples of digital panoramic image artifacts are presented in Figure 14-17.

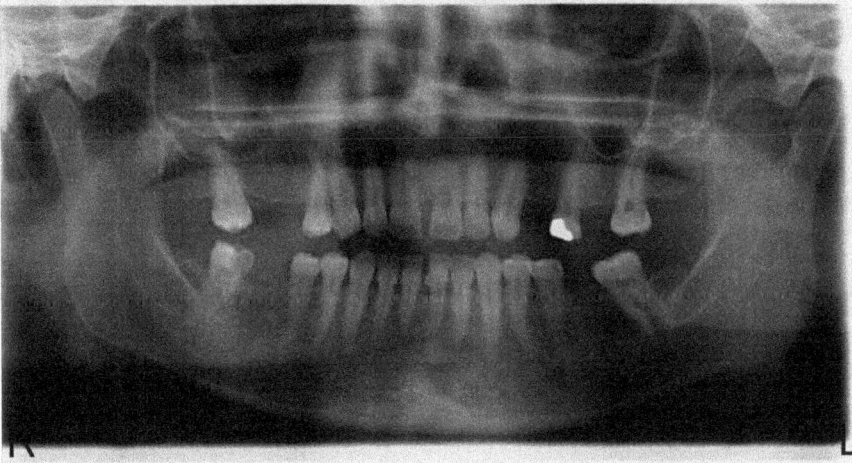

Figure 15. Digital panoramic image demonstrating radiolucency above the maxillary teeth roots due to the patient not raising the tongue against the palate.

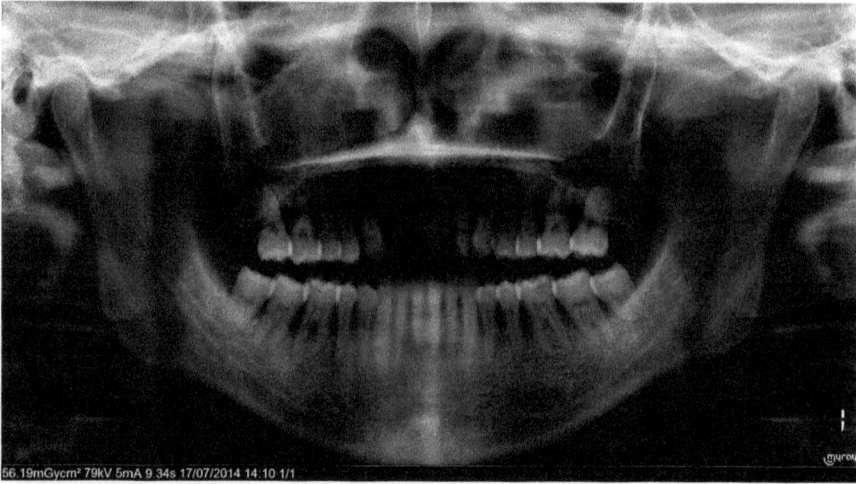

Figure 16. Digital panoramic image demonstrating narrowed anterior teeth, superimposition of the spine on the condyles or rami caused due to patients biting the bite-block too far forward and radiolucency above the maxillary teeth.

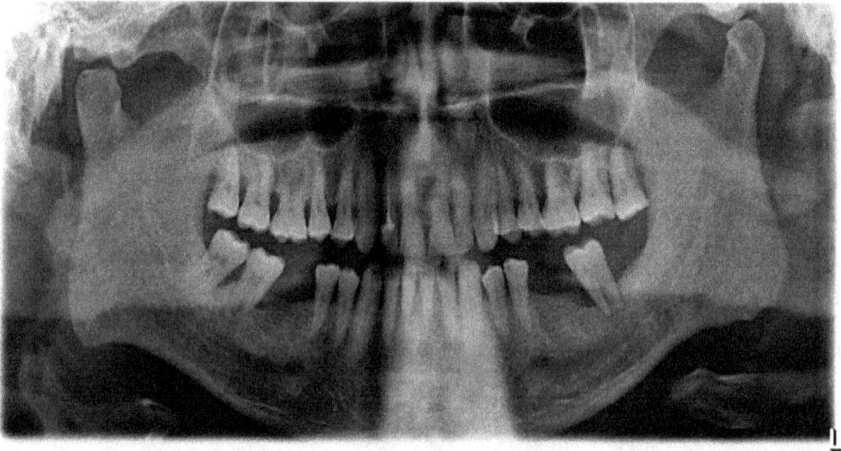

Figure 17. Digital panoramic image demonstrating vertebral column causing extreme lightness in the anterior region as a result of the superimposed shadow of the spine and noisy image.

3. Three dimensional digital imaging in dentistry

Three dimensional imaging gives the opportunity to the practitioner to examine the dento-maxillofacial region without superimposition and distortion of the image. Three dimensional imaging was acquired with conventional tomography [62] and tuned aperture computed tomography techniques in the past years [63] but, with the introduction of cone-beam computed tomography (CBCT) it left its place to this new imaging modality. Details about CBCT technique and its clinical applications are going to be discussed in this section.

3.1. Cone-beam computed tomography

CBCT is a relatively new digital imaging technology. Although, it has been given several names including dental volumetric tomography (DVT), cone beam volumetric tomography (CBVT), dental computed tomography (DCT) and cone beam imaging (CBI), the most preferred name is cone-beam computed tomography (CBCT) [55].

This technique was initially developed for angiography in 1982 and was applied to dental imaging some after. It has the advance of three dimensional imaging of the area of interest without superimposition of other structures. Multiplanar and 3D images could be achieved with this technique with lower radiation dose and higher spatial resolution relative to computed tomography (CT) providing better visualization of structures with mineralized tissue. Although CBCT images have high spatial resolution, the data from which images are created contains considerable noise caused by scattered radiation. Thus, soft tissue contrast in CBCT images is inferior to that in CT images [64]. Another problem which can affect the image quality and diagnostic accuracy of the images is the scatter and beam hardening caused by high density neighboring structures, such as enamel, metal posts and restorations [65].

The CBCT system works with a flat panel detector and special scanner using collimated x-ray source that produces a cone-or pyramid-shaped beam of x-radiation making a single full or partial circular rotation around the head of the patient. A sequence of discrete planar projection images using a digital detector is produced after exposure. Subsequently, these two-dimensional images are reconstructed into a three-dimensional volume [55,66].

Examples of multiplanar and three dimensional CBCT images are presented in Figure 19-22.

Patient positioning differs among CBCT devices (Figure 18). An image could be achieved with the patient seated, standing or supine position. CBCT is not a complex device to use and three dimensional image reconstruction can be made easily with appropriate software [55,67].

Compared with two dimensional imaging, the effective radiation dose can be higher in CBCT depending on the machine, field of view, and the resolution of the image [3,68]. The effective doses for various devices range from 52 to 1025 microsieverts [55]. This is an important issue because all imaging modalities using x-rays for the acquisition of radiographic images rely on a basic principle; 'As Low As Reasonably Possible (ALARA)'. This principle maintains the protection of patients and staff during the acquisition of images. Therefore, the selection criteria of the CBCT examination should weigh potential patient benefits against the risks associated with the level of radiation dose. This could be achieved by appropriate clinical usage and optimizing technical factors such as; using the smallest field of view necessary for diagnostic purposes, and using appropriate personal and patient protective shielding [66,69].

Although dental exposure only contributes a few percent to the populations' total medical exposure, it is curial to adopt certain measures to avoid unnecessary repeated examinations, especially with the advent of CBCT in dentistry [70].

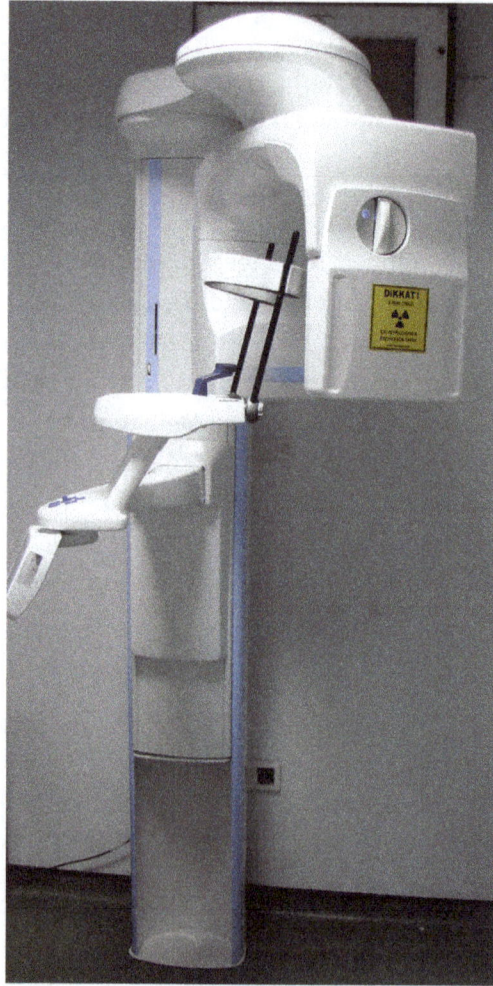

Figure 18. A CBCT unit

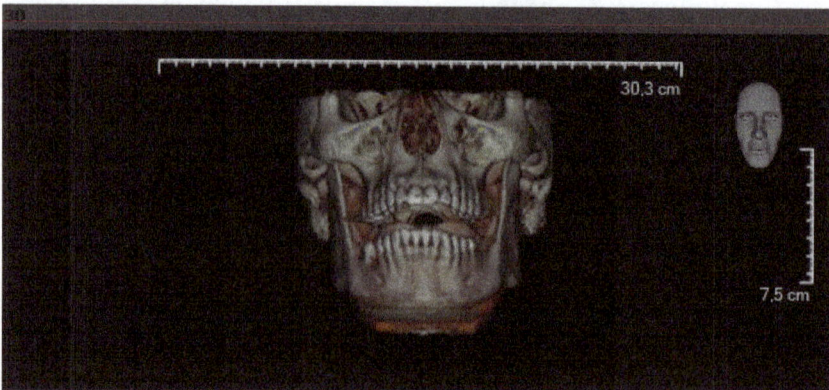

Figure 19. An example of a three dimensional CBCT image

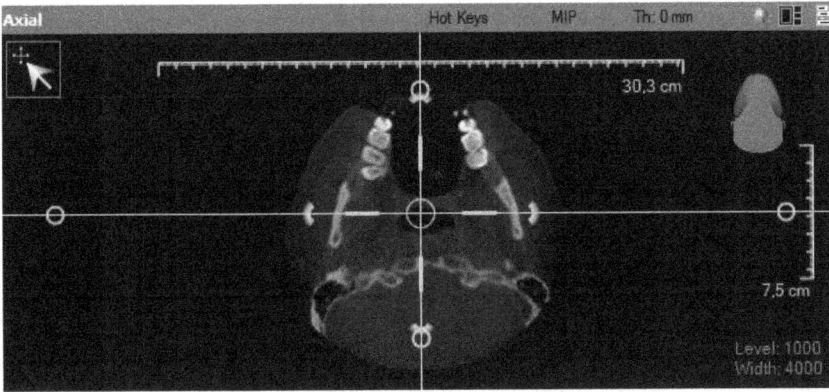

Figure 20. An example of an axial slice of CBCT image

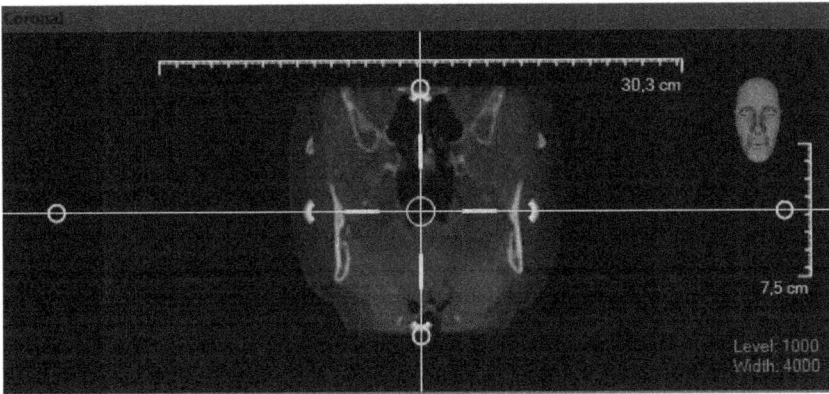

Figure 21. An example of a coronal slice of CBCT image

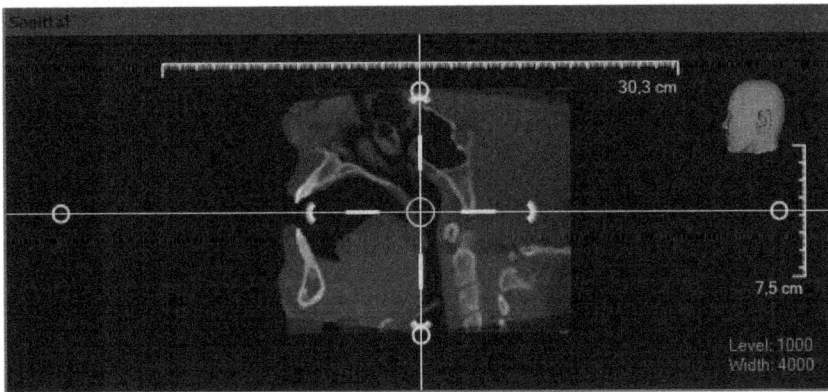

Figure 22. An example of a sagittal slice of CBCT image

3.2. Applications of CBCT in Dentistry

CBCT is used in all areas of dentistry including oral and maxillofacial surgery, orthodontics, pediatric dentistry, periodontology and endodontics. It has been recommended that the use of CBCT could benefit the diagnosis and treatment outcomes for specific cases [55,71].

3.2.1. Oral and maxillofacial surgery

Radiographic methods for the assessment of bone quantity and quality are traditionally used in preoperative planning of dental implant placement. The American Academy of Oral and Maxillofacial Radiology (AAOMR) recommended the evaluation of a potential implant site should include cross-sectional imaging, orthogonal to the site of interest [72]. CBCT is one of the techniques which could be used for cross sectional imaging orthogonal to the site of interest. It is a popular method of planning dental implant placement [73]. It provides the visualization of the alveolar bone height, width and buccolingual dimensions and spatial localization of the neighboring anatomic structures, such as inferior alveolar canal, incisive canal and maxillary sinus. Accurate measurements could be performed directly, as the images are free from distortion however; errors in patient positioning can lead to alterations in these distances. It was concluded that improper patient positioning led to imprecise measurements of bone height and width, which may cause damage to anatomical structures [74].

In addition to implant site assessment, CBCT is used in the pre-surgical evaluation of impacted teeth, supernumerary teeth, and relationship of the inferior alveolar canal to the roots of mandibular third molars, lesions localized on the jaws, osteomyelitis, and osteonecrosis etc. This will benefit to the maxillofacial surgeon to visualize the accurate location of the pathology and its relationship with adjacent structures and important anatomical landmarks [55,75].

Maxillofacial fractures could be also diagnosed with CBCT, but the limits and thus an indication for medical computed tomography exist where there is extensive fractures with suspicion of craniocerebral trauma [76].

Degenerative pathologies or abnormalities in the bony structures of temporomandibular joint, such as cortical erosion, condylar sclerosis and/or articular eminence, articular surface flattening, presence of osteophytes and ankylosis can also be visualized with CBCT [55].

Examples of CBCT images acquired for a radiolucent lesion (Figure 23), preoperative implant planning (Figure 24), TMJ (Figure 25) and a fracture in the mandible (Figure 26).

3.2.2. Orthodontics and pediatric dentistry

Radiographic assessment has always been an important aspect in orthodontics for diagnosis and treatment planning. Two dimensional radiographic techniques have been used for a long time but it has some well documented limitations such as magnification, geometric distortion, superimposition of structures, projective displacements (which may elongate or foreshorten an object's dimensions), rotational errors and linear projective transformation [77,78]. However, CBCT allows for evaluation and analysis of the area of interest without any distortion, magnification and superimposition of other structures.

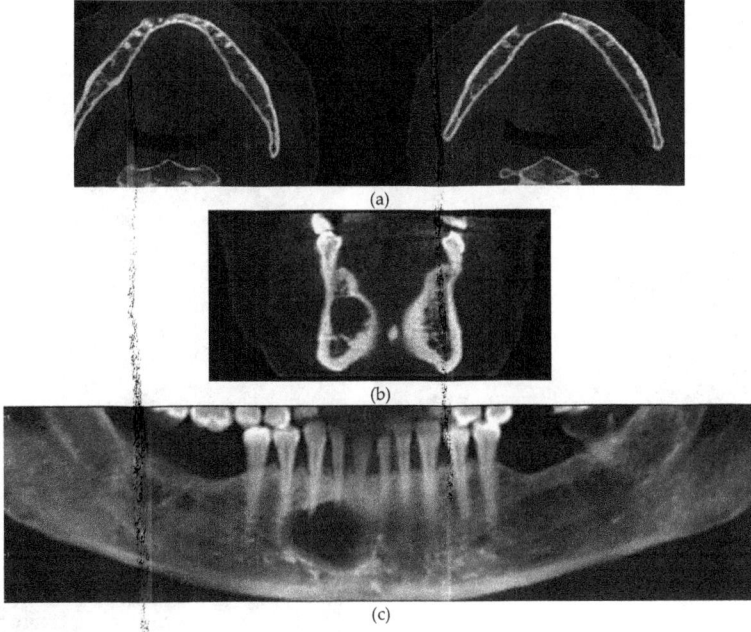

Figure 23. The axial (a), coronal (b) and panoramic (c) CBCT images of a radiolucent lesion seen in the anterior region of the mandible.

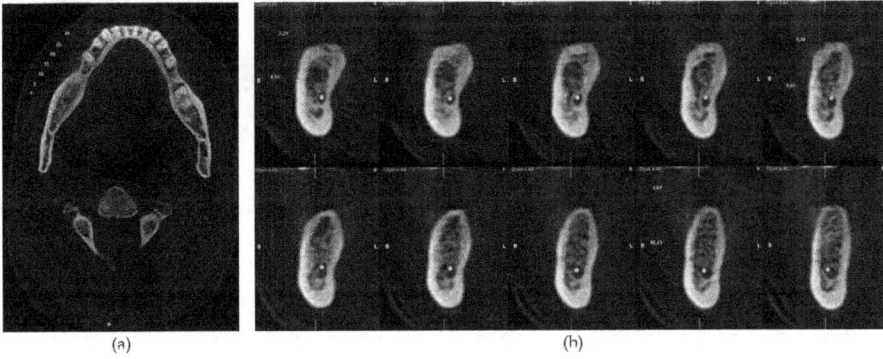

Figure 24. The axial (a) and cross sectional (b) images of a CBCT scan for preoperative implant planning.

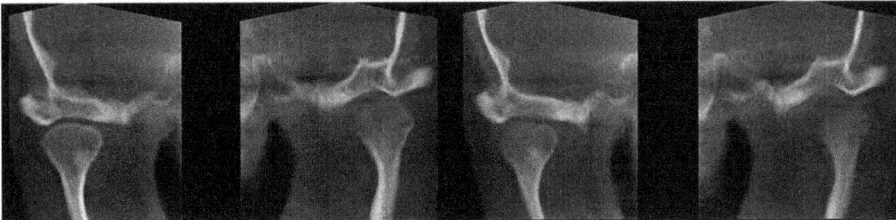

Figure 25. The coronal CBCT images of the TMJ.

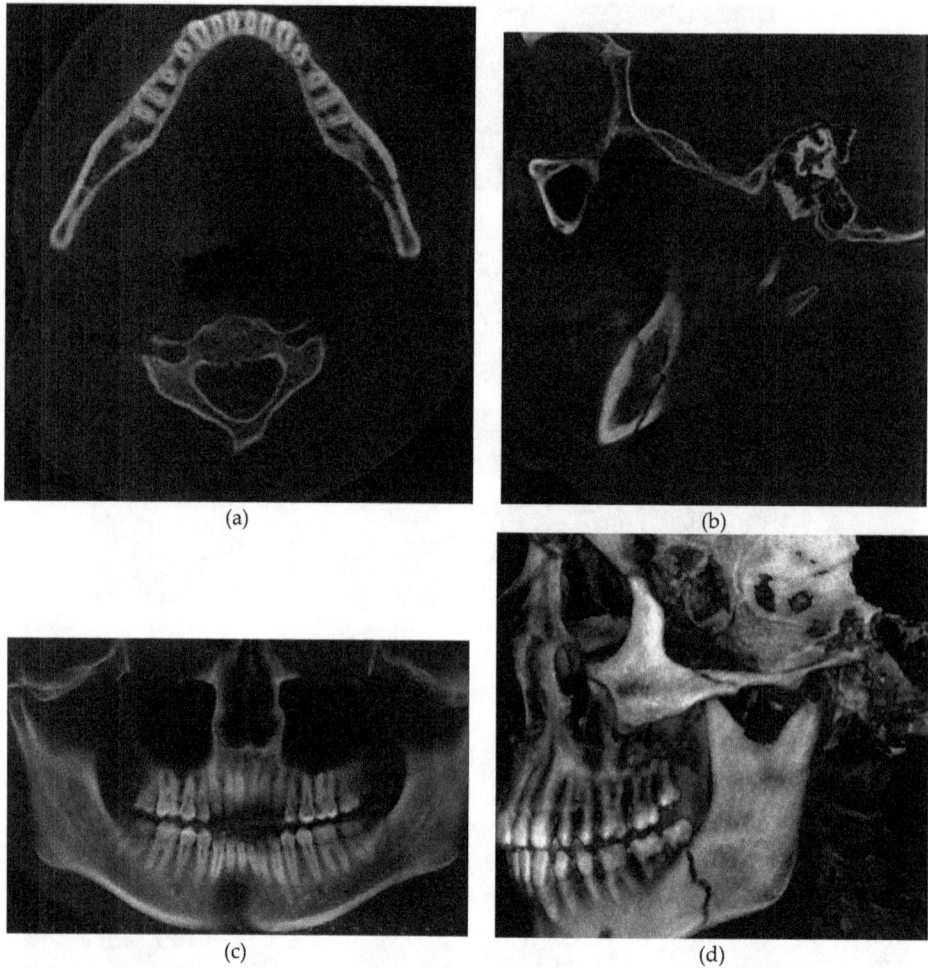

Figure 26. The axial (a), sagittal (b), panoramic (c) and 3D CBCT image (d) of a fracture in the left third molar region in mandible.

It has been suggested that information obtained from a CBCT scan has the potential to improve orthodontic diagnosis and treatment planning in airway analysis before and after orthognathic surgical planning, [79] cleft lip palate [80,81] root position and structure [82] and mini screw placement [83,84].

A study evaluated the impact of CBCT on orthodontic diagnosis and treatment planning and reported the most frequently diagnosis and treatment plan changes occurred in cases of unerupted teeth, severe root resorption, or severe skeletal discrepancies. Contrary, they found no benefit for abnormalities of the temporomandibular joint, airway, or crowding [85].

During the past decade, CBCT imaging has been a popular method in orthodontics, but the disability of showing 'minor external root resorption or not providing treatment at a micro-scopic level' still are disadvantages [86].

An example of CBCT image acquired for cleft palate is presented in Figure 27.

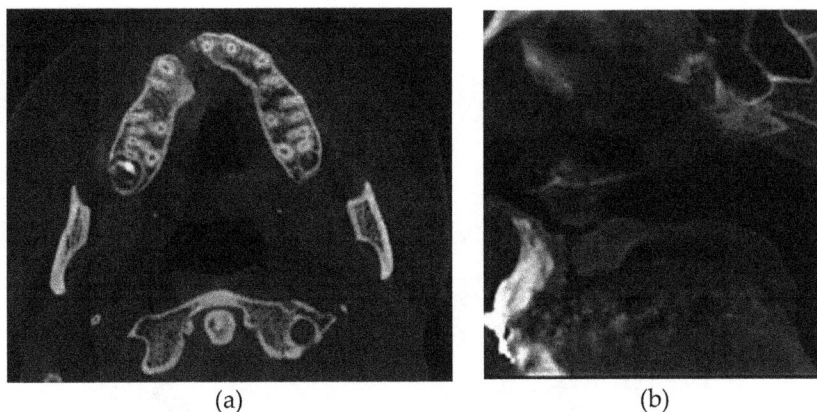

(a)   (b)

Figure 27. The axial (a) and sagittal (b) CBCT images of a cleft palate.

The use of CBCT in pediatric dentistry has been mentioned in the dental literature. A research from Korea demonstrated the most prevalent usage of CBCT among children and adolescents were for diagnosis and monitoring of the growth of cysts and other tumors, following by localization of impacted teeth, and supernumerary teeth [87].

Children are more suspicious to dental trauma on anterior teeth than adults. Thus, teeth fracture is a common sequel. From a database search it was concluded that CBCT was useful in cases in which conventional radiographic techniques yield inconclusive results or showed a fracture in the middle third of a root. CBCT may rule out or confirm an oblique course of fracture involving the cervical third in the labiolingual dimension. Although there are considerable advantages of CBCT in the diagnosis of fractures, more experimental and clinical studies are warranted to determine the exact impact on outcomes [88].

CBCT generates a higher effective radiation dose to the tissues than conventional radiographic techniques. The effective radiation dose should not be underestimated, especially in children, who are much more susceptible to stochastic biological effects [89].

Similar CBCT exposure settings are predicted to result in higher equivalent doses to the head and neck organs in children than in adults. Some CBCT scanners present in the dental market provide a pediatric option to the user. A study evaluated the equivalent radiation doses of two CBCT machines; one with a pediatric preset option and the other with an adult setting. They demonstrated significantly higher equivalent radiation dose when the child phantom was scanned with adult settings. When the pediatric preset was used for the scans, there was a decrease in the ratio of equivalent dose to the child mandible and thyroid. Thus, the practitioner must put pressure on the machine settings during scanning pediatric patients. If not, this will result in excessive radiation to children [90].

A CBCT scan must be only used in cases when the radiographic data is going to change the treatment modality and treatment outcome in orthodontics and pediatric dentistry!

An example of CBCT image acquired from a child having an impacted permanent canine and an odontoma is presented in Figure 28.

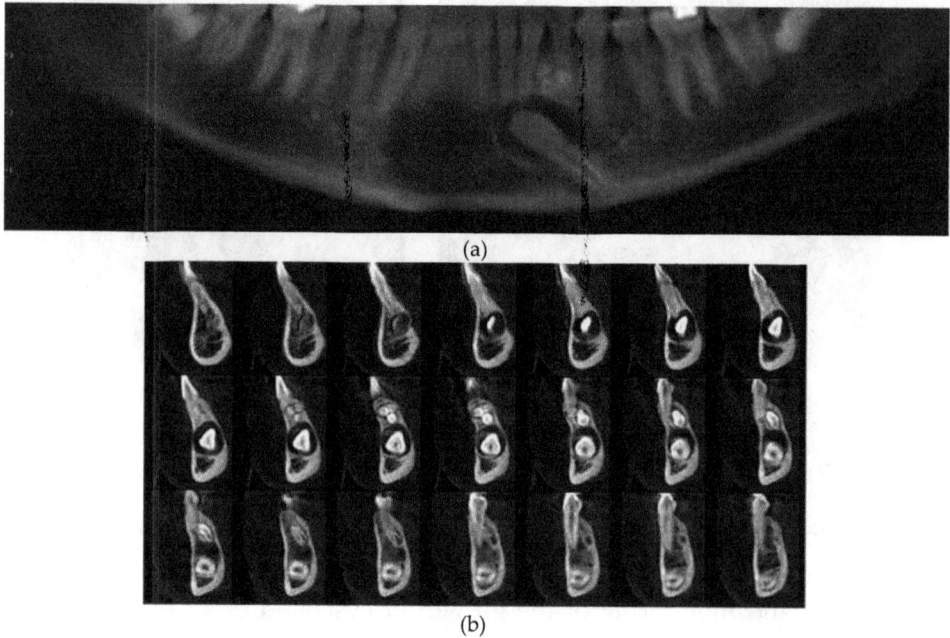

Figure 28. The panoramic (a) and cross sectional (b) CBCT image of a child having an impacted permanent canine and an odontoma.

3.2.3. Periodontology

Diagnosis of periodontal pathologies; such as, gingival hyperplasia, gingival recession and bleeding, depends on clinical signs and symptoms. However, radiographic imaging is essential in the diagnosis of pathologies related with alveolar bone. Two dimensional imaging techniques are routinely used for the assessment of alveolar bone defects in peridontology, but diagnosis of bone craters and alveolar bone support is limited by projection geometry and superimpositions of adjacent anatomical structures. CBCT has the capability of imaging these areas without the limitations of two dimensional imaging techniques [91,92].

Studies have evaluated the role of CBCT in periodontal diagnosis. In vitro studies reported the usefulness of CBCT in the imaging of periodontal defects [93-95]. A study explored the diagnostic values of digital intraoral radiography and CBCT in the determination of periodontal bone loss, infrabony craters and furcation involvements. The authors reported that the detection of crater and furcation involvements failed in 29% and 44% for the CCD, respectively. On the other hand all defects were visualized with CBCT. Besides, the panoramic reconstruction and cross sectional images of CBCT allowed comparable measurements of periodontal bone levels and defects as with intraoral radiography [96]. In a clinical study it was reported that CBCT may provide detailed radiographic information in furcation involvements present in patients with chronic periodontitis and so may have an effect on treatment planning decisions [97].

Although CBCT provide benefits in periodontal diagnosis, it should be used only in cases having the necessity of three dimensional imaging! [91]

An example of CBCT image acquired for periodontal pathology is presented in Figure 29.

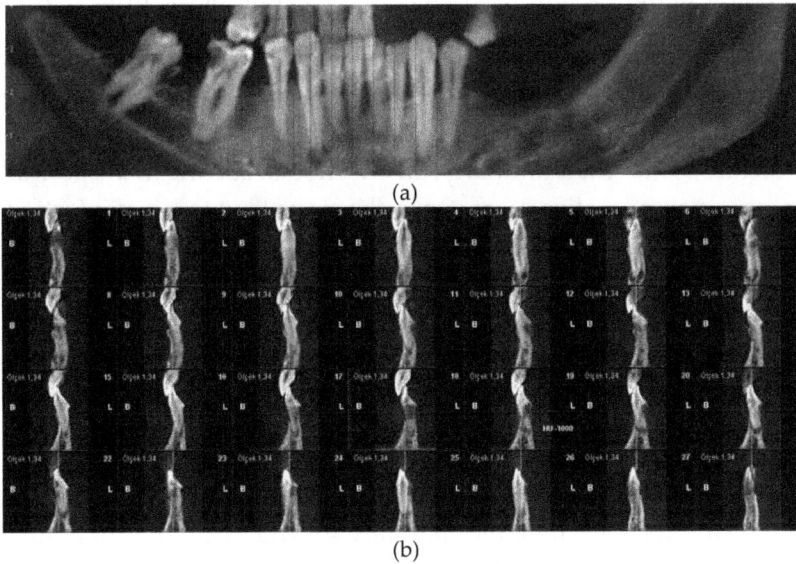

(a)

(b)

Figure 29. The panoramic (a) and cross sectional (b) CBCT image showing periodontal alveolar bone loss. Note the apical lesion and also external root resorption in the incisor.

3.2.4. Endodontics

Radiographic imaging has an important role in the diagnosis of periapical lesions and treatment procedure. Radiographic data not only helps the diagnosis of the pathology but also gives us the possibility to assess the anatomy of the tooth, such as the root number and curvature, pulp horns, coronal and radicular pulp tissue, root apex, lamina dura and periradicular alveolar bone. Until recently, the assessment of these structures relied on two dimensional radiographs. However, such images have inherent limitations in endodontics [98,99].

Endodontic applications of CBCT include the diagnosis of periapical lesions due to pulpal inflammation, identification and localization of internal and external resorption, detection of vertical root fractures, visualization of accessory canals, elucidation of causes of non-healing endodontically treated teeth, [99] and pre-surgical assessment of apical lesions for the planning of endodontic surgery [100,101].

A study evaluated the sensitivity and specificity of CBCT and digital periapical radiography in the detection of mesial root perforations of mandibular molars and demonstrated that CBCT could be used for detection of perforation *before* obturating root canals. Contrary, periapical radiography (with three different horizontal angulations) would be trustworthy in filled root canals [102].

A study compared the accuracy of CBCT scans and periapical radiographs in diagnosis of vertical root fractures and the influence of root canal filling on this issue. The results showed that the specificity of CBCT was reduced by the presence of root canal filling but its overall accuracy was not influenced. Both the sensitivity and overall accuracy of periapical radiographs were reduced by the presence of root canal filling but still CBCT showed a higher accuracy than periapical radiographs for detecting vertical root fracture [103].

CBCT is also useful for the diagnosis of the origin of pain in the maxillary posterior region. Maxillary premolar and molar teeth show a close relationship with sinus maxillaries. This may cause the periradicular infection to spread and erode the cortical border of sinus maxillaries and cause an infection in the sinus. Similarly, an infection occurring in the periradicular region of teeth having root apexes localized directly in the sinus lead to sinus infection also. In such cases the patient has both a tooth infection and sinus maxillaries infection and a correct diagnosis is essential for successful treatment. One other situation is that in some cases sinus infection leads to the posterior teeth give false positive signs and symptoms of periapical infection. It was reported that compared with periapical radiographs CBCT revealed a higher number of correct diagnosis of periapical pathology. This technique also allowed appreciate evaluation of expansion of the lesions into the maxillary sinuses, thickening of the sinus mucosa, missed canals and apicomarginal communications [104].

CBCT has become an important imaging modality for diagnosis and treatment planning in endodontics. However, the higher effective dose of ionizing radiation compared to two dimensional imaging modalities limits the routine usage of this technique. Concerning the utility of CBCT in treatment planning decisions, the gain of radiographic information with this technique has to be evaluated carefully on an individual basis. Moreover, radioopaque materials such as root canal filling and posts often create artifacts, which may compromise diagnosis [105].

An example of CBCT image acquired for periapical pathology is presented in Figure 30.

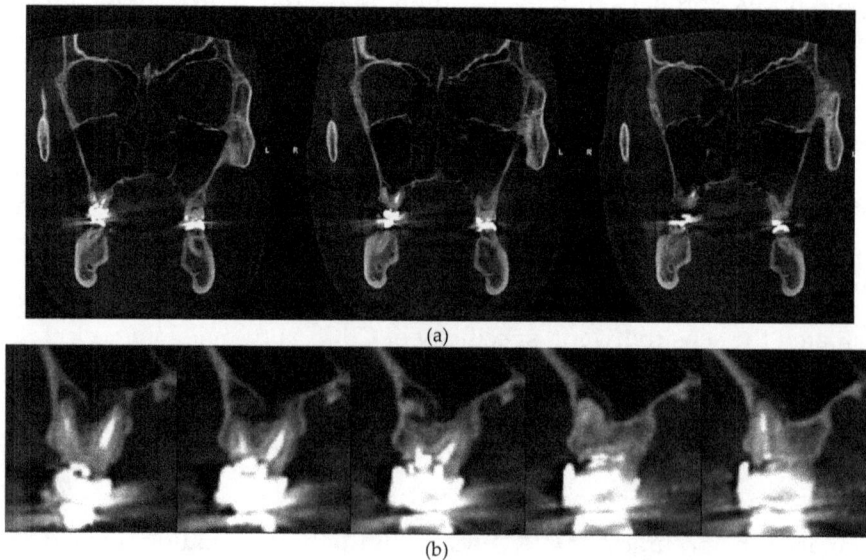

(a)

(b)

Figure 30. The coronal (a) and cross sectional (b) CBCT images of a periapical lesion present in the maxillary first molar.

4. Conclusion

Tremendous advances have been made for improvements of digital imaging systems since their initial introduction on the market and it seems that their adaption will be increasing in the future. Dentists should have knowledge of the working principles, requirements, clinical benefits and hazardous effects of these systems for proper usage.

Author details

Zühre Zafersoy Akarslan and Ilkay Peker

*Address all correspondence to: dtzuhre@yahoo.com

Gazi University Faculty of Dentistry, Department of Dentomaxillofacial Radiology Ankara, Turkey

References

[1] Ludlow JB, Mol A. Digital Imaging In: White SC, Pharoah MJ. 6th ed Oral Radiology. Principles and Interpretation. St. Louis Mosby/Elsevier; 2009. p78-99.

[2] Farman AG, Farman TT. A Comparison of 18 Different X-Ray Detectors Currently Used in Dentistry. Oral Surgery Oral Medicine Oral Pathology Oral Radiology Endodontics 2005;99(4):485-489.

[3] Eshraghi T, McAllister N, McAllister B. Clinical Applications of Digital 2-D and 3-D Radiography for the Periodontist. Journal of Evidence Based Dental Practice 2012;12(3):36-45.

[4] Erten H. Akarslan ZZ, Topuz Ö. The Efficiency of Three Different Films and Radiovisiography in Detecting Approximal Carious Lesion. Quintissence International 2005;36 (1):65-70.

[5] Castro VM, Katz JO, Hardman PK, Glaros AG, Spencer P. In Vitro Comparison of Conventional Film and Direct Digital Imaging in the Detection of Approximal Caries. Dentomaxillofacial Radiology 2007;36(3):138-42.

[6] Bottenberg P, Jacquet W, Stachniss V,Wellnitz J, Schulte AG. Detection of Cavitated or Non-Cavitated Approximal Enamel Caries Lesions Using CMOS and CCD Digital X-Ray Sensors and Conventional D and F-Speed Films at Different Exposure Conditions. American Journal of Dentistry 2011;24(2):74-78.

[7] Jorgenson T, Masood F, Beckerley JM, Burgin C, Parker DE. Comparison of Two Imaging Modalities: F-Speed Film and Digital Images for Detection of Osseous De-

fects in Patients with Interdental Vertical Bone Defects. Dentomaxillofacial Radiology 2007;36(8):500-505.

[8]   de Molon RS, Morais-Camillo JA, Sakakura CE, Ferreira MG, Loffredo LC, Scaf G. Measurements of Simulated Periodontal Bone Defects in Inverted Digital Image and Film-Based Radiograph: An In Vitro Study. Imaging Sciences in Dentistry 2012;42(4): 243-247.

[9]   Vandenberghe B, Corpas L, Bosmans H, Yang J, Jacobs R. A Comprehensive in Vitro Study of Image Accuracy and Quality for Periodontal Diagnosis. Part 1: The Influence of X-Ray Generator on Periodontal Measurements Using Conventional and Digital Receptors. Clinical Oral Investigation 2011;15(4):537-549.

[10] Paurazas SB, Geist JR, Pink FE, Hoen MM, Steiman HR. Comparison of Diagnostic Accuracy of Digital Imaging by Using CCD and CMOS-APS Sensors With E-Speed Film in The Detection of Periapical Bony Lesions. Oral Surgery Oral Medicine Oral Pathology Oral Radiology Endodontics 2000;89(3):356-362.

[11] Wallace JA, Nair MK, Colaco MF, Kapa SF. A Comparative Evaluation of the Diagnostic Efficacy of Film and Digital Sensors for Detection of Simulated Periapical Lesions. Oral Surgery Oral Medicine Oral Pathology Oral Radiology Endodontics 2001;92(1):93-97.

[12] Shintaku WH, Venturin JS, Noujeim M, Dove SB. Comparison between Intraoral Indirect and Conventional Film-Based Imaging for the Detection of Dental Root Fractures: An Ex Vivo Study. Dental Traumatology 2013;29(6):445-449.

[13] Kamburoğlu K, Tsesis I, Kfir A, Kaffe I. Diagnosis of Artificially Induced External Root Resorption Using Conventional Intraoral Film Radiography, CCD, and PSP: An Ex Vivo Study. Oral Surgery Oral Medicine Oral Pathology Oral Radiology Endodontics 2008;106(6):885-891.

[14] Kamburoğlu K, Barenboim SF, Kaffe I. Comparison of Conventional Film with Different Digital and Digitally Filtered Images in the Detection of Simulated Internal Resorption Cavities--An Ex Vivo Study in Human Cadaver Jaws. Oral Surgery Oral Medicine Oral Pathology Oral Radiology Endodontics 2008;105(6):790-797.

[15] White SC, Pharoah MJ. Oral Radiology. Principles and Interpretation. 6th Ed St. Louis Mosby/Elsevier; 2009.

[16] Wakoh M, Kuroyanagi K. Digital Imaging Modalities for Dental Practice. The Bulletin of Tokyo Dental College 2001;42(1):1-14.

[17] Pai SS, Zimmerman JL. Digital Radiographic Imaging in Dental Practice. Dentistry Today 2002;21(6):56-61.

[18] Molteni R. Effect of Visible Light on Photo-Stimulated-Phosphor Imaging Plates. International Congress Series 1256 (2003) 1199– 1205.

[19] Van Der Stelt PF. Filmless Imaging: The Uses of Digital Radiography in Dental Practice. Journal of American Dental Association 2005;136(10):1379-1387.

[20] Wenzel A, Møystad A.Work Flow with Digital Intraoral Radiography: A Systematic Review. Acta Odontologica Scandinavia 2010;68(2):106-114.

[21] Wenzel A, Frandsen E, Hintze H. Patient Discomfort and Cross-Infection Control in Bitewing Examination with a Storage Phosphor Plate and a CCD-Based Sensor. Journal of Dentistry 1999;27(3):243-246.

[22] Tsuchida R, Araki K, Endo A, Funahashi I, Okano T. Physical Properties and Ease of Operation of a Wireless Intraoral X-Ray Sensor. Oral Surgery Oral Medicine Oral Pathology Oral Radiology Endodontics. 2005;100(5):603-608.

[23] Farman AG, Farman TT. Extraoral and Panoramic Systems. Dental Clinics of North America 2000;44(2):257-272.

[24] Molander B, Gröndahl HG, Ekestubbe A. Quality of Film-Based and Digital Panoramic Radiography. Dentomaxillofacial Radiology 2004;33(1):32-36.

[25] Alan G L. Panoramic Imaging. In: White SC, Pharoah MJ. Oral Radiology. Principles and Interpretation. 6th Ed St. Louis Mosby/Elsevier; 2009.

[26] Brennan J. An Introduction to Digital Radiography in Dentistry. Journal of Orthodontics 2002;29(1)66-69.

[27] Wenzel A. Computer-Aided Image Manipulation of Intraoral Radiographs to Enhance Diagnosis in Dental Practice: A Review. International Dental Journal 1993;43(2):99-108.

[28] Van Der Stelt PF.Better İmaging: The Advantages of Digital Radiography. Journal of American Dental Association 2008;139 Suppl:7S-13S.

[29] Borg ESome Characteristics of Solid-State and Photo-Stimulable Phosphor Detectors for Intra-Oral Radiography. Swedish Dental Journal Suppl. 1999;139:i-viii, 1-67.

[30] Nair MK, Ludlow JB, May KN, Nair UP, Johnson MP, Close JM. Diagnostic Accuracy of Intraoral Film and Direct Digital Images for Detection of Simulated Recurrent Decay. Operative Dentistry 2001;26(3):223-230.

[31] Akarslan ZZ, Akdevelioğlu M, Güngör K, Erten H. A Comparison of the Diagnostic Accuracy of Bitewing, Periapical, Unfiltered and Filtered Digital Panoramic Images for Approximal Caries Detection in Posterior Teeth. Dentomaxillofacial Radiology 2008;37(8):458-463.

[32] Belém MD, Ambrosano GM, Tabchoury CP, Ferreira-Santos RI, Haiter-Neto F. Performance of Digital Radiography with Enhancement Filters for the Diagnosis of Proximal Caries. Brazilian Oral Research 2013;27(3):245-251.

[33] Kositbowornchai S, Basiw M, Promwang Y, Moragorn H, Sooksuntisakoonchai N. Accuracy of Diagnosing Occlusal Caries Using Enhanced Digital Images. Dentomaxillofacial Radiology 2004;33(4):236-240.

[34] Leonardi RM, Giordano D, Maiorana F, Greco M. Accuracy Of Cephalometric Landmarks on Monitor-Displayed Radiographs with and without Image Emboss Enhancement. European Journal Of Orthodontics 2010;32(3):242-247.

[35] Møystad A, Svanaes DB, Larheim TA, Gröndahl HG. Effect of Image Magnification of Digitized Bitewing Radiographs on Approximal Caries Detection: An In Vitro Study. Dentomaxillofacial Radiology 1995;24(4):255-259.

[36] Kositbowornchai S, Sikram S, Nuansakul R, Thinkhamrop B. Root Fracture Detection on Digital Images: Effect of the Zoom Function. Dental Traumatology 2003 19(3): 154-159.

[37] Gotfredsen E, Kragskov J, Wenzel A. Development of a System for Craniofacial Analysis from Monitor-Displayed Digital Images. Dentomaxillofacial Radiology 1999;28(2):123-126.

[38] Chen YJ, Chen SK, Chang HF, Chen KC. Comparison of Landmark Identification in Traditional Versus Computer-Aided Digital Cephalometry. Angle Orthodontics 2000;70(5):387-392.

[39] Akhare PJ, Dagab AM, Alle RS, Shenoyd U, Garla V. Comparison of Landmark Identification and Linear and Angular Measurements in Conventional and Digital Cephalometry. International Journal of Computerized Dentistry 2013;16(3):241-254.

[40] Santiago RC, Cunha AR, Júnior GC, Fernandes N, Campos MJ, Costa LF, Vitral RW, Bolognese AM. New Software for Cervical Vertebral Geometry Assessment and its Relationship to Skeletal Maturation--A Pilot Study. Dentomaxillofacial Radiology 2014;43(2):20130238.

[41] Wenzel A, Kirkevang LL. Students' Attitudes to Digital Radiography and Measurement Accuracy of Two Digital Systems in Connection with Root Canal Treatment. European Journal of Dental Education 2004;8:167–171.

[42] Horner K, Shearer AC, Walker A, Wilson NH. Radiovisiography: An Initial Evaluation. British Dental Journal 1990;168(6):244-248.

[43] Walker A, Horner K, Czajka J, Shearer AC, Wilson NH. Quantitative Assessment of a New Dental Imaging System. British Journal of Radiology 1991;64(762):529-536.

[44] Soh G, Loh FC, Chong YH. Radiation Dosage of a Dental Imaging System. Quintessence International 1993;24(3):189-191.

[45] Näslund EB, Møystad A, Larheim TA, Øgaard B, Kruger M. Cephalometric Analysis with Digital Storage Phosphor Images: Extreme Low-Exposure Images with and

without Postprocessing Noise Reduction. American Journal of Orthodontics and Dentofacial Orthopedics 2003;124(2):190-197.

[46] Näslund EB, Kruger M, Petersson A, Hansen K. Analysis of Low-Dose Digital Lateral Cephalometric Radiographs. Dentomaxillofacial Radiology 1998;27(3):136-139.

[47] Hellén-Halme K, Johansson PM, Håkansson J, Petersson A. Image Quality of Digital and Film Radiographs in Applications Sent to the Dental Insurance Office in Sweden for Treatment Approval. Swedish Dental Journal 2004;28(2):77-84.

[48] Berkhout WE, Beuger DA, Sanderink GC, Van Der Stelt PF. The Dynamic Range of Digital Radiographic Systems: Dose Reduction or Risk of Overexposure? Dentomaxillofacial Radiology 2004;33(1):1-5.

[49] Hokett SD, Honey JR, Ruiz F, Baisden MK, Hoen MM. Assessing the Effectiveness of Direct Digital Radiography Barrier Sheaths and Finger Cots. Journal of American Dental Association 2000;131:463–467.

[50] Hubar JS, Gardiner DM. Infection Control Procedures in Conjunction with Computed Dental Radiography. International Journal of Computerized Dentistry 2000;3(4): 259–267.

[51] Negron W, Mauriello SM, Peterson CA, Arnold R. Cross-Contamination of the PSP Sensor in a Preclinical Setting. Journal Of Dental Hygiene 2005;79(3):1–10.

[52] Al-Rawi W, Teich S. Evaluation of Physical Properties of Different Digital Intraoral Sensors. Compendium of Continuing Education in Dentistry 2013;34(8):E76-83.

[53] Russo JM, Russo JA, Guelmann M. Digital Radiography: A Survey of Pediatric Dentists. Journal of Dentistry for Children (Chic). 2006;73(3):132-135.

[54] Berg EC. Legal Ramifications of Digital Imaging in Law Enforcement. Forensic Science Communications 2000;2(4).

[55] Scarfe WC, Farman AG. Cone Beam Computed Tomography. In: White SC, Pharoah MJ. Oral Radiology. Principles and Interpretation. 6th Ed St. Louis Mosby Elsevier; 2009. P.225-243

[56] Peker I, Alkurt MT. Evaluation of Radiographic Errors Made by Undergraduate Dental Students in Periapical Radiography. The New York State Dental Journal 2009;75(5):45-48.

[57] Chiu HL, Lin SH, Chen CH, Wang WC, Chen JY, Chen YK, Lin LM. Analysis of Photostimulable Phosphor Plate Image Artifacts in an Oral and Maxillofacial Radiology Department. Oral Surgery Oral Medicine Oral Pathology Oral Radiology Endodontics 2008;106(5):749-756.

[58] Brezden NA, Brooks SL. Evaluation of Panoramic Dental Radiographs Taken in Private Practice. Oral Surgery Oral Medicine Oral Pathology 1987;63(5):617-621.

[59] Akarslan ZZ, Erten H, Güngör K, Celik I. Common Errors on Panoramic Radiographs Taken in a Dental School. Journal of Contemporary Dental Practice 2003;4(2): 24-34.

[60] Rondon RH, Pereira YC, Do Nascimento GC. Common Positioning Errors in Panoramic Radiography: A Review. Imaging Science in Dentistry 2014;44(1):1-6.

[61] Peretz B, Gotler M, Kaffe I. Common Errors in Digital Panoramic Radiographs of Patients with Mixed Dentition and Patients with Permanent Dentition. International Journal of Dentistry 2012;2012:584138. Doi: 10.1155/2012/584138.

[62] Frederiksen NL. Advanced Imaging. In: Oral Radiology Principles and Interprtation, 6th Ed, St. Louis, Mosby/Elsevier 2009,P. 207-224.

[63] Yamamoto K, Hayakawa Y, Kousuge Y, Wakoh M, Sekiguchi H, Yakushiji M, Farman AG. Diagnostic Value of Tuned-Aperture Computed Tomography versus Conventional Dentoalveolar Imaging in Assessment of Impacted Teeth. Oral Surgery Oral Medicine Oral Pathology Oral Radiology Endodontics 2003;95(1):109-118.

[64] Tyndall DA, Price JB, Tetradis S, Ganz SD, Hildebolt C, Scarfe WC; American Academy of Oral and Maxillofacial Radiology. Position Statement of the American Academy of Oral and Maxillofacial Radiology on Selection Criteria for the use of Radiology in Dental Implantology with Emphasis on Cone Beam Computed Tomography. Oral Surgery Oral Medicine Oral Pathology Oral Radiology 2012;113(6): 817-826.

[65] Soğur E, Baksi BG, Gröndahl HG. Imaging of Root Canal Fillings: A Comparison of Subjective image Quality Between Limited Cone-Beam CT, Storage Phosphor and Film Radiography. International Endodontic Journal 2007;40(3):179-185.

[66] American Dental Association Council On Scientific Affairs. The Use of Cone-Beam Computed Tomography in Dentistry. An Advisory Statement from the American Dental Association Council on Scientific Affairs. Journal of American Dental Association 2012;143(8):899-902.

[67] Hatcher DC, Dial C, Mayorga C. Cone Beam CT for Presurgical Assessment of Implant Sites. Journal of the California Dental Association 2003;31(11):825-833.

[68] Scarfe WC, Levin MD, Gane D, Farman AG. Use of Cone Beam Computed Tomography in Endodontics. International Journal of Dentistry 2009;2009:634567. Doi: 10.1155/2009/634567.

[69] Dawood A, Patel S, Brown J. Cone Beam CT in Dental Practice. British Dental Journal 2009;207(1):23-28.

[70] Farman AG. ALARA Still Applies. Oral Surgery Oral Medicine Oral Pathology Oral Radiology Endodontics 2005;100(4):395-397.

[71] Alamri HM, Sadrameli M, Alshalhoob MA, Sadrameli M, Alshehri MA. Applications of CBCT in Dental Practice: A Review of the Literature. General Dentistry 2012;60(5): 390-400.

[72] Tyndall DA, Brooks SL. Selection Criteria for Dental Implant Site Imaging: A Position Paper of the American Academy of Oral and Maxillofacial Radiology. Oral Surgery Oral Medicine Oral Pathology Oral Radiology Endodontics 2000;89(5):630-637.

[73] Horner K. Cone-Beam Computed Tomography: Time for an Evidence-Based Approach. Primary Dental Journal 2013;2(1):22-31.

[74] Visconti MA, Verner FS, Assis NM, Devito KL. Influence of Maxillomandibular Positioning in Cone Beam Computed Tomography for Implant Planning. International Journal of Oral And Maxillofacial Surgery 2013;42(7):880-886.

[75] Stoetzer M, Nickel F, Rana M, Lemound J, Wenzel D, Von See C, Gellrich NC. Advances in Assessing the Volume of Odontogenic Cysts and Tumors in the Mandible: A Retrospective Clinical Trial. Head And Face Medicine 2013; 20;9:14.

[76] Kaeppler G. Applications of Cone Beam Computed Tomography in Dental and Oral Medicine. International Journal of Computerized Dentistry 2010;13(3):203-219.

[77] Tsao DH, Kazanoglu A, Mccasland JP. Measurability of Radiographic Images. American Journal of Orthodontics 1983; 84(3): 212–216.

[78] Adams GL, Gansky SA, Miller AJ, Harrell WE Jr, Hatcher DC. Comparison between Traditional 2-Dimensional Cephalometry and a 3-Dimensional Approach on Human Dry Skulls. American Journal of Orthodontics and Dentofacial Orthopedics 2004;126(4):397-409.

[79] Burkhard JP, Dietrich AD, Jacobsen C, Roos M, Lübbers HT, Obwegeser JA. Cephalometric and Three Dimensional Assessment of the Posterior Airway Space and Imaging Software Reliability Analysis before and after Orthognathic Surgery. Journal of Craniomaxillofacial Surgery. 2014; Pii: S1010-5182(14)00128-0. Doi: 10.1016/J.Jcms. 2014.04.005. Article in Press

[80] Cheung T, Oberoi S. Three Dimensional Assessment of the Pharyngeal Airway in Individuals with Non-Syndromic Cleft Lip and Palate. 2012;7(8):E43405. Doi: 10.1371/Journal.Pone.0043405

[81] Garib DG, Yatabe MS, Ozawa TO, Da Silva Filho OG. Alveolar Bone Morphology in Patients with Bilateral Complete Cleft Lip and Palate in the Mixed Dentition: Cone Beam Computed Tomography Evaluation. The Cleft Palate Craniofacial Journal 2012;49(2):208-214.

[82] Baysal A, Ucar FI, Buyuk SK, Ozer T, Uysal T. Alveolar Bone Thickness and Lower Incisor Position in Skeletal Class I and Class II Malocclusions Assessed with Cone-Beam Computed Tomography. Korean Journal of Orthodontics 2013;43(3):134-140.

[83] Morea C, Hayek JE, Oleskovicz C, Dominguez GC, Chilvarquer I. Precise Insertion of Orthodontic Miniscrews with a Stereolithographic Surgical Guide Based on Cone Beam Computed Tomography Data: A Pilot Study. International Journal of Oral and Maxillofacial Implants 2011;26(4):860-865.

[84] Chang HP, Tseng YC. Miniscrew Implant Applications in Contemporary Orthodontics. The Kaohsiung Journal of Medical Sciences 2014;30(3):111-115.

[85] Hodges RJ, Atchison KA, White SC. Impact of Cone-Beam Computed Tomography on Orthodontic Diagnosis and Treatment Planning. American Journal of Orthodontics and Dentofacial Orthopedics 2013;143(5):665-674.

[86] Noar JH, Pabari S. Cone Beam Computed Tomography--Current Understanding and Evidence for its Orthodontic Applications? Journal of Orthodontics 2013;40(1):5-13.

[87] Shim YS, Kim AH, Choi JE, An SY. Use of Three-Dimensional Computed Tomography Images in Dental Care of Children and Adolescents in Korea. Technology Health Care 2014; 4. Epub Ahead of Print

[88] May JJ, Cohenca N, Peters OA. Contemporary Management of Horizontal Root Fractures to the Permanent Dentition: Diagnosis--Radiologic Assessment to Include Cone-Beam Computed Tomography. Pediatric Dentistry 2013;35(2):120-124.

[89] Aps JK. Cone Beam Computed Tomography in Paediatric Dentistry: Overview of Recent Literature. European Archievs of Paediatric Dentistry 2013;14(3):131-140.

[90] Al Najjar A, Colosi D, Dauer LT, Prins R, Patchell G, Branets I, Goren AD, Faber RD. Comparison of Adult and Child Radiation Equivalent Doses from 2 Dental Cone-Beam Computed Tomography Units. American Journal of Orthodontics and Dentofacial Orthopedics 2013;143(6):784-792.

[91] Acar B, Kamburoğlu K. Use of Cone Beam Computed Tomography in Periodontology. World Journal of Radiology 2014; 28;6(5):139-147.

[92] Corbet, EF Ho DK, Lai SM. Radiographs in Periodontal Disease Diagnosis and Management. Australian Dental Journal 2009;54(1): S27–S43.

[93] Mengel R, Candir M, Shiratori K, Flores-De-Jacoby L. Digital Volume Tomography in the Diagnosis of Periodontal Defects: An In Vitro Study on Native Pig and Human Mandibles. Journal of Periodontology 2005;76(5):665–673.

[94] Misch KA, Yi ES, Sarment DP. Accuracy of Cone Beam Computed Tomography for Periodontal Defect Measurements. Journal of Periodontology 2006;77(7):1261–1266.

[95] Mol A, Balasundaram A. In Vitro Cone Beam Computed Tomography Imaging of Periodontal Bone. Dentomaxillofacial Radiology 2008;37(6):319–324.

[96] Vandenberghe B, Jacobs R, Yang J. Detection of Periodontal Bone Loss Using Digital Intraoral and Cone Beam Computed Tomography Images: An In Vitro Assessment of Bony and/or Infrabony Defects. Dentomaxillofacial Radiology 2008;37(5):252-260.

[97]   Walter C, Kaner D, Berndt DC, Weiger R, Zitzmann NU. Three-Dimensional Imaging as a Pre-Operative Tool in Decision Making for Furcation Surgery. Journal of Clinical Periodontology 2009;36(3):250–257.

[98]   Patel S. New Dimensions in Endodontic Imaging: Part 2. Cone Beam Computed Tomography. International Endodontic Journal 2009;42(6): 463–475.

[99]   Tyndall DA, Kohltfarber H. Application of Cone Beam Volumetric Tomography in Endodontics. Australian Dental Journal 2012;57(L):72-81.

[100] Rigolone M, Pasqualini D, Bianchi L, Berutti E, Bianchi SD. Vestibular Surgical Access to the Palatine Root of the Superior First Molar: "Low-Dose Cone-Beam" CT Analysis of the Pathway and its Anatomic Variations. Journal of Endodontics 2003;29(11):773-775.

[101] Tsurumachi T, Honda K. A New Cone Beam Computerized Tomography System for use in Endodontic Surgery. International Endodontics Journal 2007;40(3):224-232.

[102] Haghanifar S, Moudi E, Mesgarani A, Bijani A, Abbaszadeh N. A Comparative Study of Cone-Beam Computed Tomography and Digital Periapical Radiography in Detecting Mandibular Molars Root Perforations. Imaging Science in Dentistry 2014;44(2): 115-119.

[103] Hassan B, Metska ME, Ozok AR, Van Der Stelt P, Wesselink PR. Detection of Vertical Root Fractures in Endodontically Treated Teeth by a Cone Beam Computed Tomography Scan. Journal of Endodontics 2009;35(5):719-722.

[104] Low KM, Dula K, Burgin W, Von Arx T. Comparison of Periapical Radiography and Limited Cone-Beam Tomography in Posterior Maxillary Teeth Referred for Apical Surgery. Journal of Endodontics 2008;34(5):557–562.

[105] Jeger FB, Lussi A, Bornstein MM, Jacobs R, Janner SF. [Cone Beam Computed Tomography in Endodontics: A Review for Daily Clinical Practice][Article in German] Schweiz Monatsschr Zahnmed 2013;123(7-8):661-668.

Dental Caries and Quality of Life Among Preschool Children

Joana Ramos-Jorge, Maria Letícia Ramos-Jorge,
Saul Martins de Paiva, Leandro Silva Marques and
Isabela Almeida Pordeus

1. Introduction

Dental caries (tooth decay) is an adverse oral condition with a multifactor etiology involving genetic, behavioral and environmental aspects (Reisine and Psoter, 2001; Petersen *et al.*, 2005). Socioeconomic factors have been associated with caries experience and the distribution of this condition among individuals (Pereira *et al.*, 2007; Traebert *et al.*, 2009). Understanding the influence of lifestyle and social aspect on the occurrence and progression of dental caries can contribute to improvements in preventive and restorative treatment (Petersen *et al.*, 2005).

Although not a fatal condition, dental caries can lead to pain as well as problems with sleeping, eating, socializing and self-esteem. Thus, tooth decay can exert a negative impact on activities of daily living and, consequently, quality of life (Patel *et al.*, 2007). Quality of life is often evaluated by means of the investigation into the consequences of an adverse health condition and its treatment from the standpoint of the affected individual (Tamanini *et al.*, 2004). The association between oral health and quality of life is considered by many researchers to be a complement to clinical indicators (Martins-Júnior *et al.*, 2012a).

There are few assessment tools for measuring the impact of oral problems on the quality of life of children. As adults are responsible for decisions involving the health of their children (Pahel *et al.*, 2007), evaluating the perceptions of parents/caregivers regarding oral health problems that affect the quality of life of children is fundamental to planning health promotion strategies.

2. Problem statement

The concept of oral health-related quality of life (OHRQoL) regards the impact that oral problems have on the performance of activities of daily living, wellbeing and quality of life (Slade, 1997). It is therefore important to assess OHRQoL in different populations to understand the oral health problems that affect individuals and design public health programs and strategies directed at prevention and treatment.

Despite the growing interest and consequent increase in the number of publications on this issue, the evaluation of the impact of dental caries in preschool children has only recently been the focus of investigation. As young children may not be capable of remembering events that occurred more than 24 hours earlier (Rebok *et al.*, 2001) and have limitations regarding the expression of emotions and anguish (Talekar *et al.*, 2005), this investigation is often performed with the aid of parents/caregivers. It is therefore important to explore the perceptions of parents/caregivers that affect the preventive care children receive at home as well as the use of dental services (Filstrup *et al.*, 2003). Moreover, the perceptions of parents/caregivers may offer insight into some of the reasons why preschool children often do not receive the dental treatment they need.

The Early Childhood Oral Health Impact Scale (ECOHIS) was developed for parents/caregivers of young children (Pahel *et al.*, 2007). The use of this questionnaire in epidemiological studies has allowed broadening knowledge on adverse oral conditions that affect the quality of life of children as well as strengthening scientific evidence on this issue and demonstrating the need for oral health programs directed at preschool children.

Based on evidence that children aged four to six years can reliably report on their own quality of life (Filstrup *et al.*, 2003), the Scale of Oral Health Outcomes for Five-Year-Old Children (SOHO-5) has recently been developed in the United Kingdom (Tsakos *et al.*, 2012). However, studies employing this instrument have been limited to evaluating its reliability and validity.

Dental caries is the oral condition most often associated with a negative impact on the quality of life of preschool children (Abanto *et al.*, 2011; Scarpelli *et al.*, 2012; Ramos-Jorge *et al.*, 2014), the consequences of which include pain, decreased appetite, difficulty chewing, difficulty eating some foods and drinking hot or cold beverages, weight loss, difficulty sleeping, changes in behavior and a poor academic performance (Abanto *et al.*, 2011; Acs *et al.*, 1992; Ayhan *et al.*, 1996; Filstrup *et al.*, 2003; Feitosa *et al.*, 2005; Oliveira *et al.*, 2008; Martins-Júnior *et al.*, 2012b). Studies carried out in China (Wong *et al.*, 2011) and Brazil (Abanto *et al.*, 2011; Scarpelli *et al.*, 2012; Martins-Júnior *et al.*, 2012b) using the ECOHIS report that dental caries has a negative impact on the quality of life of preschool children and their parents/caregivers and this impact is greater in the presence of six or more carious lesions.

A study conducted in Canada found that dental surgery is the most common surgical procedure at most pediatric hospitals (Canadian Paediatric Decision Support Network, 2004), which indicates that the treatment of dental caries in children is costly. Moreover, the need for restorative treatment can lead to the establishment of a repetitive restorative cycle (Elderton *et al.*, 1990), which further raises treatment costs (Zero *et al.*, 2011). However, caries can be detected in the early stages, when restorative treatment is not necessary. The International Caries Detection and Assessment System (ICDAS) allows the standardization and diagnosis of dental caries in different settings and situations (Pitts, 2004). The integration of criteria from other caries detection and diagnostic systems involving non-cavitated enamel lesions and the staging of the disease process (Ekstrand *et al.*, 1997; Fyffe *et al.*, 2000; Chesters *et al.*, 2002; Rickets *et al.*, 2002) led to the current system, denominated ICDAS II (Shoaib *et al.*, 2009), which contributes to the preventive management of tooth decay.

Despite the decline in the prevalence of dental caries beginning in the 1970s, the control of this condition continues to pose a challenge to public health authorities (Petersen *et al.*, 2005; Dye *et al.*, 2007). Moreover, increasing polarization is seen due to social inequalities in oral health (Sabbah *et al.*, 2007), which has led to a greater prevalence rate of dental caries in some minorities (Antunes *et al.*, 2004).

The difficulty in controlling dental caries affects both developed and developing nations. Successive national child dental health surveys in the United Kingdom have shown little change in the prevalence of caries among five-year-old children over the last 20 years (Lader *et al.*, 2004). Data from the United States of America tells a similar story, as no significant changes in the prevalence of dental caries among children aged two to 11 years was found from 1988-1994 to 1999-2002 (Beltran-Aguilar *et al.*, 2005).

The monitoring of the early stages of caries progression requires the assessment of a dentist. However, this is not a common occurrence among preschool children. Indeed, a Brazilian study found that only 13.3% of a sample of 1092 children aged zero to five years had visited a dentist at least once (Kramer *et al.*, 2008). This low rate of access to dental treatment can contribute to the greater prevalence of severe tooth decay in comparison to less advanced stages of progression (Ramos-Jorge *et al.*, 2014). Furthermore, among older preschoolers, the negative impact on OHRQoL (Ramos-Jorge *et al.*, 2014) seems to stem from the fact that these individuals have caries in more advanced stages of decay and also have a greater capacity to communicate the effect of oral health conditions on their quality of life to parents/caregivers (Ramos-Jorge *et al.*, 2014). Consequently, the prevention and management of dental caries should begin at an early age, as this is an evident public health problem among preschool children.

The diminished appetite, difficulty chewing, weight loss and difficulty sleeping stemming from dental caries can compromise growth and development. Moreover, children with severe caries appear to be at significantly greater odds of having low vitamin D status compared to their caries-free counterparts and are likely malnourished, as they display significantly lower levels of calcium and serum albumin as well as higher levels of PTH compared to a control group (reference).

OHRQoL assessment tools designed for preschool children are useful for the evaluation of public oral health strategies and interventions. Such tools should have properties that enable the detection of clinical changes following treatment. Responsiveness is a key technical property that allows researchers to choose the most appropriate measures for clinical trials, provides a basis for estimating sample sizes and facilitates the interpretation of changes occurring after treatment (Guyatt *et al.*, 2002; Malden *et al.*, 2008).

The aim of health interventions should be to improve quality of life. Despite the tendency to consider oral health as a separate concept, it is an integral part of general health (Cunningham and Hunt, 2001). Thus, the complex multidimensional interrelationship between general and oral health is essential to quality of life (Kieffe and, Hoogstraten, 2008). In this context, the use of subjective measures considering individual viewpoints has become increasingly important to the evaluation of general and oral health (Kieffer and Hoogstraten, 2008).

3. Application area

The findings of studies on OHRQoL and dental caries in preschool children are useful to the fields of pediatrics and pediatric dentistry and can be employed by public health administrators for the definition of strategies directed at improving the oral health status of this population.

4. Research course

According to a large number of the aforementioned studies, scientific evidence indicates that dental caries has a negative impact on quality of life among preschool children, especially those with six or more carious lesions or lesions in a more advanced stage of progression. The aim of the study reported herein was to evaluate the association between different stages of dental caries and the impact on the quality of life of preschool children.

5. Method used

A population-based, cross-sectional study was conducted involving preschool children. The inclusion criteria age between three and five years, enrolment in a preschool/daycare center in the city of Diamantina, Brazil, and parents/guardians fluent in Brazilian Portuguese who live with the child at least 12 hours per day. The exclusion criteria were current orthodontic treatment, systemic disease, having all carious lesions treated satisfactorily and the presence of tartar. The sample size was calculated using a 37.8% prevalence rate of impact from dental caries on the quality of life of preschool children (Martins-Júnior et al., 2013), a 95% confidence interval and 5% standard error. The minimum sample was defined as 346 preschool children. A 1.2 correction factor was applied to enhance the precision and an additional 84 children were added to compensate for possible losses, resulting in a sample of 499 preschool children. To ensure representativeness, the sample was stratified based on the type of preschool (public or private) and the distribution of the sample was proportional to the total population enrolled in private and public preschools in the city.

Parents/caregivers were asked to answer the Brazilian version of the ECOHIS (B-ECOHIS) (Martins-Júnior et al., 2012) and fill out a form addressing socio-demographic information, such as mother's schooling (years of study), whether the mother worked outside the home, monthly household income (categorized based on the Brazilian minimum wage = US$304.38), duration of salary (in weeks), family provider and number of individuals who depend on the income.

The B-ECOHIS was used to assess the negative impact of the progression stage and activity of dental caries on the quality of life of the preschool children. This questionnaire is composed of 13 items distributed in a Child Impact Section (CIS) and Family Impact Section (FIS). The former section has four domains (symptoms, function, psychology and self-image/social interaction) and the latter has two domains (parental distress and family function). The scale has five response options for recording how often an event has occurred in a child's life. The CIS and FIS scores are calculated through a simple sum of the scores on all items in each section, ranging from 0 to 36 and 0 to 16, respectively. The total score ranges from 0 to 52, with higher scores denoting greater oral health impact and poorer OHRQoL.

The clinical oral examination of the children was performed by a single dentist who had undergone a calibration exercise at a public preschool, during which inter-examiner and intra-examiner Kappa values were greater than 0.8 for all oral conditions evaluated. The examination was carried out after brushing performed by the dentist, with the aid of a head lamp (PETZL®, Tikka XP, Crolles, France), mouth mirrors (PRISMA, São Paulo, SP, Brazil), WHO probes (Golgran Ind. e Com. Ltda., São Paulo, SP, Brazil) and dental gauze for drying the teeth. During the examination, the children remained lying on a portable stretcher.

The ICDAS II criteria and Activity Lesion Assessment, which measures visual appearance, local susceptibility to plaque buildup and surface texture, were used for the determination of dental caries. Dental caries was recorded as follows: distinct visual change in enamel – ICDAS code 2 (active and inactive); localized enamel breakdown – ICDAS code 3 (active and inactive); underlying dentin shadow – ICDAS code 4 (active and inactive); distinct cavity within visible dentin – ICDAS code 5 (active and inactive); and extensive cavity within visible dentin – ICDAS code 6, without pulp exposure (active and inactive), with pulp exposure (with absence or presence of fistula and root remnants). The first visual change in enamel (ICDAS code 1, when there is no pigmentation) is detected only after drying with compressed air. As drying was performed with dental gauze in the present study, the decision was made to exclude the evaluation of this condition. When the characteristic pigmentation of this stage of carious lesion was detected on any face with the tooth either wet or dried with gauze, the tooth was recorded as "sound".

Malocclusion, traumatic dental injury (TDI) and physiological tooth mobility were evaluated as possible confounding variables. Malocclusion was recorded in the presence of anterior open bite, posterior open bite, increased overjet, deep bite, anterior crossbite or posterior crossbite. The clinical diagnosis of TDI was performed using the criteria proposed by Andreasen (Andreasen et al., 2007) and the assessment of tooth discoloration. Physiological tooth mobility was considered only when the tooth was nearing exfoliation. All confounding variables were categorized as absent or present.

Statistical analysis was performed using the SPSS 20.0 program for Windows (SPSS Inc, Chicago, IL, USA). Descriptive analysis (including frequency distribution) was performed for mean total B-ECOHIS scores. Scores for the individual domains were analyzed for differences between oral conditions and socioeconomic/demographic factors. In cases of children with a tooth exhibiting different stages of dental caries, the worst condition was considered. Poisson regression analysis with robust variance was performed to associate the mean total B-ECOHIS score with each clinical oral condition, socioeconomic factor and characteristic of the child. Prevalence rates (PR) and 95% confidence intervals (95% CI) were calculated.

6. Status

This study was completed and published in Community Dentistry and Oral Epidemiology.

7. Results

A total of 499 preschool children were initially enrolled in the study, 451 (90.4%) of whom participated through to the end of the study. The main reason for losses was the absence of a questionnaire filled out by the parents. Mean age (standard deviation) of the preschool children was 4.25 (0.83) years. The female sex accounted for 53.9% of the sample. The prevalence of untreated caries was 51.2%. A total of 60.6% of the teeth with caries exhibited severe decay. Malocclusion, TDI and physiological tooth mobility were present in 28.4%, 17.5% and 2.0% of the preschool children, respectively.

The majority of parents/caregivers reported no impact on quality of life (52.8%) (i.e., B-ECOHIS score: 0). The most frequently reported items were pain, difficulty eating and drinking, irritability, trouble sleeping and smiling.

In the final multivariate model, negative impact on quality of life was associated with the age of the child and a lower level of mother's schooling. More advanced stages of caries were associated with an increased negative impact on the quality of life of the children. Among inactive lesions, only extensive cavity without pulp exposure had an increased negative impact on quality of life (PR = 3.68; 95% CI: 1.74 to 7.81; p = 0.001).

8. Further research

Future investigations should be conducted to evaluate the results of intervention strategies on both the individual and population levels.

9. Conclusion

Dental caries exerts a negative impact on the quality of life of preschool children, especially those with a greater number of carious lesions or lesions in a more advanced stage of progression.

Author details

Joana Ramos-Jorge[1*], Maria Letícia Ramos-Jorge[1], Saul Martins de Paiva[2], Leandro Silva Marques[1] and Isabela Almeida Pordeus[2]

*Address all correspondence to: joanaramosjorge@gmail.com

1 Universidade Federal dos Vales do Jequitinhonha e Mucuri, Diamantina, Minas Gerais, Brazil

2 Universidade Federal de Minas Gerais, Belo Horizonte, Minas Gerais, Brazil

References

[1] Abanto J, Carvalho TS, Mendes FM, Wanderley MT, Bönecker M, Raggio DP. Impact of oral diseases and disorders on oral health-related quality of life of preschool children. Community Dent Oral Epidemiol 2011;39:105-14.

[2] Acs G, Lodolini G, Kaminsky S, Cisneros GJ. Effect of nursing caries on body weight in a pediatric population. Pediatr Dent 1992;14:302-5.

[3] Andreasen JO, Andreasen FM, Andersson LC. Textbook and color atlas of traumatic injuries to the teeth. Copenhagen: Munskgaard, 4 2007.

[4] Antunes JL, Narvai PC, Nugent ZJ. Measuring inequalities in the distribution of dental caries. Community Dent Oral Epidemiol 2004; 32: 41-48.

[5] Assaf AV, de Castro Meneghim M, Zanin L, Tengan C, Pereira AC. Effect of different diagnostic thresholds on dental caries calibration - a 12 month evaluation. Community Dent Oral Epidemiol 2006; 34: 213-9.

[6] Ayhan H, Suskan E, Yildrim S: The effect of nursing or rampant caries on height, body weight and head circumference. J Clin Pediatr Dent 1996;20:209-12.

[7] Beltrán-Aguilar ED, Barker LK, Canto MT, Dye BA, Gooch BF, Griffin SO, Hyman J, Jaramillo F, Kingman A, Nowjack-Raymer R, Selwitz RH, Wu T; Centers for Disease Control and Prevention (CDC). Surveillance for dental caries, dental sealants, tooth

retention, edentulism, and enamel fluorosis--United States, 1988-1994 and 1999-2002. MMWR Surveill Summ. 2005;54:1-43.

[8] Chesters RK, Pitts NB, Matuliene G, Kvedariene A, Huntington E, Bendinskaite R, Balciuniene I, Matheson JR, Nicholson JA, Gendvilyte A, Sabalaite R,Ramanauskiene J, Savage D, Mileriene J. An abbreviated caries clinical trial design validated over 24 months. J Dent Res 2002; 81:637-40.

[9] Cunningham SJ, Hunt NP. Quality of life and its importance in orthodontics. J Orthod 2001; 28:152-8.

[10] Dye BA, Tan S, Smith V, Lewis BG, Barker LK, Thornton-Evans G, Eke PI, Beltrán-Aguilar ED, Horowitz AM, Li CH. Trends in oral health status: United States, 1988-1994 and 1999-2004. Vital Health Stat 2007; 11:1-92.

[11] Elderton RJ. Clinical studies concerning re-restoration of teeth. Adv Dent Res 1990; 4:4-9.

[12] Ekstrand KR, Ricketts DN, Kidd EA. Reproducibility and accuracy of three methods for assessment of demineralization depth of the occlusal surface: an in vitro examination. Caries Res 1997; 31:224-31.

[13] Feitosa S, Colares V, Pinkham J: The psychosocial effects of severe caries in 4-year-old children in Recife, Pernambuco, Brazil. Cad Saude Publica 2005;21:1550-6.

[14] Filstrup SL, Briskie D, da Fonseca M, Lawrence L, Wandera A, Inglehart MR: Early childhood caries and quality of life: child and parent perspectives. Pediatr Dent 2003; 25:431-40.

[15] Fyffe HE, Deery C, Nugent ZJ, Nuttall NM, Pitts NB. Effect of diagnostic threshold on the validity and reliability of epidemiological caries diagnosis using the Dundee Selectable Threshold Method for caries diagnosis (DSTM). Community Dent Oral Epidemiol 2000; 28: 42-51.

[16] Guyatt G, Osoba D, Wu A, Wyrwich K, Norman G: Methods to explain the significance of health status measures. Hamilton, Ontario: Clinical Significance Consensus Meeting Group, Unpublished paper; 2002.

[17] Kramer PF, Ardenghi TM, Ferreira S, Fischer LA, Cardoso L, Feldens CA. Use of dental services by preschool children in Canela, Rio Grande do Sul State, Brazil. Cad. Saúde Pública 2008;24:150-6.

[18] Kieffer JM, Hoogstraten J. Linking oral health, general health, and quality of life. Eur J Oral Sci. 2008;116:445-50

[19] Lader D, Chadwick B, Chestnutt, Harker R, Morris J, Nuttal N, Pitts N, Steele J, White D: Children's Dental Health in the United Kingdom, 2003 London: Office for National statistics; 2004.

[20] Malden PE, Thomson WM, Jokovic A, Locker D: Changes in parente assessed oral health-related quality of life among young children following dental treatment under general anaesthetic. Community Dent Oral Epidemiol 2008, 36:108–117.

[21] Martins-Júnior PA, Ramos-Jorge J, Paiva SM, Marques LS, Ramos-Jorge ML: Validations of the Brazilian version of the Early Childhood Oral Health Impact Scale (ECOHIS). Cad Saude Publica 2012a;28:367-74.

[22] Martins-Júnior PA, Vieira-Andrade RG, Corrêa-Faria P, Oliveira-Ferreira F, Marques LS, Ramos-Jorge ML. Impact of early Childhood caries on the oral health-related quality of ife of preschool children and their parents. Caries Res 2012b;47:211-8.

[23] Oliveira LB, Sheiham A, Bönecker M: Exploring the association of dental caries with social factors and nutritional status in Brazilian preschool children. Eur J Oral Sci 2008;116:37-43.

[24] Pahel BT, Rozier RG, Slade GD. Parental perceptions of children's oral health: The Early Childhood Oral Health Impact Scale (ECOHIS). Health Qual Life Outcomes 2007; 5:6.

[25] Patel RR, Tootla R, Inglehart MR. Does oral health affect self perceptions, parental ratings and video-based assessments of children's smiles? Community Dent Oral Epidemiol 2007; 35: 44-52.

[26] Pereira SM, Tagliaferro EP, Ambrosano GM, Cortelazzi KL, Meneghim MC, Pereira AC. Dental caries in 12-year-old schoolchildren and its relationship with socioeconomic and behavioural variables. Oral Health Prev Dent 2007; 5: 299-306.

[27] Petersen PE, Bourgeois D, Ogawa H, Estupinan-Day S, Ndiaye C. The global burden of oral diseases and risks to oral health. Bull World Health Organ 2005; 83: 661-69.

[28] Pitts NB. Are we ready to move from operative to non-operative/preventive treatment of dental caries in clinical practice? Caries Res 2004; 38: 294-304. Review.

[29] Ramos-Jorge J, Pordeus IA, Ramos-Jorge ML, Marques LS, Paiva SM: Impact of untreated dental caries on quality of life of preschool children: diferent stages and activity. Community Dent Oral Epidemiol 2014; 42:311-22.

[30] Rebok G, Riley A, Forrest C, Starfield B, Green B, Robertson J, Tambor E. Elementary school-aged children's reports of their health: a cognitive interviewing study. Qual Life Res 2001;10:59-70.

[31] Reisine ST, Psoter W. Socioeconomic status and selected behavioral determinants as risk factors for dental caries. J Dent Educ 2001; 65: 1009-16.

[32] Ricketts DN, Ekstrand KR, Kidd EA, Larsen T. Relating visual and radiographic ranked scoring systems for occlusal caries detection to histological and microbiological evidence. Oper Dent 2002; 27:231-7.

[33] Sabbah W, Tsakos G, Chandola T, Sheiham A, Watt RG. Social gradients in oral and general health. J Dent Res 2007;86:992-6.

[34] Scarpelli AC, Paiva SM, Viegas CM, Carvalho AC, Ferreira FM, Pordeus IA: Oral health-related quality of life among Brazilian preschool children. Community Dent Oral Epidemiol 2012;41:336-44.

[35] Schroth RJ, Levi JA, Sellers EA, Friel J, Kliewer E, Moffatt ME. Vitamin D status of children with severe early childhood caries: a case-control study. BMC Pediatr 2013;13:174.

[36] Shoaib L, Deery C, Ricketts DN, Nugent ZJ. Validity and reproducibility of ICDAS II in primary teeth. Caries Res 2009;43:442-8.

[37] Slade GD. Derivation and validation of a short-form oral health impact profile. Community Dent Oral Epidemiol 1997; 25:284-90.

[38] Tamanini JTN, Dambros M, D'ancona CAL, Palma PCR, Netto Jr NR. Validation of the International Consultation on Incontinence Questionnaire – Short Form" (ICIQSF) for Portuguese. Rev Saude Publica 2004; 38:438-444.

[39] Talekar BS, Rozier RG, Slade GD, Ennett ST. Parental perceptions of their preschool-aged children's oral health. J Am Dent Assoc 2005;136:364-72.

[40] Traebert J, Guimarães LA, Durante EZ, Serratine AC. Low maternal schooling and severity of dental caries in Brazilian preschool children. Oral Health Prev Dent 2009; 7:39-45.

[41] Tsakos G, Blair YI, Yusuf H, Wright W, Watt RG, Macpherson LMD. Developing a new self-reported scale of oral health outcomes for 5-year-old children (SOHO-5). Health Qual Life Outcomes 2012;10:62.

[42] Wong HM, McGrath CP, King NM, Lo EC: Oral health-related quality of life in Hong Kong preschool children. Caries Res 2011;45:370-6.

[43] Zero DT, Zandona AF, Vail MM, Spolnik KJ: Dental caries and pulpal disease. Dent Clin North Am 2011;55:29-46.

Permissions

List of Contributors

Javier de la Fuente Hernández, Fátima del Carmen Aguilar Díaz and María del Carmen Villanueva Vilchis
Escuela Nacional de Estudios Superiores Unidad León – UNAM, León, Gto, México

Dongliang Zhang
Beijing Stomatology Hospital affiliated to Capital University of Medical science, Beijing City, P.R. China

Lei Zheng
Clinical director, Xinya dental, Changchun City, P.R. China
The department oral maxillofacial surgery, Jilin University, Chaoyang District, Changchun City, P.R. China

Ana Pejcic
Department of Periodontology and Oral medicine, Medical faculty, University of Nis, Serbia

Elena Preoteasa, Marina Imre and Ana Maria Tancu
Department of Prosthodontics, Faculty of Dental Medicine, Carol Davila University of Medicine and Pharmacy, Bucharest, Romania

Henriette Lerner
Private Practice, Baden-Baden, Germany

Cristina Teodora Preoteasa
Department of Oral Diagnosis, Ergonomics, Scientific Research Methodology, Faculty of Dental Medicine, Carol Davila University of Medicine and Pharmacy, Bucharest, Romania

Mariana Minatel Braga, Isabela Floriano, Fernanda Rosche Ferreira, Juliana Mattos Silveira, Alessandra Reyes, Tamara Kerber Tedesco and Daniela Prócida Raggio
Dental School, Department of Pediatric Dentistry, University of São Paulo, São Paulo, Brazil

José Carlos Pettorossi Imparato
University Camilo Castelo Branco, São Paulo, Brazil and CPO São Leopoldo Mandic,

Fausto Medeiros Mendes
Dental School, Department of Pediatric Dentistry, University of São Paulo, São Paulo, Brazil University Camilo Castelo Branco, São Paulo, Brazil and CPO São Leopoldo Mandic, Campinas, Brazil

Cecilia Santiago Araujo de Lima and Rafael da Silveira Moreira
Department of Public Health. Oswaldo Cruz Foundation. Aggeu Magalhães Research Center Recife. Pernambuco, Brazil

M. Larrea, N. Zamora, J. L. Gandia and V. Paredes
Department of Orthodontics. Faculty of Medicine and Dentistry, University of Valencia, Spain

R. Cibrian
Department of Physiology. Faculty of Medicine and Dentistry, University of Valencia, Spain

Zühre Zafersoy Akarslan and Ilkay Peker
Gazi University Faculty of Dentistry, Department of Dentomaxillofacial Radiology Ankara, Turkey

Joana Ramos-Jorge, Maria Letícia Ramos-Jorge and Leandro Silva Marques
Universidade Federal dos Vales do Jequitinhonha e Mucuri, Diamantina, Minas Gerais, Brazil

Isabela Almeida Pordeus and Saul Martins de Paiva
Universidade Federal de Minas Gerais, Belo Horizonte, Minas Gerais, Brazil

Index

A
Ageusia, 54
Angular Cheilitis, 55, 61
Aphthous Stomatitis, 49, 55
Asathiopurine, 49

B
Black Hairy Tongue, 53, 60
Bone Atrophy, 26
Burning Mouth Syndrome, 49, 58-59

C
C-oidp, 15
Candidosis, 53-54
Cleft Lip, 48, 186, 197
Corticosteroid, 54
Crest Module, 33-34
Crevicular Fluid Analysis, 138-139, 142, 152, 155
Crohn's Disease, 55

D
Dental Caries, 6, 17, 19, 99, 102, 111-112, 115-117, 122, 200-206, 208-209
Dental Disease, 1, 8, 20
Dental Floss, 86, 93-95, 101-102
Dental Fluorosis, 1, 6
Dental Impact Profile, 9, 13
Dental Implant, 26, 30, 47, 62, 64, 66-67, 79, 81, 84, 184, 197
Dental Injuries, 1, 122
Drug Therapy, 49, 56
Dysgeusia, 54, 61

E
Edentulism, 5, 29, 40, 62-64, 73, 75, 82, 123, 131-132, 207
Endodontic, 164, 189, 196, 199
Epithelial Necrosis, 50
Erythema Multiforme, 49-51, 59-60

G
Generic Prosthetic Component, 31

G
Gingival Crevicular Fluid, 143, 159-162
Gingival Enlargement, 53
Glossitis, 49-50
Gohai, 8-9, 13, 20-22

H
Halitosis, 56-57, 61
Hemorrhage, 57
Hydroxyapatite, 32, 87
Hypodontia, 6

I
Implant Body, 32-37, 41, 70
Implant Surgery, 30, 35, 39, 84
Interdental Papillae, 41, 43-44

L
Lichen Planus, 49-52, 59
Losartan, 49
Lupus Erythematosus, 50, 52

M
Malocclusion, 6-7, 20, 204-205
Mandibular Overdenture, 38, 46, 64, 79
Maxillary Denture, 38, 62
Maxillofacial Surgery, 46, 84, 184, 197
Modern Dentistry, 26

O
Oral Candidosis, 54
Oral Health, 1-5, 7-17, 19-26, 54, 57-58, 61, 64, 122-124, 128, 132-133, 135-136, 200-204, 206-209
Oral Infection, 49, 57
Oral Medicine, 48, 58, 84, 191-193, 195-197
Oral Mucosa, 48, 50-52, 64, 84
Oral Ulcerations, 50
Orthodontic, 6, 12, 63, 67, 97-99, 138-142, 154, 157-162, 186, 198, 203
Orthodontic Treatment, 138-140, 142, 157-160, 203
Osteonecrosis, 56, 61, 184
Osteotomy, 33-34, 69-70, 76

P

Pain Evaluation, 138
Pain Level, 141-142, 145-153, 157
Pediatric Dentistry, 110, 112, 115, 184, 187, 198, 203
Pemphigoid, 50-51, 60
Pemphigus, 49, 51-52, 60
Pemphigus Vulgaris, 49, 51-52
Periodontal Disease, 1, 6, 30-31, 57, 122, 162, 198
Prophylactic Antibiotherapy, 69
Prostaglandin, 139, 150-151, 155, 157-162
Prosthesis Fabrication, 36

Q

Quality of Life, 1, 3-10, 12-13, 16-17, 19-24, 80, 133, 200-209

S

Salivary Gland, 56, 60-61
Severe Fluorosis, 6
Sialorrhoea, 56
Stomatitis, 49, 55, 61, 64
Surgical Treatment, 6

T

Temporomandibular Joint, 184, 186
Tooth Loss, 1, 5-6, 27, 29, 31, 41, 122-125, 128, 130-133, 135-137
Total Pain, 141-142, 145-146, 151, 156-157
Traumatic Dental Injury, 204

X

Xerostomia, 53-56

www.ingramcontent.com/pod-product-compliance
Lightning Source LLC
Chambersburg PA
CBHW061958190326
41458CB00009B/2903